BUILDING THE WORLDS THAT KILL US

Praise for *Building the Worlds That Kill Us*

"This book shows why public health needs to learn history. Beginning with the European settlement of what became the United States, it addresses the seizure of indigenous lands, the adoption of a labor system that relied on enslaved workers, and nineteenth-century industrialization, continuing up to the present day. The authors ask the larger question of what accounts for exploitative working conditions and environmental degradation. The answer lies in how the particularly predatory form of capitalism in the United States can win out over healthful lives. History also offers hope. The call to protect health can be unifying, and social arrangements can be changed."

—Mary Travis Bassett, Harvard University

"In *Building the Worlds That Kill Us*, the renowned historians of public health David Rosner and Gerald Markowitz offer a sobering and compelling account of the critical and persistent health disparities so characteristic of the United States. Addressing the fundamental question of who gets sick and why, they powerfully demonstrate that existing social and economic structures account for—and augment—existing health inequities. In this sweeping historical narrative, they offer a clarion call for revitalizing public health to serve social justice and health equity."

—Allan M. Brandt, author of *The Cigarette Century: The Rise, Fall, and Persistence of the Product That Defined America*

"Rosner and Markowitz have gifted us with an industrial and literary history that focuses on the poisons we eat, the pollutants we inhale, the economic systems that render them possible, and the political movements that challenge their dominance. Deeply researched and vividly written, this brilliant chronicle— from chemicals and infectious disease to occupational health and clean water— is filled with stunning insights. Everyone will benefit from reading this dazzling, most significant book."

—Blanche Wiesen Cook, City University of New York

"*Building the Worlds That Kill Us* does not simply demonstrate the many ways in which we (and our industries, legislatures, and courts) are responsible for the diseases that kill us. It also reveals the history of people fighting back to protect their health. This book is the culmination of decades of research by Rosner and Markowitz: it assembles their key arguments into an invaluable and comprehensive overview."

—David S. Jones, author of *Broken Hearts: The Tangled History of Cardiac Care*

"To understand a society deeply, to reveal who has powers to shape how people work and live, look to its patterns of disease and health inequities—and who fights for health justice. Rosner and Markowitz's rich history of the United States offers solidaristic hope in a time of deep peril."

—Nancy Krieger, author of *Epidemiology and the People's Health: Theory and Context*

"For four decades, Rosner and Markowitz have been among the nation's leading historians of public health. Now in this magisterial work, they examine public health in America from the 1600s to the present, documenting that for four hundred years structural inequalities based on race, history, economics, and social class have shaped disparities in health and disease to a previously unimagined extent, determining which Americans' lives are long and healthy and whose are marked by disease, suffering, and premature death. The book also describes the work of labor unions, civil rights activists, and brave individuals like Greta Thunberg and U.S. senator Sheldon Whitehouse who have fought for justice and countered the forces of greed and exploitation. It shows that inequality is not inevitable. This book is essential reading not only for physicians, nurses, and public health workers but also for ethicists, historians, policymakers, and all concerned with advancing health and bending the arc of moral justice."

—Philip J. Landrigan, Boston College

"After collaborating for more than fifty years, Rosner and Markowitz have written a sweeping book that traces devastating patterns in American public health history. Again and again, they show that economic and social forces determine the distribution of disease and suffering. Even as the particular health threats change over time—from smallpox, tuberculosis, cholera, and typhoid through lead, tobacco, PCBs, endocrine-disrupting chemicals, and even climate change—they take their toll on the poorest and most vulnerable. The esteemed elders of public health history leave little question that sickness and death often result from the decisions we make as a society. It's a dark truth, though one they leaven with the reminder that we always have the power to make better choices."

—Sharon Lerner, reporter at *ProPublica*

"Every few decades a major study emerges that shines a vital new light on the appalling health inequalities in our society. *Building the Worlds That Kill Us* is one such book. Eminent historians David Rosner and Gerald Markowitz probe deeply into the socioeconomic roots of persistent health disparities and medical neglect. Covering the collective struggles against health injustices from America's birth to the present, *Building the Worlds That Kill Us* provides an invaluable roadmap to social changes needed to improve the nation's health care for its most vulnerable segments."

—David McBride, author of *Caring for Equality: A History of African American Health and Healthcare*

"*Building the Worlds That Kill Us* is a great read and a historical tour de force. It is a fascinating, thorough, and terrifically important exploration of the social factors that have driven the health and disease of Americans from the nation's earliest days to the present."

—David Michaels, George Washington University School of Public Health

"This book must be read by all fighting for a healthy world. The authors draw a clear picture of how people's health is socially determined by worlds being built to kill us. We will avoid this existential threat to our survival when we success-fully organize enough power to build worlds that are sustainable, at peace, and where social justice is the law of the land."

—Linda Rae Murray, University of Illinois Chicago School of Public Health

"Say the word 'illness,' and most of us envisage bacteria and viruses—or maybe genes—and we think that who gets sick is mostly a matter of bad luck or bad choices. In this path-breaking work, Rosner and Markowitz show how the pat-terns of disease and death in America have been largely the result of social conditions produced by conscious choices. Not by the sick person, however, but by people in positions of corporate power to profit at the expense of others, and by people in positions of social or political power to allow the sacrifice of some people's health for other people's wealth. By calling attention to these choices across the sweep of American history, Rosner and Markowitz remind us that, just as we have built worlds that foster disease, injury, and death, we can also build worlds that keep us safe—or at least substantially safer. This is a powerful and important book."

—Naomi Oreskes, coauthor of *The Big Myth: How American Business Taught Us to Loathe Government and Love the Free Market*

"The discussion of health disparities has needed an overview book for a long time that links the social and institutional reasons for ill health. This book will be critical to anyone in public health or the health professions as well as to a general audience. Historians of American health care will welcome it into their syllabi. I wish I had it when I was teaching."

—Susan M. Reverby, author *of Examining Tuskegee: The Infamous Syphilis Study and Its Legacy*

"*Building the Worlds That Kill Us* offers an incisive, sobering, and critically important new history of health in the United States, revealing how capital-ism, commercial greed, and social injustice have worked to produce unequal suffering and disease across generations and the concerted work of reformers across time to right those wrongs. A brilliant, capacious, and instructive study by leading scholars of health and society."

—Keith Wailoo, author of *Pushing Cool: Big Tobacco, Racial Marketing, and the Untold Story of the Menthol Cigarette*

Building the Worlds That Kill Us

Disease, Death, and Inequality
in American History

David Rosner
and Gerald Markowitz

Columbia University Press   New York

Columbia University Press
Publishers Since 1893
New York   Chichester, West Sussex
cup.columbia.edu

Library of Congress Cataloging-in-Publication Data
Names: Rosner, David, 1947– author. | Markowitz, Gerald E., author.
Title: Building the worlds that kill us : disease, death and inequality
    in American history / David Rosner and Gerald Markowitz.
Description: New York : Columbia University Press, [2024] | Includes
    bibliographical references and index.
Identifiers: LCCN 2024006837 (print) | LCCN 2024006838 (ebook) |
    ISBN 9780231200844 (hardback) | ISBN 9780231200851 (trade paperback) |
    ISBN 9780231553803 (ebook)
Subjects: MESH: History of Medicine | Disease—history | Health Inequities |
    Social Determinants of Health | United States
Classification: LCC R151 (print) | LCC R151 (ebook) | NLM WZ 70 AA1 |
    DDC 610.973—dc23/eng/20240618
LC record available at https://lccn.loc.gov/2024006837
LC ebook record available at https://lccn.loc.gov/2024006838

Printed and bound by CPI Group (UK) Ltd, Croydon, CR0 4YY

Cover design: Julia Kushnirsky
Cover image: Shutterstock

Contents

Contents

Preface and Acknowledgments

One evening in February 2000, the two of us pulled into a motel off Route 10 between Baton Rouge and New Orleans, Louisiana. We had spent the day traveling along River Road, the local two-lane route that parallels the Mississippi River. Cancer Alley, as it is known, was to be one focus of a chapter in *Deceit and Denial*, the book we were then working on about the lead and chemical industries. It had been a long few days. We had visited Convent, a small, largely African American community along the east bank of the river whose residents had organized to fight a proposed vinyl chloride plant, as well as an area along the west bank, in Plaquemine, that had once been the largely African American community of Reveilletown where residents had been forced to abandon their homes some time earlier because of groundwater contamination. We had also visited the Holy Rosary Cemetery (see figure P.1), the last remnant of the town of Taft, which had vanished as Union Carbide's giant cracking towers engulfed it. The river, once the site of sugar and cotton plantations, was now the home to scores of polluting chemical plants. The human suffering of the agricultural and slave economy of the past had been replaced by new forms of death, disease, displacement, and suffering associated with the petrochemical industry.

We were both troubled and inspired by what we had seen. In our conversations, the residents of Convent explained their political and legal efforts that had stymied Shintech, the Japanese chemical giant that wanted to build a huge vinyl chloride plant in their midst. Theirs was a David and Goliath story. The trip to Plaquemine, however, had been depressing: residents of the once vibrant Reveilletown had literally been uprooted by the Georgia Gulf Company. To escape the costs

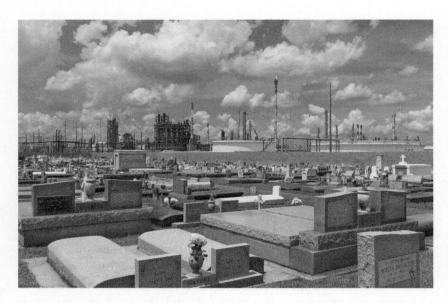

FIGURE P.1 "Taft, Louisiana—June 20, 2014: View of the Holy Rosary Cemetery in Taft, Louisiana, with a petrochemical plant on the background." The site of the former town now engulfed by a chemical plant. Courtesy of Shutterstock.

of its pollution of the groundwater and the inevitable lawsuits that would follow, the company gave the residents two bad options: either be bought out by the company or forcibly be removed. We were exhausted by all we had seen and called out to the local pizza shop for a large pie with pepperoni.

When a knock announced the arrival of our dinner about a half hour later, we were startled to see at the door a Louisiana state trooper, bedecked in full regalia with gun and badge, holding a pizza box in his hands. He had "been in the store" when our order had been called in and offered to deliver the pizza to us. Smiling quizzically, we thanked him, paused, and then invited him in for a slice. Surprisingly, he accepted, came in, looked around the motel room, and sat down.

After a couple of moments of awkward chit chat, it became clear that he already knew a lot about our movements: he had been following us as we meandered up and down River Road snapping pictures of cemeteries and manor houses, as well as the chemical plant entrances, cracking towers, conveyer belts, and tankers that lined the Mississippi to collect and deliver chemicals. He had been called by security at several plants, he said, and had been tracking us all afternoon.

After we explained that we were there as historians, he settled in for about a half hour, drinking Coke and talking freely about the history of the river and the chemical plants that had transformed it during the previous few decades. With little prompting, and in between romantic remembrances of a "simpler" time, he bemoaned the flares of the Gulf and Chevron cracking towers that now lit up the evening skies, the shelter-in-place alerts that told locals to remain indoors when the air became too toxic to breathe, and the complaints of water pollution and cancers that had led to tensions between the companies, residents, and environmentalists.

While we answered truthfully that we were historians writing a history of the plants along the river, not "agitators" working with local environmental or community groups, we did not acknowledge that our sympathies were certainly with those who were. Over the previous decades, we had published a number of books and articles that specifically addressed the history of occupational and environmental health in America and had become increasingly disturbed by the impact of industrial practices both within and outside of the workplace on the health and well-being of workers, their families, and communities. In the late 1980s we had published *Dying for Work*, a collection of essays on the history of workers' health. Another, *Slaves of the Depression*, was a collection of letters to Eleanor Roosevelt, Secretary of Labor Frances Perkins, and President Roosevelt from the families of workers who had been disabled, diseased, and often destroyed by working conditions during the Depression. This second book took us deep into working people's experience of often horrific jobs that had barely sustained them. The arenas they were working in, the forms of exploitation that these men, women, and children experienced, and the impact of this work on their lives deeply affected how we came to see history and our work.

In 1991 we published *Deadly Dust*, a short book on silicosis, then seen as an obscure disease of the past. It was written originally with other historians in mind, and it detailed how the introduction into the workplace of steam-, water-, and, ultimately, electrically driven high-speed drills, chisels, sandblasters, and other machinery to workplaces had created an epidemic of silicosis among skilled and unskilled workers. By pulverizing rock and sand, the new power tools created huge clouds of dust that slowly strangled and killed foundry workers and steelworkers, miners, quarrymen, stonecutters, glassblowers, construction workers, and others who had little or no access to protective equipment.

The book's reception quickly introduced us to the considerable contemporary relevance of this history: although the book dealt primarily with events of the first half of the twentieth century, our findings proved of interest to lawyers working on behalf of workers in court cases around the country. For years, workers who were suffering and dying silently and invisibly from silicosis in far-flung reaches of the nation had tried to sue their employers and suppliers, only to be told by company lawyers that what they suffered from was a "new" disease that their company had never heard of, and therefore "no one was to blame." Soon we were meeting workers and their families in Odessa, Texas, and other places where dust was an issue and testifying in court cases regarding the long history of documented corporate knowledge about the devastating effects of silicosis.

In the ensuing years, we have written extensively about other corporate products, the conditions of their manufacture, and the history of controversies over their health effects, ranging from lead poisoning, asbestosis, mesothelioma, occupational lung cancer, and chemical exposures to PCBs. But, as we wrote, testified in court, and taught our students about the history of public health, it became increasingly clear that what we had been describing were just the most obvious examples of a much broader and even more troubling story of life and death in the United States: the worlds we as a society have created at different periods of our history and the racial, economic, political, and social inequalities that have lain at the heart of so much of American history have determined to a surprising extent who have gotten what disease and when, who have lived long lives, and who have died sooner, often after years filled with pain.

While there are certainly limits to human life, and while accidents do happen despite precautions, much disease, disability, and death result from willful negligence, inattention, and the pursuit of more and more production and profit at the expense of those doing the producing, as well as from the refusal by those with power to arrange adequate care for people they deem unworthy or unimportant. History is replete with examples of this problem. Chaining fire doors closed at the Triangle Shirtwaist Factory in 1911 New York, spraying pesticides on migrant workers in the grape orchards of California in the post–World War II decades, refusing to properly ventilate mineshafts in the coalfields of Pennsylvania—all are examples of actions taken, or not taken, that have resulted in the deaths of countless people. Our earlier work demonstrates that often the responsibility for suffering lies not with some panoramic collective "we," but rather with specific corporations or government inactions. Conversely, responsible corporations, government policy, regulation, and union and public health mobilizations can positively affect people's health.

In this book, we also show that, from the beginning, the conditions of work and life have been, to varying extents, contested ground. We document the efforts on the part of unions, legislators, public health advocates, and others to address unhealthy, unsafe, and oppressive conditions in field and factory, residences and communities at large, efforts that are also very much part of the account of disease and death in America.

The history we relate in this book is that of health and disease in America from colonial times to the present. Much of that story reflects inequalities in who suffers disease and death, inequalities that are so often determined by those in power. We begin with what every public health student learns in example after example and what every thoughtful person at least suspects: the best predictors of who lives and who dies and who differentially bears the pain of building and maintaining this society are in large part determined by income, wealth, race, gender, sexuality, and social position. We make use of this lens in looking at suffering from the time when Europeans first invaded North America to today, when Covid-19 epidemics and global warming threaten all our lives. Throughout this history, those who have been most affected—working people, African Americans, immigrants, women, and the poor more generally—have, when in a position to do so, called out the systems that have led to their early death and the unequal burdens they have suffered from disease and disabilities. In some instances, these demands from below have resulted in movements that pushed for dramatic reforms that have benefited everyone.

What we're confronting today is an existential crisis over the survival of many species, our own included, but, as with many calamities that Americans have encountered in the past, those concerned about short-term profits have mounted determined resistance to the changes needed to cope adequately with looming disaster. With regard to climate change, for example, many first denied that global warming was taking place, then that if it was, human activity was not the primary cause of it, and more recently, that, yes, it may be occurring, but proposed remedies are too expensive and disruptive of business-as-usual to implement. However, broad segments of the population have been mobilizing to counter these entrenched forces. Greta Thunberg has inspired millions of people throughout the United States and the world to demand action. Nongovernmental organizations such as Greenpeace, Earth Justice, and the Environmental Defense Fund and academics like Naomi Oreskes, Michael Mann, Richard Jackson, and others have documented the machinations of fossil fuel companies and their supporters and have mobilized scientists and other academics to use their expertise and authority to demand politicians' attention. National figures like Al Gore and Senator Sheldon Whitehouse have confronted special corporate interests that have stymied action. This dynamic of crisis, reform, and reaction has been true throughout U.S. history.

But we are also attempting to provide a new lens through which to view the history of the country. By looking at the social, political, and economic history of the country while focusing on death and disease, we believe that we have revealed fundamental aspects of our national history. The changing rates and kinds of diseases and deaths the nation experiences at different moments of its history are in large part reflections of the social, political, and economic worlds that have emerged. The deep inequalities of those worlds are reflected in the different health experiences of rich and poor, Black and white, men and women, immigrant and native born, Native Americans and colonial settlers. We recognize that there are many areas that we are not covering in this book, and there is much more work to be done by historians and other scholars. But we hope that this book stimulates others to take up the task.

Of course, there is also a more hopeful aspect to the general rule that we as a society construct the worlds that kill us: we also as a society can build worlds that don't, or certainly that do so less gratuitously. While death and disease may always be with us, we as a people can create institutions and movements that save lives, ameliorate disease, and build a safer and more healthful world. As a nation, we have done so in the past. We can do so again.

Many people have played a role in the creation of this book. Our colleagues at Columbia University and John Jay College have been helpful throughout. The faculty, staff, and students at Columbia's Center for the History and Ethics of Public Health were helpful in numerous ways. Merlin Chowkwanyun, through his creation of toxicdocs.org and commentary, provided us with the technology and intellectual support to sort through and integrate many of the documents that form the core of chapter 6. Kavita Sivaramakrishnan, James Colgrove, Gerald Oppenheimer, and Ronald Bayer, also at the center, are the best colleagues one could ever hope for. Nitanya Nedd deserves a special shout-out for her unwavering good cheer and calm even when we were our worst selves. At the Mailman School of Public Health and elsewhere, other colleagues were supportive of this effort: Dean Linda Fried, Jeremiah Barondess, Lisa Bates, Leslie Davidson, Melissa Dupont-Reyes, John Santelli, Bob Klitzman, Steven Morse, Peter Messeri, Daniel Giovenco, Christian Gloria, Jeff Fagan, Helen-Maria Lekas, Mary Clare Lennon, Waffa El-Sadr, Charles Branas, Kathy Sikkema, Connie Nathanson, Bob Fullilove, Joseph Graziano, Daniel Giovenco, Heather Butts, Diana Hernandez, Wendy Chavkin, Yasmin Davis, Kim Hopper, Lisa Rosen-Metsch, Karolynn Siegel, Rachel Shelton, Marni Sommers, Gina Wingood, Ezra Susser, Sally Conover, Jennifer Hirsch, and Angela Aidala. In Columbia's History Department we want to thank Elizabeth Blackmar for her untiring, selfless efforts on behalf of our students and program. Pablo Piccato, Caterina Pizzigoni, Professor Manan Ahmed, Rashid Khalidi, Amy Chazkel, Frank Guidry, Hillary Hallett, Hannah Farber, Mae Ngai, Marwa Elshakry, Samuel Roberts, Barbara Fields, Casey Blake, George Chauncey, Karl Jacoby, Rebecca Kobrin, Natasha Lightfoot, Eugenia Lean, Gregory Mann, Mark Mazower, Stephanie McCurry, Kim Phillips-Fein, Michael Stanislawski, Alma Steingart, Rhiannon Stephens, Michael Witgen, and Madeleine Zelin have all been wonderful colleagues over the years. Our doctoral students, past and present, particularly Valentina Parisi who patiently collected the illustrations in this text, sought the permissions and generally aided us throughout. Sadie Bergen, Kathleen Bachinsky, Sarah Vogel, Nick Turse, Sarah Samuels, Marianne Sullivan, Megan Wolff, Kristen Meister, and Michael Yudell have all produced important books and articles that prove to us that both historians and public health practitioners benefit greatly by talking to one another.

At John Jay College, President Karol Mason and Provost Allison Pease were very supportive of this work. Colleagues in the Department of Interdisciplinary Studies and the broader college have been terrific friends over many years: Chair Susannah Crowder, Richard Haw, Amy Green, Adriana Perez, Katie Gentile, Lisandro Perez, Nina Rose Fischer, Bibi Calderaro, Michael Blitz, Kofi Scott, Meghan Duffy, Sarah Meister, Sandra Leftoff, Carol Groneman, Betsy Gitter, Dennis Sherman, Jessica Gordon Nembhard, Lissette Delgado-Cruzata, Schevaletta Alford, Edward Paulino, Allison Kavey, Michael Pfeifer and Caroline Reitz. Blanche Wiesen Cook "hired" Jerry over fifty years ago and has been a constant source of support ever since. And Jerry's union colleagues have never stopped fighting for a better university "for the whole people": John Pittman, Zabby Hovey, Nivedita Majumdar, and Rulisa Galloway-Perry.

We especially want to thank those who read and commented on the manuscript and gave us valuable commentary and encouragement: Susan Reverby and David Jones were especially helpful, providing page-by-page comments and suggestions. Michael Meeropol, Ruth Heifetz, and Nick Freudenberg provided useful reflections on portions of the manuscript.

Two people were critical in the creation of this book: Jonathan Cobb, friend and editor extraordinaire, worked with us to shape many of chapters and to provide critical feedback, encouraging us to avoid academic jargon. Kathy Conway did multiple edits of the manuscript, clarifying our prose and arguments. This is an immeasurably better book for their insights. We also want to thank Jim O'Brien, who indexed the book, and Susan Zorn, who carefully and intelligently copyedited it.

We are grateful to Columbia University Press for publishing this manuscript, and particularly to our editor at the press, Stephen Wesley, for his insights and care for this work. He gently and efficiently moved this project forward from inception to completion. The production team with the press, Wren Haynes and Kathryn Jorge, were outstanding.

Of course, none of this would have been possible without the support and love of our families. Throughout our careers writing together, our wives, Kathy Conway and Andrea Vasquez, have always been there for us. We love you dearly. Our children and their mates, Zachary and Emilie Rosner, Molly Rosner and Paul Anderson, Tobias Markowitz, Elena and Steve Kennedy, and Isa Vasquez, are our pride and joy. We also remember Billy Markowitz and Anton Vasquez, who are always in our hearts. This book is dedicated to our grandchildren, who, despite the miserable world we are leaving them, still give us hope: Owen and Margot Rosner, Zach Rosner Anderson and Joey Rosner Anderson, and Mason and Ceeb Kennedy.

We have been writing together since 1973 and have published between us 15 books and scores of articles. The books and articles were generally close studies. Here we place the themes of those books and articles in the broader historical context of the history of the United States. Hence, sections of this book have appeared elsewhere. Specifically, some material in chapter 3 appeared in Rosner's book, *Hives of Sickness*; some material in chapter 5 appeared in our book *Deadly Dust*; some material in chapter 6 appeared in our book *Deceit and Denial*; some material in chapter 7 appeared in the article, "America is Poisonous to Your Health" which appeared in tomdispatch.com. In addition some material was previously published in the *Milbank Quarterly*, the *American Journal of Public Health*, and the *Journal of Public Health Policy*.

BUILDING THE WORLDS THAT KILL US

Introduction

"Sick and Tired of Being Sick and Tired"

"I'm sick and tired of being sick and tired." So declared Fannie Lou Hamer, the iconic organizer of the Mississippi Freedom Democratic Party, in her famous December 1964 speech at a Harlem rally with Malcolm X. The speech, which captured the frustration and anger that she and millions of others felt about white southern resistance to racial integration in general and more specifically to the Mississippi Democratic Party's segregationist policies, detailed the exploitation of Blacks as they worked ten- or eleven-hour days picking cotton for a mere 3 dollars per day. And it detailed how the consequences of such treatment in disease, suffering, and death were woven into the fabric of the state's history.[1] As Jack Geiger, the physician-activist who went to Mississippi with the Medical Committee on Human Rights during the "Freedom Summer" of 1964, later summed up the conditions he found, African Americans "lacked medical care . . . lived in poverty . . . had huge burdens of illness and premature mortality and [had] limited or no access to medical care."[2] It was a history that, in Hamer's words, was more than "a little sickening."[3]

Attentive observers writing about the experiences of workers in the United States of whatever race, ethnicity, gender, or geographic region have, with good reason, similarly remarked on the often-enormous disparities in health and well-being found among different classes, races, and other social groups. Studs Terkel, in *Working*, his now-classic 1972 book of interviews of American workers and their families, begins by saying that the "book, being about work, is, by its very nature, about violence—to the spirit as well as to the body. It is about ulcers as well as accidents . . . fistfights, about nervous breakdowns . . . about daily humiliations. To survive the day is triumph enough for the walking wounded among the great many of us."[4] That so much of Terkel's book uses the language of bodily harm, physical and psychic wounds, and even disease to describe the experience of workers is itself "no accident" or even a metaphor.

The argument that Terkel uses to describe exploitation in work can be used to help us reconceptualize health. After all, at their core, disease, disability, death, and psychic distress of all sorts that may have physical manifestations entail violence done to the human body. The story of ill-health is the story of damage done, by bacteria and viruses like Covid-19, by another disease attacking the body, by exposure to toxic chemicals in the workplace or in the wider environment, or by the physical harm done to people by machinery, automobiles, guns, or the whip.

There are, of course, aspects of death, disease, and suffering that lie outside human control and that have varied across time. We all die; certain genetic mutations that lead to debilitating effects are, at least so far, beyond human control; we can end up in the wrong place at the wrong time (such as by getting caught in an earthquake, volcanic eruption, or a lightning strike); or we can unwittingly be exposed to dreadful diseases for which effective treatment anywhere is not available.

To a surprising extent, however, disease, suffering, and premature death are a function of the worlds that we as a society have constructed for ourselves and for others over time. They are, more particularly, often a function of specific people and groups of people making decisions that create or maintain conditions in which ill-health and suffering can flourish. Some instances of unnecessary suffering are glaringly obvious: for example, the exploitation and often premature death of Africans who were enslaved and transported to the New World under conditions so inhumane that approximately 10 to 20 percent perished during the Middle Passage; or the suffering and early death of those who survived and were consigned by whites to forced labor in the houses and fields of the American South, where the average life expectancy of a newborn slave child was less than twenty-two years, about half that of a white infant of the same era. To take another example, Crystal Eastman, feminist cofounder of the American Civil Liberties Union and social reformer, in her famous 1906–1907 study of Pittsburgh, *Work-Accidents and the Law*, wrote of 526 men who were killed in accidents in the steel mills of Pittsburgh and another 509 who suffered serious injuries in just one year, arguing cogently that many of these accidents would have been preventable if work conditions had been different. "Seven men lost a leg, sixteen men were hopelessly crippled in one or both legs, one lost a foot, two lost half a foot, five lost an arm, three lost a hand, ten lost two or more fingers, two were left with crippled left arms, three with crippled right arms, and two with two useless arms. Eleven lost an eye, and three others had the sight of both eyes damaged. Two men have crippled backs, two received internal injuries, one is partially paralyzed, one feebleminded, and two are stricken with the weakness of old age while still in their prime," she reported.[5]

Even aspects of the inevitable, such as death and disease, that appear to lie outside human control are also affected by how societies care for their members. That in turn may affect the outcomes of a person's experiences with health and disease. Race, social class, geographic location, gender, age, immigrant status, and the like all have been shown to have a tremendous impact on access to medical care and the quality of care received, which in turn shape Americans' length and quality of life.[6] These and many other situations are a function of the decisions of some human beings to construct conditions, or allow such conditions to persist, that are clearly detrimental to the well-being of others, and often in ways that were perfectly obvious at the time.

This book focuses on how the social and economic arrangements Americans have created and maintained have shaped patterns of disease occurrence, prevalence, distribution, and recovery over the course of the country's history. Most obviously, an economic and social system dependent on slavery produced untold suffering and death among those most exploited; a commercial economy involving trade between various regions of the country and the world enabled easy transmission of diseases brought by mosquitoes, rats, and other vectors of infection; and the development of cities with large immigrant populations from the countryside and overseas allowed landlords to profit from rents of

airless tenements without adequate sewerage or pure water and produced epidemics of tuberculosis, cholera, and other diseases of poverty.
Similarly, the disfiguring accidents and diseases caused by toxic chemicals were often produced by the rampant expansion of a laissez-faire
industrial system that put profit over human life. And decisions today
to ignore the impact of fossil fuels on the climate and on the potential
destruction of the health and well-being of the world's population are
perhaps the most glaring examples of the construction and maintenance
of a world that is killing us.

We argue here that the relationship of socioeconomic forces to
death and disease is true not only of obvious forms of exploitation such
as the massive deaths resulting from the slave trade and the forced
migrations of native peoples. Often, we as a people also create the conditions within which disease takes hold. Among infectious diseases,
smallpox in the eighteenth century; the typhoid, typhus, yellow fever,
and cholera epidemics in the nineteenth century; and the childhood diseases through much of the twentieth were all exacerbated by the squalid
conditions in which people lived. The growing and harvesting of indigo
and rice in the mosquito-infested swamps of South Carolina during
the colonial era and beyond promoted yellow fever and malaria among
the enslaved and indentured people who were forced to do that work.
Exploitative working conditions during nineteenth-century industrialization created conditions for epidemics of silicosis, lead poisoning,
and asbestosis. Recently, America's collective environmental practices
have contributed disproportionately to global warming and consequent
extreme droughts, more severe hurricanes, and rising sea levels that
threaten to flood entire nations, and these events in turn have frequently
resulted in compromised resistance to disease. Endocrine disruptors
such as bisphenol A, phthalates, PCBs, and dioxins manufactured in the
twentieth century turn out to cause a variety of cancers, birth defects,
and other developmental disorders. Hundreds of chemicals manufactured in recent decades may also have resulted in increased deaths,
diseases, and neurological damage, as well as developmental problems,
reproductive problems, brain damage, immunity suppression, and other
problems all over the world.

Often, as already suggested, it is particular individuals or groups of
people who have built a world or created the conditions that adversely

affect many others. Tycoons of the Cleveland, Pittsburgh, and Buffalo steel mills of the late nineteenth century kept their factories going twenty-four hours a day, and workers on twelve-hour shifts there suffered horrendous accidents and diseases; women working in the match industry in the early twentieth century experienced disfiguring and deadly phossy jaw from their exposure to phosphorus. In more recent decades, agricultural workers in the vineyards of California and elsewhere were regularly showered with pesticides while harvesting the food that agricultural companies packaged and sold to the nation. In this process, millions of people have suffered diseases and deaths that could have been avoided.

The Covid-19 pandemic provided an example of how unequal are the effects of disease on a population.[7] Over the course of the pandemic's first few years, Covid-19 killed more than one of every three hundred Americans. The burden of these deaths was hardly distributed evenly through the population, however. At virtually every turn, the biological reality of a virus that coursed through the society revealed that biological action, social conditions, and values are inextricably linked. Those already in a weakened state or without access to adequate health care were more likely to become seriously ill or die. According to data from the Centers for Disease Control and Prevention (CDC), "American Indians and Alaskan Natives are 3.1 times more likely to be hospitalized, Black or African Americans are 2.5 times more likely to be hospitalized and 1.7 times more likely to die, and Hispanic or Latino persons are 1.5 times more likely to get Covid and 2.3 times more likely to be hospitalized."[8] In stark graphs, the Poor People's Campaign documented that "people living in poorer counties died at nearly two times the rate of people who lived in richer counties." During the early Omicron phase of the epidemic, from December 2021 through February 2022, counties with the lowest median income "had a death rate nearly three times higher . . . compared to those with the highest median incomes," differences that could not be explained by disparities in vaccination rates.[9]

This book, then, as noted in the preface, is an effort to examine American social history through the lens of death and disease, looking at how morbidity and mortality are so often reflections of how some, throughout history, have treated others and how structures, institutions, and processes have been constructed around forms of exploitation that over time have put vast numbers of people in peril. Unlike other books that have looked at health and have posited that diseases and disabilities are largely a result of biological agents, natural acts of God, or personal choices, here we explore how social, economic, and political decisions in the United States have shaped different experiences with human suffering, including susceptibility to harmful biological agents. The history of disease in the United States can only be truly understood by analyzing how "history," or human constructions, have affected biological manifestations of disease.

Americans, like people elsewhere, have created worlds that foster disease and early death, but many among them have also fought to alter those worlds, to repair and to prevent damage to human life, sometimes to great effect. So, in this book we also describe individual, community, and government efforts to counter those forces creating damage. Historically, various groups have attempted to counter violence done to the body by protesting exploitative conditions, developing public health or preventative procedures, and advocating for governmental reforms. Some very real structural changes have greatly improved the health of the vast majority of people in the United States. The building of reservoirs and pipelines to deliver clean water to homes and the construction of sewerage systems in every part of the growing cities in the nineteenth and early twentieth centuries were public investments that clearly and dramatically improved the health of people regardless of social and economic status. The building of dams and power stations during the Depression of the 1930s allowed for the provision of electricity and raised the living standards of millions in the rural South and West. Soon refrigerated food, pumps capable of providing water from deep wells, and indoor plumbing became widespread throughout many rural areas, improving living conditions and health and allowing for the flowering of previously arid and poverty-stricken areas in the southern and western states, among other regions. The creation of Medicare and Medicaid in the 1960s, along with other antipoverty programs, gave millions of poor and elderly access to medical care. These were significant reforms that curtailed disease and human suffering.

But throughout North American history, there have been real limits on how far or how deep these reform efforts could go before they met strong headwinds from an economic and social system deeply rooted in structural inequalities and unequal power relationships between classes and races. In the colonial era, when Caribbean planters saw their slaves die at extraordinary rates, they calculated that it was often cheaper to import more Africans than to keep them healthy and alive once here. When the United States found that the Industrial Revolution was being paid for with lost eyes, arms, legs, and fingers, states in the early twentieth century created workers' compensation systems to provide monetary benefits to injured workers, but they failed to reorganize how work was done. Speed-ups, scientific management techniques, and high-speed, often dangerous machinery remained the preferred means of producing mass-manufactured goods.

When experiments with rats in the 1920s showed that the introduction of lead into gasoline would result in massive air pollution that would damage human beings as well as rats, the auto and chemical industry successfully argued that "human progress" should not be stopped just because "a few rats die."[10] When paint manufacturers argued that systematically removing the lead paint that had been poisoning homes was simply too complex—and too expensive—to accomplish, they in effect were writing off future generations of predominantly Black and Puerto Rican children.[11]

It wasn't only overt corporate or individual greed that led to such social injustice. The state has often enforced the inequalities at the root of ill-health. When the first federal laws establishing the Occupational Safety and Health Administration were passed in 1970, OSHA was required to establish regulations to protect the health and safety of American workers—with the caveat that any regulation had to be "technologically and economically feasible," leaving OSHA to weigh the interests of companies against the health of the American workforce. Similarly, public health workers and the broad public recognize that the poor nutritional quality of the food many Americans eat causes a variety of health problems such as diabetes, heart disease, and antibiotic-resistant bacterial diseases. But it has been difficult for those demanding change to counter the economic interests that lie at the root of Americans' dependence on meats and milk injected with hormones, prepared foods that contain chemical preservatives, and high levels of salt, high-fructose corn syrup, and pesticides. These products are deemed necessary to maintain the profits of a food manufacturing and distribution system that is largely controlled by a few giant agricultural businesses. While few would argue against the idea that real reform of this system would benefit health, the entrenched interests that have promoted this industrial food production are, in the absence of a strong social movement, virtually immune to serious restructuring. Indeed, there seems little resistance at present to the continuing growth of the agricultural sector and few challenges to the rights of Monsanto, McDonald's, Perdue, Campbell's, Smithfield Foods, and others to conduct their businesses in ways that threaten the health of tens of millions of Americans.[12]

Readers will see that we tend to have an expansive, social definition of the public's health. We include in this definition not only biological disease, but also human suffering more broadly because that too affects well-being and longevity, and we also include the impact of stress on mental and physical health. We begin with the position that maximizing lifespans and minimizing disease and suffering should be the goal any just society and is a fundamental human right. Further, although we acknowledge the role that public health institutions play—hospitals, departments of health, and unaffiliated medical and public health professionals—we attempt to broaden the scope to account for what affects the health and ill-health of the population. In doing so we look at, in addition to medical professionals and institutions, colonial invaders, slaveholders, factory owners, corporate executives, philanthropists, workers, activists, and government officials. All of these have played a role in creating the worlds that help or harm us.[13]

There have been other books that aim to trace the importance of disease in American social history.[14] But they often present disease as an independent actor. In that view, either plagues, pandemics, or germs have shaped the demography of a nation or a continent, or some ecological or geographical accident has shaped the success or the failure of different societies, as if the nature of those societies and their response to these encounters were incidental. This book specifically rejects these arguments. It is not that biology is unimportant, but that the human experience with biology—and thus disease—is determined by the societies and communities within which it occurs.[15] Humans create the conditions within which disease and death flourish—or don't.

When one reads basic public health texts, whether Harry Stoll Mustard's *An Introduction to Public Health*, published in five editions from 1935 through 1969, or modern epidemiology books, one typically finds a story of ever-greater improvement. They begin with brief historical introductions, sometimes only a paragraph or two, that tell a seemingly self-evident story that "back then," in an ambiguous past, the world was dark, dreary, and depressing, people lived only a short time, and during the few decades when they could expect to survive they were plagued by illnesses, disabilities, and pain. This is typically followed by a discussion of how lives have improved: we learn, for example, that the average life span of a white boy born in 1900 in large U.S. cities was only 46.3 years—33 years for African Americans—but, by the second decade of the twenty-first century, the average life expectancy for most Americans, white and Black, was closer to 78 years.[16]

The story of progress toward greater health does, of course, have real truth in it. The United States, for example, has reduced the number of deaths that used to plague children and women giving birth, and it has largely controlled cholera and other water-borne diseases through the introduction of relatively safe water supply and sewerage systems. The last 150 years, writes one historical demographer, have seen the "average life span" more than double globally from twenty to forty years at the turn of the last century to somewhere between sixty and eighty years today.[17] Others have trumpeted the control of diseases that were once considered uncontrollable, as measured by shifting epidemiological and mortality statistics. And certainly, medical care and technologies have had a dramatic impact on all of our lives. One need only consider the impact of antiretrovirals on the AIDS epidemic. Tens of millions of lives have been saved by their use, both in this country and in Africa, Asia, and the rest of the world.

Nonetheless, these achievements are fragile, and circumstances can easily increase disease rates. Since 2014–2019 (when life expectancy peaked), life expectancy has actually decreased to 76 years, or to 1996 levels, ostensibly because of the Covid and opioid epidemics, with a huge drop in life expectancy among Native Americans followed by whites living in Republican states who opposed vaccination and mask mandates and were particularly hard hit by opioids and Covid.[18]

While averages of national and international mortality statistics tell an important story, they often hide wide variation of what makes up those averages. A closer look, for example, at the life spans of industrial workers, women, Native Americans, African Americans, and Hispanics reveals vast differences in Americans' disease experience. The persistence of disparities in health and longevity between races, classes, and different ethnic groups is perhaps the most enduring health reality of American society over time. Despite overall increases in life spans, over the course of American history, disparities in length of life between the rich and the poor, the industrial worker and the factory owner, the white and the Black, the immigrant and the native, as well as the Native American and all other groups, underscore the point we are making. In a society characterized by inequalities in income, wealth, education, and opportunities, there will be disparities in the health outcomes of different groups. Although new discoveries in medical science, impressive technological interventions, and modest policy initiatives have improved Americans' health and narrowed the gaps already described, these disparities have now persisted for over four centuries. There have always been rationalizations for the inequalities that mark the life spans and general health of Americans. For African Americans biology was often used to justify differences. For much of the nineteenth and twentieth centuries physicians focused on the frailty or hysteria of women which, in effect, was used to justify the neglect of their health.

In a paper detailing the continuing yet fluctuating gap between Black and white mortality between 1960 and 2002, the epidemiologist Nancy Krieger and her colleagues illustrated both the possibilities and limitations of reform without structural change. For the period between 1960 and 1980, the disparity between minority and white infant mortality rates declined significantly, an observation the authors ascribe to dramatic efforts at addressing the yawning gaps in economic and environmental inequalities, as well as in health service provision, that were started during the 1960s "War on Poverty." The civil rights and other social movements addressing racial discrimination and inequality had a tremendous impact on the health disparities that had long plagued American society. Yet, by the early 1980s with the end of the federal War on Poverty, the advent of Reagan-era policies, and the growth of conservative, antiregulatory ideologies, the gap between white and minority health status once again began to widen before narrowing again in the 2000s.[19] This ability to narrow the gap with the sustained effort of a massive investment, followed by a once-again widening of that gap, tells us several things: first, that reform is possible by concerted efforts to address the underlying inequalities that lead to differentials in health, and second, that factors such as the power and influence of specific entrenched interests limit how far reforms can go in the absence of major structural change.[20]

The notion of continuous improvement in health thus must be qualified: many have experienced improvements, but the disparities based on race, ethnicity, and income remain. Technological progress in medical treatment plays a role, but who you are, where you live, what you do, and what you earn have always been the central factors in determining your life span, the quality of your life—and your health. The narrative of ever-more substantial improvement that has been the bread and butter of so much of public health's self-congratulatory history needs to be modified to acknowledge the millions of years lost through early death that African Americans, Native Americans, the poor, and working-class whites have given up since the colonial era—centuries of life that can never be repaid.

As many epidemiologists, historians, anthropologists, and sometimes bench scientists have made clear over the last half century, how health and disease are defined determines how they are addressed. For much of American history, disease was understood by those relatively free of it through a particular social lens, that disease was the result of local custom, personal behavior, politics, economics, and morality. Designations of the "worthy" and "unworthy," the "deserving" and "undeserving poor," explained to those in power why some people suffered and others did not; why some "deserved" to be treated to the best medical care and others did not; why some "belonged" in private institutions and other were shunted to the poorhouse or underfunded public hospitals; why elderly who had worked all their lives deserved federally supported Medicare in their old age and why others who had not "contributed" enough to Social Security no matter what their labors had been might receive Medicaid, a system linked to public welfare programs whose benefits are often defined by the prejudices of the legislators in individual states. Racist biological ideas and eugenical notions of which lives were more or less valuable—even worth living—and social Darwinian ideas of the "natural" reasons that southern European immigrants and African Americans were doomed to shorter and less healthy lives all combined to provide a powerful intellectual and seemingly objective legitimacy and rationale for the observed differences in health and well-being—and for the refusal of the society to redress these inequities.

The nineteenth-century emphasis on the supposed failures of individuals or groups as the source of disease informed actions to improve health. Because illness was understood as a reflection of your place in a community, the type of work you did, your economic and social status, your race, your embrace of local religious and moral beliefs, and your personal habits, stress was often placed on reforming the individual rather than on reforming the society. With the nineteenth and early twentieth centuries' mass immigration of Irish Catholics, Italians, and eastern Europeans and Jews, along with the accompanying urbanization, industrialization, and physical and environmental effects, reformers recognized that the problem was bigger than supposed individual failings and that they needed to figure environmental conditions into the equation of what determined a healthful population. To control disease, they needed to attend to the physical, economic, and social worlds within which humans lived. Street sweeping, improved housing conditions and urban reform, clean water, and adequate sewerage systems were seen to address disease as much as medical or professional measures.[21]

The advent of bacteriology in the late nineteenth century also slowly shifted professional understanding of disease. The "germ theory," the view that a specific bacterium was the immediate source of a specific disease, was integrated into older notions of causation. The 1880s and 1890s saw a shift from a multicausal, social model of causation to a unicausal, specifically biological model based on the germ, with enormous consequences for the evolving field of public health. "Before 1880 we knew nothing," declared William Sedgwick, a prominent bacteriologist of his era. "After 1890, we knew it all. It was a glorious ten years."[22]

Over the course of the nineteenth century, then, efforts to improve health went through various phases. Initially, moral reform was seen as a way to improve the health of the poor, whose way of life was identified as the source of disease. Structural changes were also made in the physical environment, including housing reform, the development of a sewerage system and pure water supply, and systematic street cleaning. But in the waning decades of the nineteenth century and the early decades of the twentieth century, the emphasis again shifted. Philanthropists associated with the new industrial order, who were influenced by the discovery of the germ, poured a great deal of money and attention into medical education, laboratories, and professional medical groups and organizations, believing that this approach would find cures for disease.[23] Concurrently, public health, historically focused on prevention and improving the general health of populations, was by the early twentieth century seeing itself as a subspecialty of medicine, which increasingly defined disease as the result of a germ, either a bacterium or, perhaps, an invisible virus, that could be linked specifically to a clear set of symptoms.

There was a special attraction to looking for a unitary, biological "cause" of disease. Disease specificity, the idea that there is one microbe, virus, or, later, one or a group of genes responsible for a specific disease, is comforting. It provides, in theory at least, possible solutions in the form of antimicrobial agents, antitoxins, or genetic manipulations—solutions that do not require any reorganization of society. If a disease-specific entity can be found and technologically neutralized, there will be little impetus to solve difficult, systemic problems associated with the inequalities, oppression, or violence that Studs Terkel, Jack Geiger, Fannie Lou Hamer, and others saw as at the heart of suffering.[24]

There were those who, over the course of the twentieth century, saw the limits of attributing disease primarily to a microbe, virus, or gene. C.-E. A. Winslow, an American bacteriologist and seminal figure in public health, the renowned microbiologist and environmentalist René Dubos, and others identified the limits of the single-germ paradigm. Dubos, who coined the phrase "think globally, act locally," described the unicausal germ theory as a "cult—generated by a few miracles, undisturbed by inconsistencies and not too exacting about evidence." Bacteria, he suggested, were only "opportunistic invaders of tissues already weakened by crumbling defenses."[25] The Harvard epidemiologist John Gordon observed in 1952 that disease was a product of instability in the social as well as environmental ecology in which populations lived.[26]

By the 1970s, few would deny the validity of the "ecological perspective" regarding causes of disease, but, increasingly, the politics of the various explanations surfaced in discussions of multicausality and where the stress should lie. How much emphasis should be placed on individual, personal life choices, and how much should focus on broader socioeconomic forces outside of individual control: poverty and class inequality, racism, conditions of work, and pollution from industrial sources? Some felt that structural, societal factors should be emphasized. Social epidemiologists in South Africa, England, and the United States such as Mervyn Susser, Zena Stein, and Sidney Kark, and even more recently, Michael Marmot and George Davey Smith, pressed for a return to focusing on class and poverty as critical factors in identifying the "fundamental causes" of disease.[27]

Our thesis in this book is that disease is largely the product of human decisions about the way society is built and organized. Building on this perspective, we will look at how the prevalent diseases and conditions of health in different historical eras reflect the changing physical, economic, social, and political realities of American culture. For example, we consider the standard account that the destruction of Native American populations in the early colonial period resulted from epidemics that ravaged their communities because they had not built immunity to them. But we see this through the lens of colonialism in which European settlers displaced native populations, disrupting their social, economic, and ecological relationships, leaving them vulnerable to disease. In the nineteenth century, the incidence of classic infectious and communicable diseases—typhoid, cholera, smallpox, tuberculosis, and others—need not be seen as the inevitable product of an abstract urban, industrialized society, but just as often as the product of decisions, for example, by landlords for the sake of their own profit to jam people into tenements and leave them with outdoor plumbing and a polluted water supply. That is, rather than see people's suffering as the inevitable product of urbanization and industrialization, we see it as the product of dominant ideologies that reinforced a particular laissez-faire economic system with profit as its goal. There were, in fact, ways to urbanize and industrialize that would not have entailed such large-scale squalid conditions, terrible wages, and massive pollution—and consequently such considerable disease. Why did few question the logic of crowding so many together when there was nearly unlimited space in which to live in a still sparsely populated nation? Who determined that some people's health could be sacrificed for the wealth of others, even though there were often no objective reasons why conditions could not have been different?

In effect, leaders at the time made social and political decisions about who should live and who should die. But those decisions were hidden behind Victorian (and older) ideas about personal or community "worthiness" and who were the "truly" needy and who were "unworthy" or "undeserving," which led to the creation and maintenance of worlds that differentially killed the wealthy and the poor, the immigrant and the native-born American, the Black and the white, and Indigenous populations and those of European backgrounds.

From the very first moments when English and Spanish colonizers, as well as the French and Dutch, landed on the American continent, the worlds, both material and social, that they created were rooted in inequalities that produced different disease outcomes and different patterns of life and death. This was devastatingly true, of course, for Native Americans, whose lands and livelihoods were stolen from them. In the first 150 years following the British and Spanish colonization of the eastern seaboard, for example, one can see very different disease and mortality outcomes depending on the character of the communities that were established. As we discuss in chapter 1, for example, the early New England colonists experienced relative healthfulness, while the colonists in Jamestown experienced extraordinarily high death rates. In the North the organization of stable farming communities produced relatively healthful conditions, while the exploitative, unstable cash-crop economy of the South based on slavery produced higher rates of disease and death. In chapter 2 we trace the development of a southern economy built around cotton and commerce that created massive suffering and exploitation of Africans as well as the forced removal of the remaining communities of Native Americans from east of the Mississippi. We trace the links between this exploitative system and the beginnings of the northern industrial economy.

While the slave economy created its own patterns of suffering through the plantation system, it also fed the expansion of industrial capitalism in the North. New textile mills in New England and a national economy of trade and commerce built around the export of cotton to England and Europe transformed the lives of laborers, both Black and white. As workers were drawn to the factories of New England and the trading cities of New York, Philadelphia, and Boston, growing poverty, changing diets, and increased crowding nurtured an environment where infections were ready to spread among a weakened, more vulnerable community of laborers and their families. Chapter 3 explores the declining health status and life spans of the urban poor as epidemic diseases took an ever-increasing toll.

Similarly, in later chapters, we examine how a growing complex of chemical and petroleum industries in the twentieth century promoted new diseases among workers and consumers alike. It could have been different. Had companies acted more responsibly and government regulated chemicals, banning those that were deadly, far fewer would have died. Or, when it became apparent that their products sickened workers or damaged flora and fauna, they could have found ways not to pollute the environment outside the factory. For example, the petrochemical industry presented the country with a host of new threats from cancers and chronic conditions from diabetes, heart disease, and endocrine disruptions through climate change and environmental destruction. Similarly, the creation of huge markets for tobacco and processed foods pushed by national brands and marketing firms contributed immeasurably to chronic epidemics of heart disease and cancer.

The industrial capitalist economy as it developed in the United States left its mark not only on workers and adult consumers, but especially on children. Lead, for example, once primarily a danger to a small group of miners and industrial workers, was already a well-known toxin when, in the early twentieth century, companies such as Sherwin Williams and National Lead marketed paint manufactured with this poisonous metal throughout the nation. This was despite the fact that nonleaded, zinc-based, nontoxic paints had been available since the early nineteenth century. Lead paint, leaded gasoline, leaded plumbing fixtures, pipes, and solders—staples in the new housing of early-twentieth-century America—introduced "industrial" diseases to a mass audience. See figure 0.1.

Now, as policymakers confront the dangers of low-level exposures caused by pollution of the nation's waterways and air, new concerns have arisen about endocrine disruptors: certain chemicals found in soaps, shampoos, and other personal care products. Bisphenol A, found in some

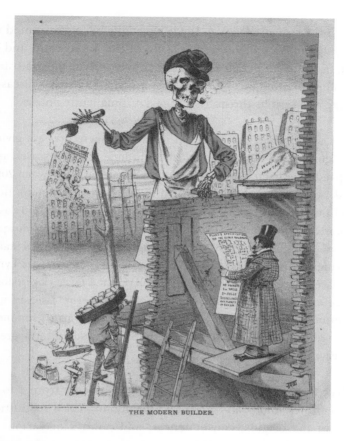

FIGURE 0.1 James E. Wales, "The Modern Builder," *Puck*, January 7, 1880. Box 8, Folder 11., Ms Coll 67, Bert Hansen Collection of Medicine and Public Health in Popular Graphic Art. Historical Library, Harvey Cushing/John Hay Whitney Medical Library, Yale University.

containers such as water bottles, has been linked to gender imbalances, behavioral change, and subtle neurological impairments. These and other hazardous chemicals in synthetic consumer products are typically introduced into the environment with little or no independent testing or, if needed, regulation. They have contributed to the development of new biological conditions such as autoimmune disorders, behavioral changes such as hyperactivity and attention deficit disorder, and possibly forms of autism or even lowered intelligence, even though many question whether we need many of these products.

With the spread of Covid-19 we have now been confronted with a highly infectious epidemic reminiscent of the nineteenth- and early-twentieth-century experience. New conditions such as those attributable to climate disruption increase the likelihood that infectious diseases will reemerge as a serious threat.[28] As the CDC poignantly notes:

> Mild winters, early springs, and warmer temperatures are giving mosquitoes and ticks more time to reproduce, spread diseases, and expand their habitats throughout the United States. Between 2004 and 2018, the number of reported illnesses from mosquito, tick, and flea bites more than doubled, with more than 760,000 cases reported in the United States. Nine new germs spread by mosquitoes and ticks were discovered or introduced into the United States during this period. The geographic ranges where ticks spread Lyme disease, anaplasmosis, ehrlichiosis, and spotted fever rickettsiosis have expanded, and experts predict that tickborne diseases will continue to increase and perhaps worsen. Longer, warmer summers have also given mosquitoes more time to reproduce and spread diseases.[29]

Over the decades, our work has ranged broadly from a focus on medical professionals and hospital and public health institutions to studies of the origins, consequences, and politics of various occupational and environmental diseases. In our study of the history of work and disease, we have developed a growing appreciation of how extensive social and economic factors have been in the generation and spread of disease. In *Building the Worlds That Kill Us*, we shift our focus from particular industries and the health consequences of their practices to explore what we see as a continuing theme—that throughout American history, different worlds have been created that reflect decisions about whose lives can be compromised or cut short. Simply put, the message that we can learn from the past is that we need not continue to build worlds that kill us but can, collectively, make more life-affirming decisions.

CHAPTER ONE

Disease and Exploitation During the Colonial and Revolutionary Eras

"I am now to relate some strange and remarkable" events, wrote William Bradford, the longtime governor of the Plymouth Colony in his diary entry of June 1634. A colony of one thousand white settlers had moved into an area along the Connecticut River in a region populated by native peoples. Bradford observed that the settlers were "enimise of those Indeans . . . and of whom they stood in some fear." A smallpox outbreak had hit during a particularly harsh winter when both food and wood for heat were scarce.[1] He estimated that 950 of the 1,000 native peoples had perished, in contrast to approximately 500 of the 1,000 white settlers.[2]

But the impact on the Indian population in the area was even worse because they "died most miserably; for a sorer disease cannot befall them." Bradford described their terrible suffering:

> . . . The poxe breaking and mattering, and runing one into another, their skin cleaving (by reason therof) to the matts they lye on; when they tume them, a whole side will flea of at once, (as it were,) and they will be all of a gore blood, most fearfull to behold; and then begin very sore, what with cold and other distempers, they dye like rotten sheep. The condition of this people was so lamentable, and they fell downe so generally of this diseas, as they were (in the end) not able to help on another; no, not to make a fire, nor to fetch a little water to drinke, nor any to burie the dead; but would strivie

as long as they could, and when they could procure no other means to make fire, they would bume the woden trayes & dishes they ate their meate in, and their very bowes & arrowes; & some would crawle out on all foure to gett a little water, and some times dye by the way, & not be able to gett in againe.[3]

By 1634, the incidence of deaths from smallpox and other diseases among everyone living in New England was pronounced, but the devastation of native peoples by disease was particularly profound. The smallpox epidemic of 1633–1634 afflicted the communities of Mohegans, Abenakis, Pocumtuks, Massachusetts, Pequots, and other peoples who lived on the land, and accounts of the time tell of villages that one year were seemingly healthy, even robust, but the next were virtually deserted, populated only with the sick and dying.[4]

The suffering that Bradford described was not the first time that disease would wreak havoc on the native population, but it was a harbinger of the terrible toll that it would take in future decades. In fact, the crisis in health and longevity that Native American peoples still experience is eerily similar to early encounters in which white settlers disrupted, destroyed, and dismantled native cultures, leaving the population especially vulnerable to the ravages of viruses, bacteria, and every other form of assault on their bodies.[5]

This chapter explores the toll that disease and suffering took on all those living in America before the Revolution—on the native population, whose lives were greatly impacted by the arrival of colonists; on the colonists themselves, whose survival depended on the nature of the communities they created; and on the enslaved people who were imported in chains to produce much of the wealth of the New World, whose lives were devastated as a result of the conditions of the slave system. The chapter also examines slavery and the toll it took on the Africans it exploited, and finally the state of affairs in the Revolutionary period.

THE ECOLOGICAL CONSEQUENCES OF SETTLER EXPANSION AND THE IMPACT ON THE NATIVE POPULATION

Wherever Europeans landed in the New World, they encountered people living in diverse communities with established ways of providing for themselves, sometimes adequately, sometimes not. Large numbers of people lived along the coast, inland, and on the islands off the North and South American continents. They fished, farmed, and hunted, went to war, and experienced famines and disease, as did most of the world's people. The Indigenous people of the North American coasts comprised a wide range of linguistic and tribal groups—including the Algonquin and Iroquoian peoples of the Northeast and Great Lakes, the Powhatans of the mid-Atlantic, the Siouans and Muskogeans of the southern East Coast, the Seminoles, Creeks, and Apalachees of what is now Florida, and many more.[6]

Estimates of the numbers of Indigenous people living in the Western Hemisphere before the Europeans arrived have differed widely. Early-twentieth-century estimates were often low, between 8 and 15 million people, partly because of the methodologies used and the limitations of the archaeological evidence. But these low estimates may also reflect the biases of scholars who believed that native peoples were too primitive to have established viable societies capable of sustaining large populations or that the European colonists could not possibly have displaced or destroyed so many.

Contemporary archaeologists and demographers have raised those early estimates substantially. Today, some estimate that there were between 60 and 100 million people in the Americas in 1492, though other recent estimates are substantially lower. One estimate is that there were 44 million Indigenous people in the Americas and some 2 million in North America.[7] Estimates of the number of Indigenous peoples living in what is now New England before the arrival of Europeans in the early 1600s also vary.[8] We will never know the precise number, but if the early accounts approximate reality, native populations lined the coast of North America from today's New England all the way down through the Florida Keys and the islands of the Caribbean. Native populations far outnumbered Europeans for at least a century following Columbus's arrival, and they outnumbered the British in North America for another century after the first enduring English settlement in 1607.

Life in North America before the Europeans arrived was not easy, and like all societies, those of Native Americans had their share of illness and disease. Archaeological and genetic studies indicate that there was wide variation in the native experience with malnutrition, infant mortality, and infectious diseases such as tuberculosis. Other studies have revealed episodic cycles of nutritional crises caused by droughts and the deleterious effects of parasites, infections, and even syphilis. Skeletal remains have revealed injuries from wars and evidence of dental cavities.[9] Native Americans were not a "virgin" population, as some Europeans described them, living in a paradise without disease or premature death.[10] The New World before the Europeans arrived was not an Eden, and its mix of populations, ecologies, and economic and social relations was as complex as any other set of societies.

As with every culture throughout world history, infectious disease and even epidemics were an ever-present threat, and, as with other epidemics that had swept through populations, Native Americans were more susceptible to pathogens previously unknown in their region. Yet, like their European counterparts and people everywhere, they did have natural defenses that could react to biological invaders when their bodies were in full health. We now understand that the human immune system, when not compromised by malnutrition or conditions that undermine its biological defenses, will develop antibodies that will give it a chance to recover. In generally well-fed, healthy populations, even the most severe epidemics will typically affect a minority of the population. As a population, groups can adapt, survive, and, over time, regain their numbers. Just as they did everywhere around the globe, epidemics in the New World came and went, leaving temporary depletions of populations whose numbers would one day rebound.[11]

Along the southern New England coast, native peoples typically built small structures for one or two families for summer use, while in the winter, further inland, they used longhouses that could shelter many families, conserving heat and resources.[12] Warmer weather and longer growing seasons supported a more robust agricultural society. In the inland areas, grains and other crops made up a much larger proportion of the diet, replacing venison, since the grains were easily stored.[13] By the early decades of the seventeenth century, the native peoples had cleared vast amounts of land for agricultural production.[14] To escape the winter storms, populations that fished in ocean waters in the summer trekked inland to hunt, often approaching near starvation during the harsh months of January and February. During these difficult times, native peoples were more subject to disease, including bacterial infections from common microorganisms, perhaps staphylococcus and streptococcus.[15]

Even in the most remote northern communities, Native American populations moved from inland areas to the coast in spring in anticipation of the spawning runs and the bounty of cod, trout, striped bass, flounder, sturgeon, scallops, clams, mussels, and crab. For some, more than half the yearly food supply came from these waters. The environmental historian William Cronon writes, "In late March, the smelt arrived . . . in such quantities that one could not put a 'hand into the water without encountering them.'"[16] With the fish and shellfish came the animals that fed upon them. Ducks and other migratory fowl were said to be so abundant that one could easily hunt them with bow and arrow. And with the ducks came a ready supply of eggs to be gathered by the village children. Nuts, berries, and fruits added to a rich and healthful diet in the spring and summer months. In September, as winter approached, families moved inland again, and there they found beaver, moose, caribou, and bear to hunt.[17]

In the Southeast, according to studies that rely on examination of human bones and teeth, native peoples in the centuries before contact with Europeans and Africans gradually became farmers. They cultivated a range of plants like knotweed and sunflowers but ultimately came to depend on maize as the mainstay of their diet, along with beans and squash. But, as the historian Paul Kelton explains, this reliance presented a "paradox." On the one hand, a diet based on the cultivation of maize "enhanced female fertility" in part because the agricultural system allowed for a steady diet, freed from the instability and periods of deprivation characteristic of a hunting-gathering society. This steadiness allowed the native population to expand, but it also led to "higher rates of infant mortality and shorter life expectancies than their hunting and gathering ancestors," in part because nutritional deficiencies made populations more vulnerable to infectious disease. Although native communities attempted to diversify their diets beyond maize by hunting game and cultivating beans as well as gathering nuts and berries, Kelton writes that "the archeological evidence . . . indicates that among some populations compensatory strategies were not enough to stave off anemia; many people depended too much on maize."[18] Further, the turn to farming meant that populations were more concentrated, which itself led to increased susceptibility to disease and a greater likelihood that diseases could spread more easily.[19]

But after the colonists had grown in numbers, established settlements, and taken control of land, their presence in many places began to have an appreciable effect on Native American movements, farming, fishing, and hunting, which in turn affected natives' ability to cope with adversity. In addition, the physical assaults on native peoples—including attacks on specific villages and all-out wars—clearly had an impact on the growing mortality rates. All of these together—war, social disruption, restricted ability to hunt and fish—had dramatic effects on both Native Americans' immediate health and their ability to recover from epidemics. "Had Indians simply experienced new pathogens," the historian David Jones explains, "their populations would have declined and recovered, as happened in Athens (after the plague in 430 BCE), Rome (after smallpox in the second and third centuries), and medieval Europe (after the bubonic plague)."[20] But this was not to be the experience of the Indigenous people of North America.

There are plentiful descriptions that ascribe the decimation of local Indian groups after the initial arrival of Europeans to smallpox, measles, flu, and other diseases that were common in the crowded, often urban environments of Europe but unknown in the Americas and that therefore had a particularly devastating effect on previously nonexposed Indigenous populations. But this portrayal obscures different experiences with first contact. Along the Massachusetts coast, even before the arrival of the Pilgrims, there was an epidemic, probably smallpox, that was apparently caused by episodic contact with explorers from Greenland and Norway, who, upon landing in North America, had stopped along the New England coast. But other early encounters in the sixteenth century did not have the same outcome, whether they were Ponce de León's expeditions in what is now Florida or the arrival of early traders who traversed the Ohio or Illinois River valleys. As the historian George R. Milner suggests, "a dispersed settlement pattern and uneasy social relations provided a protection of sorts against epidemics." There could be local outbreaks of disease as a result of sporadic contacts, but they were limited even if sometimes devastating.[21]

As more and more settlers arrived, increasing restrictions on Native American movement and access to fishing, hunting, and land for planting transformed native diets and the ability to resist disease. As Milner explains, it would require greater numbers of Europeans, including men, women, and children and more sustained contact, "before repeated and widespread epidemics in the interior were likely to occur."[22] Such was the case with the devastating smallpox epidemic of 1633–1634, described earlier, which involved the Connecticut River valley and all of interior New England.

As early as 1632, one year before the epidemic hit and just a dozen years after the *Mayflower* had landed, William Bradford, governor of Plymouth colony, described the process that would later lead to considerable disease and death, particularly among New England's Native American population. After describing the initially friendly relations with the Indians who greeted the Pilgrims' arrival, Bradford discussed the large numbers of other British people who followed the Pilgrims to Plymouth and their impact on his colony and the ecology of the region. He related how "the people of the plantation begane to grow in their owtward estats, by reason of the flowing of many people into the cuntrie, especially into the Bay of the Massachusett; by which means corne & catle rose to a great price."[23] From the first landings of about 100 Pilgrims in 1620, the colony grew to approximately 1,500 in the next three decades.[24]

While this population growth led to general prosperity in the short run as diets improved with the greater availability of meat and grains, Bradford worried that the colony's foundation as a tight-knit community built around church and common purpose, a "peaceable kingdom" of self-imposed exiles from England, was being undermined. The original cohesion, only two decades after its founding, was beginning to fray, for as individual fortunes increased, "ther was no longer [much] holding them together." The population expansion created new demands for land further and further afield. Bradford described the impact of new farms and settlers eager to expand acreage to accommodate cattle and agriculture. "No man now thought he could live, except he had catle and a great deale of ground to keep them," he observed, "all striving to increase their stock." New settlements "were scattered all over the bay" and "[h]aving oxen growne," he observed, "they must have land for plowing & tillage."[25]

At first, the original colony attempted to counter the splintering of their community by giving out special grants of land to select members that would "tye the lands to Plimoth . . . and retain their dwellings here," Bradford wrote. "But, alas! this remedy proved worse than the disease; for within a few years those that had thus gott footing . . . partly by force, and partly by wearing the rest with importunitie and pleas of necessitie," challenged the hierarchy "so as they must either suffer them and goe, or live in continuall opposition and contention." Bradford feared that this process "will ber the ruine of New-England, at least of the churches of God."[26] As the historian A. C. Swedlund simply points out, "the rapid intrinsic growth, coupled with the high rates of English immigration, flooded the region with families looking for more land."[27]

This population growth was not limited to the original Plymouth plantation but extended to a host of new settlements that dotted the Cape Cod peninsula, as well as to new settlements to the west and north of Plymouth. The Massachusetts Bay colony was established in 1629 by arriving Puritans; only seven years later, the Connecticut colony was born, as was the New Haven colony in 1638, along with numerous other settlements in the seventeenth century. Until the early 1640s, the population increase was the result of massive migration from England. After the 1640s, the population increased mainly through a high birthrate, relatively low infant mortality, and an increased life span. For the New England colonies, the population was about 3,000 in 1630, 14,000 in 1640, 33,000 in 1660, and 68,000 in 1680.[28]

Bradford was wrong about geographic and demographic expansion being the ruin of settler New England, but the explosion of population, the demand for new land, and the use of force to get that land certainly were major reasons for the steep decline of the native population and a major reason for a failure to recover from earlier epidemics. Indian communities that traditionally migrated during warm weather to the ocean to fish were cut off by the settlements that grew along the eastern seaboard, generally in the very harbors where the waters were calmer and thus safer for ships and commerce as well as for fishing. Similarly, the creation of private property and fences in the inland settlements limited the ability of native peoples to hunt on traditional lands. Tribes that migrated across regions found their entire way of life disrupted, if not destroyed, leading to hunger and even starvation. As the historian Alan Swedlund argues, "malnutrition, relocation, disruption of community and family life, and depression of fertility, not to mention war and conflict all came together to suppress the Native population of Massachusetts and New England until at least the mid-nineteenth century."[29] Native Americans were left weakened, sometimes starving, and ultimately susceptible to viruses that, in a healthier population, would not take such a toll. Epidemics of smallpox, influenza, scarlet fever, dysentery, pneumonia, and other named and unnamed plagues swept through native populations, killing huge numbers deep into the nineteenth century.[30]

A. C. Swedlund gives some vivid accounts of how the sweep of Europeans into New England coastal areas and their movement into arable lands farther west severely disrupted and undermined Native American agricultural, hunting, and fishing practices, leaving villages isolated, often unable to fish, hunt, or even harvest lands that they once had free access to. In 1675, for example, at the beginning of what became known as King Philip's War, the area in what is now Rhode Island and southern Connecticut and Massachusetts was "given" by the crown to the English settlers, which led to attacks by the Pocumtucks, who were then joined by the Wapanoags, Nipmucks, Narragansetts, and Abenakis in a war with the English. After a series of losses to the native peoples spanning a few years, the English regrouped and sent a considerable force into the area, slaughtering about three hundred natives, mostly women, children, and elderly. They forced a migration of the remaining native communities north and west into Vermont and New York, leading them to conflicts with Indigenous peoples already in those areas. After various attempts of the Pocumtucks and other Indian peoples to return and to reconstitute their communities, the English settlers prevailed, leaving numerous remaining Native Americans homeless, with no means of self-support and doomed to perpetual forced migrations.[31] The war extended throughout southern New England, and, as the Society of Colonial Wars put it, the conflict "resulted in the virtual extermination of tribal Indian life in southern New England."[32] By 1700, demographers estimate that the Native American population in that area had declined anywhere from 50 to 90 percent.[33] "With each encroachment," Swedlund argues, "the ability for Native settlements to maintain their own fertility and family structure was severely compromised."[34]

By 1700 the various conflicts in North America between the English and French over control of territory also left many native populations forced to choose sides and ultimately lose homelands and means of support if they happened to select the losing side in their region. In the first century after the colonists' arrival, much of the Massachusetts Native American population was, according to Swedlund, indiscriminately "killed, sold, or made to serve as indentured servants" or "sold into slavery to other colonies as far as the West Indies."[35] The Hurons of what is today northern New York State along the St. Lawrence River sided with the French during the French and Indian War (1754–1763) and abandoned their villages because of attacks from other native peoples as well as the British. As a result, they were vulnerable to malnutrition and "a contagious malady," and, according to one librarian and historian writing in 1899, they were reduced to "dying skeletons eking out a miserable life."[36]

Of course, encounters between colonists and Native Americans and the resulting disease effects were not confined to New England. What the historian Paul Kelton calls the "Great Southeastern Smallpox Epidemic" (1696–1700) devastated a wide range of native peoples from Virginia to the Gulf Coast and even up the Mississippi River, including the Creeks, Siouans, Natchez, Chickasaws, Biloxis, and Quapaws, among many others.[37] Kelton acknowledges that the virus spread through a "virgin population," but the "explosiveness and devastation" that it wrought on all but the most remote villages happened because "English trade dramatically changed the social landscape and disease ecology of the region." The British in the Southeast "flooded" the region with a wide variety of goods that were traded with the native population, one of the most prominent of which was guns. What had been formerly self-sufficient communities were now intimately tied into "the larger Atlantic World." The British were especially interested in buying native captives who could work their lands, and this desire "dramatically increased the volume of human traffic, as traders, raiders, slaves and refugees crisscrossed the region." These violent and disruptive raids led native peoples to barricade themselves in settlements where disease outbreaks were more prevalent. In many of these "fortified, compact, and unsanitary towns," natives experienced malnutrition (and hence greater susceptibility to disease) because they were reluctant to leave their compounds to hunt or gather food for fear of being captured and enslaved.[38]

The narrative that Jones, Swedlund, Kelton, and others tell, compared to the simple disease/immunity model, is thus more complex and nuanced, demanding both biological and historical explanation and analysis. The Indigenous peoples' special vulnerability lay in the disruptions to the social organization of their lives brought on by invasion, appropriation, trade, and war. The European arrival and settlement destroyed Indigenous migratory patterns. The Europeans created systems of private ownership of land along the coast, denying fishing rights or even acreage to the native peoples. The bays and coves were the settlements of choice because they provided safe harbor for the ships that carried settlers and supplies and later rum, molasses, and slaves from Europe, Africa, and the West Indies, thereby cutting off native peoples from easy access to fish and shellfish. The forced movements of the Indigenous peoples from their lands and the inevitable consequences on their farming, fishing, and hunting created severe nutritional and social problems. As Jones summarizes: "It was the turbulence of colonization and not genetic liability that created Indians' devastating susceptibility to imported pathogens."[39] Questioning the "virgin soil" hypothesis, he posits that it was not genetic susceptibility to European viruses and bacteria that accounted for the devastation. What if the epidemics of smallpox that ravaged the Mohawk Nation in 1634, the native peoples in the Lake Ontario area in 1636, the Iroquois tribes in 1679, or the Quapaw Nation of Arkansas in 1698 had not taken place in the context of the introduction of guns and iron and brass arrowheads that made conflicts between native peoples and incoming French and English settlers much more deadly and devastating to native societies? As the historian Daniel Richter said, "European diseases and firearms intensified Indian conflicts." In addition, the growing integration of trade between colonists and native peoples "made economic motives central to American Indian conflicts for the first time. Because iron tools, firearms, and other trade goods so quickly became essential to Indian economies, struggles for those items and for furs to barter for them lay behind numerous seventeenth-century wars." Such disruption by war and the new technologies that made conflicts more deadly left remaining populations more susceptible to the ravages of disease.[40]

The epidemics themselves were of course devastating, but germs alone do not explain why native populations did not fully recover over the course of the following century or more. The historian Alan Taylor estimates that by 1670 there were about 17,000 native people in New England and that that number went even lower by the end of the century, a dramatic drop from the 60,000 estimated to be there in 1630.[41] Even the worst large-scale epidemic in world history, the bubonic plague, "only" wiped out anywhere between a third and a half of Europe's population in 1348–1349, yet the population eventually recovered to pre-epidemic levels by the early 1500s. This is in contrast to the experience of Indigenous populations of North America and specifically the United States, where the populations of Native Americans in parts of the United States have never fully recovered. As Kelton, Swedlund, and other historians succinctly argue, a fuller explanation lies in the "warfare, enslavement, land expropriation, removals, erasures of identity and other non-disease factors" that set the conditions for the impact of disease.[42]

But we should remember that, despite the frequency of assaults on native people and the epidemics of disease that devastated certain tribes, many native peoples were able to maintain their cultures. They often did this even on vastly restricted parcels of inferior land and difficult terrain. In New England, for example, there is evidence, in Swedlund's words, of "large settlements and populations of Native groups living along the coast and in the interior of Massachusetts after 1634," even after the devastating epidemic of that year.[43] Even the Hurons, who were overwhelmed by war and disease in the seventeenth century, had been able to reestablish themselves in communities in Michigan and northern Ohio by the mid-eighteenth century. In Georgia, Alabama, and elsewhere in the South and in the mid-Atlantic colonies, some tribal communities found ways of surviving, even thriving, through armed resistance or through accommodation and even integration into the settler economies. Other times survival depended on negotiation and treaties.[44] In certain parts of the Midwest and Great Lakes, through much of the colonial period, Native American culture and political and social dominance marked the economic and social lives of French and English traders and settlers. Michael Witgen, in his magisterial study of the relations between Native Americans and European settlers in the Great Lakes region, argues that Native American peoples outside the Atlantic coast largely controlled their economic and social fate for the first two centuries after Europeans arrived and did so well into the nineteenth century. What Witgen describes as the "infinity" of native identities—the flexibility of their social groupings, the resistance to identities formed around the idea of nations defined by geography, and the shifting alliances based upon linguistic, geographic, and social relationships rather than nationality alone—allowed for a continuing coherence that avoided dominance by colonial powers.[45] The full conquest of native peoples would wait until their planned removal and genocide by the U.S. government in the 1800s.

DIVERGENT PATTERNS OF DISEASE AND DEATH AMONG THE SETTLER POPULATION

The worlds created by the English in the North American colonies to a large extent also dictated their own health and mortality outcomes, and they varied considerably depending on the region. Consider the cases of three of the earliest English settlements: Jamestown, Virginia, and the Massachusetts settlements of Andover and Plymouth, both of which have particularly good documentation of the settlers' experience in the early years and exemplify the story we are going to see developing throughout this book. Superficially, one might think that these settlements—populated by people who spoke the same language, came from the same homeland, and practiced variations on the same religion—would have had relatively equivalent health and mortality experiences. Yet this was hardly the case. At least for the first three generations, their experiences would contradict some common assumptions about what determines health and disease.

One would think, for example, that the Virginia settlement would have fared the best because it was set in a more hospitable climate, with mild winters, long growing seasons, and rich soil. In Massachusetts, by contrast, 700 miles to the north, settlers landed in a harsh, cold, and uninviting land. The weather foreshortened their growing seasons, the soil was sandy and rocky, and the hilly terrain made agriculture difficult even where the soil was fine. Think of wandering the New England woods, coming across stone fences made from the rocks that had to be pulled from the ground before crops could be planted.

Plymouth and Andover: Early Demographic Success

The climate and environment of New England in the seventeenth century would seem hardly conducive to good nutrition or endurance. But, in fact, New Englanders thrived, living comparatively long, relatively healthy, and prosperous lives. Their communities grew dramatically in size, first by migration and later by natural increase. Women married young, they had many children, and those whose lives were not cut short by complications of childbirth could expect to see most of their children grow to adulthood. Men who reached the age of twenty-one could expect to live into their sixties, seventies, and even eighties, often marrying younger women if their first wives died. Infant mortality was low by the standards of the time, birthrates were high, and the average age of death compares favorably to the life spans of Americans through much of the twentieth century. The average age of death for the first generation of Andover settlers who reached the age of twenty-one was a remarkable 71.8 years for men and 70.8 years for women.[46] Unlike in the few larger communities like Boston, New York, and Philadelphia, epidemic disease was generally not a major cause of death among the European and small African populations in the rural areas of New England and the middle colonies.[47]

We can see this story told in the old New England cemeteries. In a family plot, there is often one large headstone surrounded by slightly smaller ones. The largest is the patriarch of the family, and at his side are his wives, whose deaths often predated his own. In front are a number of small headstones of children who died at birth or in infancy. In Andover, Massachusetts, for example, an extraordinarily high birthrate and low infant mortality led to a population explosion that ultimately created social tensions over land use, land distribution, inheritance, and family structure.[48] From our perspective today, these gravestones seem to tell a depressing story of early death. Certainly, some New England deaths reflected epidemics of smallpox, the disfiguring disease that Europeans introduced to the colonies, and diphtheria, the terrifying children's disease that choked its victims to death and that killed approximately five thousand children in Boston during outbreaks in the first decades of the eighteenth century. Other epidemic diseases killed and sickened children as well: measles, chin cough (whooping cough), bloody flux (dysentery), influenza, and mumps were prevalent. Yellow fever, whose symptoms were sudden high fever, debilitating headaches, vomiting, exhaustion, and jaundiced skin, became endemic throughout the New England area (as well as in the Caribbean and the American South), and there were even occasional outbreaks of cholera, the diarrheal disease that dehydrated and killed its victims often in a matter of hours. But these were generally confined to local communities and rarely affected the overall death rate of the Massachusetts Bay colony as a whole until the mid-eighteenth century.

In the seventeenth century, while New England settlers were enjoying a revolutionary change in their length of life, if not well-being,[49] their relatives who remained in England were typically dying in their thirties and forties. Men there who reached the age of forty often saw themselves as at the end of their lives, not the middle. Women could not expect to see their children grow up. Plague still struck down huge numbers of English before 1665.[50] Childhood mortality was astronomical: more than 70 percent of children died before the age of five. How extraordinary it would have seemed to hear that in New England nine of ten children survived at least until age five.

New England colonists in the seventeenth century had left behind a world of crowded cities, feudal patterns of land ownership, and oppressive social norms. Largely populated by families permanently leaving Europe behind, many saw the New World as, in the words of one settler, a "place that God has opened . . . for their deliverance . . . for here all that a man works for is his own; and there are no revenue hounds to take it from us . . . no one to take away yer corn, yer potatoes, yer lint or yer eggs."[51]

In New England and the mid-Atlantic colonies, the abundance of land, the self-contained nature of many of the early settlements, the organization of governance and everyday life—all augured a relatively healthy population. For much of the eighteenth century, historical demographers have shown, British settlers and their descendants were substantially taller than their European brethren.[52] In contrast to the English, there were no height differences based on class or occupation. From this fact we can assume that good nutrition and clean water were more or less equitably distributed.[53]

In the seventeenth century, the typical New England farm family owned between 100 and 200 acres of land, about 10 percent of which was harvested. Because of technological limitations and the intensity of labor required, the New England family had historically tilled only about 10 to 12 acres of land: the difficulties inherent in the use of mule-pulled plows, rough terrain, and walking made more efficient cultivation impossible. So, for much of the seventeenth century, approximately 90 percent of the family's land went unplowed, lying fallow, replenishing its nutrients sometimes for as long as a decade. Much of the land could be used for grazing livestock, milk cows, oxen, and sheep, all of which provided plentiful supplies of milk, meat, cheese, wool, leather, and fertilizer for the relatively self-sufficient farm.[54] This abundant and diverse use of the land allowed the family to live on a varied diet of vegetables that could be preserved and meat that could be slaughtered and then smoked or salted for the long winter months.

Jamestown: A Society Based on Death

In contrast to the northern colonists, the British who landed in Virginia, found terrain that was much more amenable to agriculture and the establishment of permanent settlements. In fact, early colonists wrote of the extraordinary contrast of the cold English weather and the warm, welcoming, lush world that they had found. The summers were long and falls mild, the topsoil deep, and the rivers stocked with sturgeon and other fish. "The country is excellent and pleasant," began "I. H." in an introduction to a description of Virginia by John Smith, founder of the original colony at Jamestown in 1607. "The clime temperate and healthful, the ground fertill and good." All seemed ready for an existence "whereby those that shall succeed, may at ease labour for their profit, in the most sweete, coole, and temperate shade."[55]

John Smith recounts the first encounters with the Indigenous inhabitants of the region. After unloading their supplies and developing fortifications, the colonists began an exploration that took them upriver about 60 miles. They went along "plains high ground, with many fresh springs, the people in all places kindely intreating us, daunsing and feasting us with strawberries, Mulberries, Bread, Fish, and other . . . provisioned whereof we had pleanty." The explorers "kindly requited their least favours with Bels, Pinnes, Needles, beades, or Glasses, which so contented them that [Smith's] liberalitie made them follow us from place to place, and ever kindely to respect us."[56]

Soon, however, those writing back home told of an irony between the plentiful land and the suffering they experienced. "This torrid sommer bene visited with great sickness and mortality; which our good God (his name be blessed for it) hath recompensed with a marvelous plenty, such as hath not bene since our first coming into the lande," wrote John Pory, the Crown's secretary of Virginia, in 1619.[57] Soon the native peoples on whom the colonists depended for corn during their early months turned hostile, and the disease and starvation in this plentiful land had the settlers, in the words of the historian Edmund Morgan, "living with death."[58]

The first eighty years in colonial Virginia were, demographically speaking, a disaster. Death and disease, not long life and health, were its hallmarks. While many men in New England would sometimes live to see their seventies, the Virginia settlers often lasted less than a year before disease and death struck them down. The first boats to arrive in 1607 brought 108 English settlers to Jamestown. The boats returned to England with word of wondrous conditions in the colony, but when they returned a year later bringing many new settlers, they found only 38 of the original colonists—all sickly and starving—still alive.[59] The following year was equally disastrous. A colony now of 500 settlers was reduced to 60 in a mere six months. In the early years following the first landings at Jamestown, dysentery, nutritional deficiencies, and starvation accounted for the dramatic increase in mortality. (Yellow fever and malaria did not become factors until later in the 1600s with the expansion and growing dependence of Virginia on the slave trade.)[60] Nor did things improve in the years thereafter. Between 1619 and 1622, the British sent almost 4,000 people to Virginia to supplement the 700 who were there at the time; 3,000 of the newcomers died. One historian estimates that about 6,000 English left for the Virginia colony between 1607 and 1624, but only 1,200 were still alive by 1625.[61] By 1640, approximately 15,000 immigrants had arrived on Virginia's shores, yet the colony was only 8,000 strong.[62]

The second half of the century was also bleak. Men who reached the age of twenty in Virginia could not, on average, expect to live past the age of forty.[63] In general, during the seventeenth century, the death rates for southern colonists were twice those of New Englanders. While southern women tended to marry earlier than those in New England, maternal mortality and higher infant mortality led to lower fertility rates than those in the mid-Atlantic and New England colonies.[64] In New England, roughly one in ten children died before adulthood, approximately half the death rate of children in Virginia.[65] As the historian Edmund Morgan observed, "No matter how one reads the figures, they show that Virginians had to cope year after year with a death rate comparable only to that of severe epidemic years in England."[66]

In those early years, biological, environmental, social, and political forces in Virginia converged into a sustained catastrophe. Typhoid and dysentery, poor water quality, drought, an imbalance between men and women, childhood diseases, extreme isolation, and malnutrition combined to create a society that lived with death.[67] The historian Karen Ordahl Kupperman has likened the attitude and psychological depression of the early Jamestown settlers to those of prisoners of war.[68] What accounts for the disastrous experience in Virginia? Some scholars have blamed supply shortages, tensions with the native population, greed, and competition among colonists as they searched for gold and silver— and even "neglect of the crucial business of growing food to stay alive."[69] They may have all played a role, but there is certainly some truth as well in the explanation that the cause was disease, demographics, and environmental realities.

One reason the colony could not increase its population, immigration aside, was its skewed ratio of men to women. While the Massachusetts colonists arrived in boats filled with entire families leaving to establish for themselves a New World and never to return to England, those who settled Virginia were not nearly as varied a lot. Men outnumbered women almost four to one, and there were very few children aboard. These demographics made it virtually impossible for the population to naturally increase, and it seems unlikely that many of those who came voluntarily planned to stay longer than a few years.

The very purpose of the colony helped to define its failure. From the first, it was intended as an exploitative enterprise, founded for the enrichment of the Crown. The colony was there to exploit mineral and agricultural products and establish new commercial relationships, not to settle the land, escape oppression, or fulfill the vision of a new society.

Like the Spanish and Portuguese monarchs who encouraged colonization of Central and South America, the British Crown expected untold
riches, gold and silver bullion easily mined or purchased for a song from
native peoples. But in Jamestown the gold and silver failed to material-
ize; within a few years, the cultivation of tobacco instead became the
center of Jamestown's economic life. Whatever economic value tobacco
had as a source of profits, dependence upon it carried risks. It was per-
ishable, and the uncertainties of shipping made it a gamble: shipping
delays or bad weather could destroy an entire crop. More importantly
for the long-term survival of the colony, tobacco was of little nutritional
value, and the absence of nutritional crops made the colony dependent
on trade with Native American populations. At the same time, the colony had been mandated to impose Christianity on the native population, a mission that required fealty to the Crown, undermined friendly
relations, and hampered trade. The colonists set out, according to the
aforementioned "I. H.," "erecting of true religion among the Infidels,
to the overthrow of superstition and idolatrie, to the winning of many
thousands of wandering sheepe, unto Christ's fold, who now, and until
now, have strayed in the unknown paths of Paganisme, Idolatrie, and
superstition." Hardly goals that would encourage mutual respect and
peaceful interactions.[70]

The physical, social, and economic worlds of the colonists of
Jamestown and Massachusetts thus led to profoundly different experiences with health and disease. The Jamestown colony, despite its salubrious natural environment, was marked by death and disease for much
of the first century of its existence, while the Massachusetts colonists,
despite a challenging natural environment of short growing seasons,
sandy soil, and cold winters, generally thrived, on land they comman-
deered from the native population. This difference between the two
cultures in disease experience was largely due to the way each group
constructed their world.

THE HEALTH AND HUMAN CONSEQUENCES
OF A SLAVE ECONOMY

From early on, slavery was the signature element of the emerging southern economy, and with it came disease, abuse, and death. Since the

colony's beginnings in Jamestown, Virginia and the rest of the South largely depended on single-crop agriculture. That system, in turn, depended on the exploitation and suffering of white indentured servants and, increasingly, African slaves to do the backbreaking labor required for the production of cash crops for export—rice, indigo, tobacco, and eventually cotton.[71]

Slavery was the South's answer to the broad need to find human beings to labor in the harsh conditions that were imposed to extract as much profit as possible from the land. Initially, land was plentiful but people willing to do the work were scarce, so the Crown offered huge tracts of land to those willing to settle in the Virginia colony. But even this was not enough to secure the Crown's purposes. So the Crown gave 40 hectares (about 100 acres) to English settlers who sponsored passage of someone—indentured servant, slave, or voluntary immigrant—to the Virginia colony, thus encouraging the indentureship of some and the enslavement of others.[72]

In the 1600s, approximately 300,000 indentured servants, mostly young men between the ages of fifteen and twenty-five from Britain, Ireland, and Germany, came to North America—more than half of all Europeans who came to North America in that period. Of the indentured servants, about 220,000 went to the mainland colonies, with the rest going to the islands of the Caribbean.[73] These servants essentially mortgaged four to seven years of their lives to work in the colonies, receiving food, clothing, and housing in return; if they survived that period, they received 50 acres of land at the end of their term of service. According to the historian Alan Taylor, "English servants composed at least three-quarters of the emigrants to the Chesapeake during the seventeenth century: about 90,000 of the 120,000 total."

In the first half of the century, planters preferred indentured servants to enslaved Africans largely because the rate at which the indentured died on the voyage over was about 3 percent, far less than the estimated 10 to 20 percent of Africans, who were kept in horrific conditions on the slave ships. In addition, few of the Africans survived more than five years in the colony. Overwhelmingly male (women represented only 14 percent of indentured servants who left from one port in 1635 and only 25 percent over the entire colonial period), the indentured worked, Taylor tells us, primarily "in the intense labor of tobacco cultivation," enduring "the blistering sun, soaring temperatures, thick humidity, and voracious mosquitoes of the long, hot Chesapeake summer."[74]

In the economy that developed in the following years, it was deemed cheaper to purchase kidnapped Africans and import indentured servants than it was to provide free laborers with the necessities for a life that lasted more than a few years. Acceptance of death at an early age—at least the death of others—was essential to Virginia's early labor-intensive agricultural system. Human lives were measured in the number of sacks of rice and bundles of indigo hauled out of the swamps of South Carolina and the bales of cotton and stacks of tobacco harvested in the fields of Virginia and Georgia. Pain, shortened lives, and the threat of death were essential tools of repression for the young and able-bodied, whose overseers depended upon them to do the work, and for the elderly, rebellious, or disabled who could not.

The agricultural system devised in the American South, based on slave labor, cheap land, and production of crops such as rice, tobacco, and cotton, changed the environment, eventually depleting the soil and therefore the capital of the planters and their families. Rather than developing a system of crop rotation and allowing depleted lands to remain fallow, plantation owners found it cheaper to exhaust the land and steal the lands of native Americans or move to fertile grounds farther west or south. The plantation system thereby disrupted the natural ecologies of the region. Cultivating swamplands to grow rice and clearing woodlands to grow tobacco fostered the spread of mosquito-borne diseases such as yellow fever and malaria, diseases that would plague those who did the work as well as those who profited from their labor in southern communities from the 1600s through the early twentieth century.

Ultimately, though, the vast majority of unfree labor was provided by enslaved Africans, beginning in 1619 in Jamestown itself. For much of the 1600s, the number of enslaved people brought to the colonies was relatively small, in the hundreds every year, in comparison to what would occur in the 1700s.[75] While by 1700 there were 27,000 enslaved Africans in the colonies, by 1770 there were some 462,000 people of African descent there. Each decade of the eighteenth century, tens of thousands of men, women, and children were transported by slave ship from Africa to Charleston, Baltimore, and other seaports. The boats were generally funded by northern merchants and European traders. In continental North America, the historian Jennifer Morgan argues, "in the period prior to the eighteenth century, women and men arrived in near-balanced numbers to many parts of the Americas." Almost none were children, since they had little value before the advent of the cotton trade, when their small fingers became useful for picking the bolls from the fragile plants. But "as slave traders shifted toward the import of children in the waning years of the trade, adult men ultimately constituted a minority of all those transported." [76]

The political economy of the slave trade was not limited to the few ports and auction blocks of the American South. Rather, the trade was organized through the shipping, trading, and financial centers initially of European powers like Britain, Spain, and Portugal, along with Africa itself and, later, New York, Boston, and other ports. In fact, the history of the trade in slaves illuminates a complex set of financing and agricultural and trade relationships among the European powers that predates the slave trade's rapid expansion. By the seventeenth century, a robust market in slaves had developed between various African kingdoms and European traders supplying not only Europe but, even more importantly, the developing sugar and tobacco plantations of the Caribbean and the Americas.

In the eighteenth century, with much of the country still firmly rural, nascent urban coastal centers in Rhode Island, Massachusetts, and New York became the financial centers and points of departure for many "slavers," ships used to move people from Africa to the Caribbean and mainland North America.[77] Newport and Bristol, Rhode Island, were centers for much of that time, launching close to a thousand ships to Africa that would transport more than a hundred thousand slaves to the United States.[78]

The financial calculus of the first slave ships included the price of disease and death. The historical demographer Herbert Klein estimates that approximately 15 percent of all enslaved Africans died during the voyage to North America, as well as 10 percent of the white crew, while others have placed the death rate for Africans at over 20 percent.[79] British slave ships often packed up to 450 people lying prone side by side in separate levels below deck; the ships leaving from Bristol and Newport were considerably smaller in size, capable of transporting only between

75 and 150 slaves at a time. The smaller size of these American slave ships enabled quicker loading and unloading of people, potentially limiting the danger from endemic diseases to crew and slave alike.[80] Planning for trips involved considerations related to disease as well. Boats left Rhode Island from May through November, for example, so they wouldn't arrive along the African coasts during the hot, humid months when mosquitoes carrying yellow fever and malaria seemed most prevalent. Likewise, planners calculated the "worth" of healthy or sick "cargo" to planters, as well as the perceived different susceptibility of the Rhode Islanders and the Africans they transported.[81]

Disease was a constant on-board threat to the enslaved Africans, who were chained together and forced to lie prone below deck for up to sixty days, the length of a typical voyage. Hygienic conditions were rudimentary at best. There were no changes of clothing, no toilets, and hardly any disposal of human waste. The accounts that exist describe what were considered good practices: crew were said to "attend" to slaves every day and to conduct a "major" cleaning with vinegar and water once every two weeks or so.[82] When a slave became ill during a trip, the captain calculated the threat of the loss of one diseased slave against the potential loss of the entire cargo. A case of dysentery could be impossible to contain in slave quarters. One account told of a slave woman suspected of smallpox on the slave ship *Polly*. She was tied to a chair and thrown overboard; the captain grieved for the lost chair.[83]

The medical treatment of sick slaves in transit was typically perfunctory. Even though many ships had physicians on board, they could do little other than isolate the sick or give concoctions of rum, turpentine, or calomel. Some boats might be able to find dry land to dock, but the human "cargo" was valuable, and time spent on an island might or might not provide a cure. According to the historian Richard B. Sheridan, the slave boats brought together in one cramped, unsanitary, and airless space three disease environments, those of "north Europe, Africa south of the Sahara, and tropical and subtropical parts of the Americas." He relates that "included among the long list of diseases and ailments suffered on the Middle Passage were dysentery, diarrhea, ophthalmia [eye inflammation], malaria, smallpox, yellow fever, scurvy, measles, typhoid fever, hookworm, tapeworm, sleeping sickness, trypanosomiasis [sleeping sickness transmitted through tsetse flies], yaws [a chronic skin infection], syphilis, leprosy, and elephantiasis [a parasitic disease that causes gross inflammation of body parts]."[84] Fevers, dysentery, and smallpox could destroy the value of a shipment of slaves that traders had spent months collecting from ports along the African coast.[85]

Diseased or sickly slaves fetched a depressed price, and traders also faced the possibility that slaves would revolt if not heavily guarded or chained. "Disease and revolt were the two biggest killers aboard the slavers," reports the historian Jay Coughtry. "Therefore, health and security were the captors' principal preoccupations," as slave mortality determined the size of profits and losses. One Rhode Island slave ship owner reported losing 101 slaves to disease and rebellion in 1765, costing him 2,000 pounds sterling. Another Rhode Island trader, operating in 1786, returned with only seventy slaves; the other eighty had died during the voyage.[86] On a more profitable trip, the trader celebrated losing "only" five lives. Another bragged that his ship had arrived in Charleston with "eighty-nine prime negroes and no slaves lost on passage." According to one account, from 1752 through 1807, about one in six slaves lost their life aboard a transatlantic slave ship.[87]

Graphic descriptions of the horrors of these transatlantic voyages sometimes appeared at the time, including this one: "The change which negroes undergo, from the open air . . . to the pestilential atmosphere, stagnating between the decks of a Guinea-ship, debarred the free use of their limbs, oppressed with chains, harassed by sea-sickness, and the incessant motion of the vessel; sometimes stinted in provisions, and poisoned with corrupted water, is . . . great"; it was a wonder that so many survived the passage. Even so, "under the most favorable circumstances . . . a great many are delivered at the end of the voyage, with indispositions . . . which manifest themselves soon after their landing."[88]

A writer named Olaudah Equiano, who had been stolen from his village and sold into slavery at age eleven, described his boarding the slave ship: "A multitude of black people of every description chained together, every one of their countenances expressing dejection of sorrow. . . . I no longer doubted my fate; and, quite overpowered with horror and anguish, I fell motionless on the deck and fainted. . . . I was soon put down under the decks, and there I received such a salutation in my nostrils as I had never experienced in my life." His summation of his experience was as clear as it was simple: "The white people looked and acted . . . in so savage a manner; for I had never seen among any people such instances of brutal cruelty."[89]

Many on the slave ships suffered and died from the "flux"—a bloody discharge with a severe diarrhea—brought on by the putrefying foods, which were stored in open bins and delivered in communal troughs. But the list of sicknesses produced by the Middle Passage seems endless: fevers, inflammations of eyes, venereal diseases, itch, scurvy, ague, yaws, Guinea worms, and smallpox—in addition to the bloody flux, all were a constant threat throughout the colonial period.

Added to the bodily complaints was the mental anguish of those stolen from their homelands. "To the disorders above enumerated of the body, may be added another, of the mind," one Caribbean planter noted. It "contributes to some degree to the mortality soon after arrival; and that is despondency, produced by causes scarcely to be guessed at." The enslavement and Middle Passage "work so strongly on their imaginations, as to determine these to quit their existence" once they landed in the New World.[90] He estimated that in the approximately two weeks between landing and sale, nearly five slaves per hundred killed themselves. He concluded that many more than that would die—presumably by their own hand—a few months after auction.[91]

MASTERS, SLAVES, AND THE STRUCTURE OF CRUELTY

The plantation system, whether in the coastal rice-growing regions of South Carolina, the tobacco regions of Virginia and Maryland, the sugar plantations of Barbados and Jamaica, or "the [later] cotton plantations of the South," was a closed system with the masters and foremen having absolute power over the life and labor of sometimes thousands of enslaved people. The system was run on the backs of Black laborers and designed to extract as much toil as possible. The Africans who arrived in the Americas faced ever-present threats of violence, cruelty, and death. Not only was the whip used to enforce discipline and labor, but women were regularly subjected to rape at the hands of white masters. At its base, the plantation was a profit center, and slaves were disposable if they did not contribute adequately to that profit. Little care was given to their well-being. Whatever the superficial similarities the plantation had to feudal estates, the plantation masters were not lords with inherited rights and status and corresponding responsibilities. Paternalism and customary obligation may have had a role in maintaining the stability of the older feudal estates of England, but not so in the rice and sugar fields of the American South and Caribbean in the eighteenth century. Here, power and violence were the primary tools to control an enslaved population.

The hierarchy that formed the governing structure of the larger plantations allowed the masters to insulate themselves from the everyday drumbeat of pain. To manage the enslaved, they hired white overseers, managers, foremen, superintendents, and "under-overseers" young men who were generally drawn from the local poor or displaced yeomen farmers or from the ranks of former indentured servants. These layers of bureaucracy imposed work discipline and order on a labor system based on the threat of violence, the threat of familial separation, the threat and reality of rape, the threat of imprisonment in locked hovels, shackles and chains, and the denial of food.[92] These middle managers who stood between the master and the slave decided who would clear the forests to plant tobacco in Virginia, dig the trenches to drain the swamps and grow rice in the marshlands of South Carolina, and plant the indigo and cotton in Georgia, as well as how they were to be treated.

The slave system was far from being a benign, or even benevolent, institution, as was depicted in post–Civil War revisionist history books and popular movies like *Gone with the Wind*. The planting and harvesting of rice, indigo, and sugar along the marshy shores of South Carolina or the planting of tobacco in North Carolina and Virginia was brutal and deadly work: plantations were, in the words of historian Edward Baptist, "slave labor camps."[93]

The cruelty of the plantation system was reinforced by the masters' fear of insurrection among the enslaved populations, especially in areas of the South where Blacks often outnumbered their white overlords. In South Carolina, for example, through the latter part of the seventeenth and the early eighteenth centuries, enslaved persons working the rice regions vastly outnumbered whites. This was especially true in the summers, when the planters left the mosquito-infested coastal marshlands and traveled to Charleston and farther north and inland if they could.[94]

All enslaved people—whether they worked the fields or worked in the boiling houses or kitchens or with children in the big house—were subject to the whims of whites who believed it essential to assert their power over them, including by whipping, torturing, lynching, and providing inadequate food and ramshackle housing—all of which was deleterious to their short-term and long-term health. Especially in the mosquito-infested marshes of South Carolina, where rice was first culti-vated in huge amounts, the power of the plantation manager was unbri-dled, partly because masters feared the many ways that resistance to this terrible work could be manifested.[95] For those working the marshes, as well as the whites who oversaw the work, assorted fevers and the venom of rattlesnakes complemented the diseases that mosquitoes carried as things to fear.[96]

In 1755, Alexander Garden, a physician in South Carolina, detailed the extraordinary toll that processing the rice harvest took on African American slaves: "Some task their slaves at more, but often pay dear[ly] for their Barbarity, by the Loss of many . . . Valuable Negroes," he remarked. "And how can it well be otherwise, the poor Wretches are obliged to Labour hard," leading to death, which, he continued, "rid them of Cruel Masters, or more Cruel Overseers" and "End[ed] their Wretched Being here."[97]

In 1803, a man calling himself "Dr. Collins," a self-described "pro-fessional planter" in the Caribbean, wrote a 500-page tome entitled *Practical Rules for the Management and Medical Treatment of Negro Slaves in the Sugar Colonies* that apparently was popular with plant-ers in the United States.[98] With incredible attention to detail, Collins described what provisions should be made to preserve the health and life of slaves for the purpose of deriving the most labor and, therefore, the most profit from them. He detailed the "costs" in human life associ-ated with the Middle Passage and arrival on the sugar plantations of the region: "Experience has demonstrated that a great number of negroes exported from the coast of Africa to the West Indies, die within three or four years after their arrival," he wrote in chapter 2, "On the Season-ing of Negroes." He continued: "I believe the most moderate calcula-tion cannot rate the loss at less than one fourth, upon an average." So great a "waste of the species," he went on, "for a purpose merely com-mercial, though perhaps justifiable enough on those principles," was, he allowed, of concern morally as well.[99] Whatever the moral qualms, Collins's advice had one overriding purpose of maximizing profit, for which the slave was but the means. Any advice that benefited the slave was purely secondary.

If Africans survived their capture and their sale to European slavers, as well as the trip across the Atlantic, a new set of tribulations awaited them at the slave auction and on their subsequent trip to their new owner's plantation. This period was commonly referred to as the "seasoning," as if the person enslaved were merely a block of wood. Collins warned his readers that they should not mistake the seeming similarities between the African and Caribbean climates and think those similarities boded well for the arriving slave. Despite the similarities in temperature, differences existed that were not immediately apparent and to which the enslaved might react poorly. "Even when the temperature is perfectly equal," he explained, "seasoning is required to negroes that are carried from one island to another." Collins, among others, believed that differences in altitude, sea winds, and the resulting temperature drops at night could result in dramatic increases in disablement and disease. "When they turn out in the morning, even in the lowlands, they embrace their bodies closely with their wrappers, to defend them from the cold. In the mountains, even wrappers are insufficient for that purpose." "Seasoning" of the newly enslaved required an understanding of physiology because "the effect of a greater degree of cold, particularly when united with moisture, is to close the pores of the skin, and to check perspiration, which descends in torrents when negroes are in health, and at work." Such conditions led them, he argued, to be "thrown into fluxes [bloody stools or what might later be called dysentery], and dropsies [what we might call congestive heart failure], two of the worst diseases, and almost the only fatal ones, with which they are afflicted."[100] Of course, in reality it was undoubtedly overwork, malnutrition, heat exhaustion, and other forms of exploitation that were the root causes of these ailments, not susceptibility to the cold.

Even Collins acknowledged that labor and how it was extracted were "the most frequent cause of the mortality of new negroes."[101] White plantation owners explained away any resistance to the ten- to fourteen-hour days toiling in hot fields as a product of the "natural laziness" of the enslaved accustomed to the paradises of their African villages. "To press for sudden and unremitted exertion, is to kill them, which many unfortunately do every year."[102]

Every aspect of the enslaved person's existence was measured against the return on investment, even eating. Collins devoted an entire chapter to diet, beginning with the simple observation that many in the planter class were not necessarily convinced that the immediate cost of feeding the enslaved would be paid back eventually in higher productivity and greater profits. But, he argued in his chapter "On Diet," that it is "necessary a man should eat, as that he should work, is a proposition from which few, I think, can withhold their assent." "Yet, I am afraid this was a speculative truth only . . . there having been many . . . who seemed to think the one productive of profit, whilst the other begets only expense."[103] He went to pains to explain how much "a well-fed negro is capable of executing, in proportion to one who is half starved."[104] A common diet of the enslaved worker was six or seven pints a week of flour along with salt herring, reported Collins, "a scanty pittance" that might "hold soul and body" together long enough to earn a profit on his or her purchase price. But that was hardly enough to support any labor at all. "How is the body to support itself? What is there to enrich and thicken the fluids? What to strengthen the solids, to give energy to the heart, and to navigate its pulsations?" Appealing to the self-interest of his fellow planters, he argued that underfed "negroes crawl about with feeble emaciated frames." Their "attempts to wield the hoe prove abortive, they shrink from their toil, and . . . you are soon obliged to receive them in the hospital, whence . . . they depart but to the grave." Could they not be given "little vacant spots" where they could grow their own food? he asked.[105]

Indeed, Collins advised masters to provision their enslaved laborers with small plots of land so they might grow their own food. When it was provided, the small plot, located often on the most depleted portion of the plantation's land, was inadequate to maintain health year-round. Hence, "pilfering"—taking food from the kitchens or the storehouse, or stealing an occasional chicken from the coop—was also part of the nutritional economy of the plantation, and Collins encouraged slave owners who wanted to maintain their workforce to look the other way when the food was stolen, if that stealing was merely to maintain their own strength and health.[106] "Such conduct is perfectly natural," Collins declared. "I was going to say, justifiable," he continued, "yet, when the delinquent is detected," he was often severely whipped and then chained and confined. Collins warned owners that such punishment would prove ineffective because it would not extinguish hunger and only lead to more surreptitious acts, or even to escape. When found, the escapee would be so weakened and possibly ill from "scanty nourishment" and exposure to the weather that "it is ten to one but he falls into a distempered habit, which soon hurries him out of the world."[107]

The starvation diets imposed by the owners inevitably led to increased susceptibility to disease and death. The sporadic early epidemics, most notably of yellow fever and smallpox, that claimed the lives of colonists and the enslaved alike in the mid-eighteenth century show how disease was imbedded in the slave economy. Yellow fever outbreaks before the 1790s in particular appear to have been a direct result of the growing slave trade: it is suspected that the disease was of African origin and entered the Caribbean and the American South with mosquitoes that found fertile territory in which to expand in humid, swampy environments, as the historian Rana Hogarth points out. The mosquitoes spread along the trade routes, infecting and feeding off the blood of the diseased.[108] Unlike how they saw smallpox, which was endemic in Europe, mainland planters and their physicians often saw yellow fever in racial terms, rationalizing that Africans appeared relatively immune from its effects. While Africans may have had a particular immunity because of previous exposures, their higher survival rates when compared to whites during epidemics were explained at the time in biological, rather than in environmental, terms—as a quality inherent in them, not the result of a different environmental experience. The irony, of course, is that the creation of a slave economy led to the spread of virulent epidemics of the disease throughout the eighteenth and nineteenth centuries among white and Black populations who lacked earlier exposures. For example, in 1793 outbreaks occurred in Charleston, New Orleans, and even in northern Philadelphia and New York; in 1800 there was an epidemic in Baltimore, and then in Memphis and other cities primarily in the South, but also in the North.[109]

It is clear that disease and death during the colonial era were not simply the result of biological events but were also the result of a social and economic system that created the conditions for disease to thrive among Indigenous peoples, the colonists themselves, and enslaved Africans.

THE POLITICAL AND SOCIAL DISRUPTIONS OF THE REVOLUTIONARY PERIOD

The changes that occurred during the colonial period created new conditions that led to new patterns of disease and death. The increased population and also the growth in trade meant that more people lived in densely populated cities and that contact increased among people moving up and down the coast. In 1751, twenty-five years before the American Revolution, Benjamin Franklin wrote a short treatise titled *Observations Concerning the Increase of Mankind*, describing the dramatic demographic changes that were overtaking Britain's northern American colonies, especially their extraordinary population growth. Over the previous century, the population had seemingly doubled every two decades. In England and in Europe more generally, he observed, each marriage produced an average of four children, of whom only two survived to adulthood. In the colonies, by contrast, women married earlier, and each union produced an average of eight births, of which at least four typically survived to adulthood. In a little over a century, the colonial population of British background had grown from zero to nearly "One Million English Souls in North America." Of these, it was later estimated, only one-quarter had been born abroad. He accurately intuited that natural increase, or the number of births over deaths or out-migration every year, and to a lesser extent immigration, largely accounted for this exponential growth.[110]

Franklin predicted that the social and political consequences of such large demographic increases would be tremendous. For one, if such population increase continued at the same rate for a century, the number of Americans of British descent would outnumber the people of England itself. Not yet anticipating the revolution that would establish a new state, he predicted that within a few generations the "greatest number of Englishmen will be on this side of the water." The economic implications of this growth in the size of the colonies were overwhelming for the home country and Britain's colonies as a whole. "What an Accession of Power to the British Empire by Sea as well as Land! What Increase of Trade and Navigation! What Numbers of Ships and Seamen!"[111]

What accounted for this extraordinary population growth and concomitant expanding economic opportunity that Franklin anticipated?

He pointed to the unique environment and the seemingly unlimited possibilities for new inhabitants on a vast continent. Focusing primarily on New England, Franklin ascribed these unlimited possibilities to the moral and racial characteristics of peoples of British descent; he was suspicious not only of the impact of Africans who were brought to the southern colonies in chains but also of the German and Dutch colonists of the mid-Atlantic colonies, particularly Pennsylvania. In European societies, the urban poor or agricultural peasantry could never gain control over scarce land, which was instead held fast by aristocratic elites, dooming many to lives of perpetual poverty as peasants or underpaid urban wage earners. The people in the colonies had no such limitations, Franklin argued. Land was "plenty in America, and so cheap as that a labouring Man, that understands Husbandry, can in a short Time save Money enough to purchase a Piece of new Land sufficient for a Plantation, whereon he may subsist a Family." This abundance had broad implications, he went on, as men "are not afraid to marry; for if they even look far enough forward to consider how their Children when grown up are to be provided for, they see that more Land is to be had at Rates equally easy, all Circumstances considered."

The dynamic was clear to Franklin. Expanding farther across the continent meant prosperity. In anticipation of Frederick Turner's "frontier thesis," he saw the availability of cheap land as providing an outlet for the growing population in cities and also as a means of keeping labor relatively scarce and therefore keeping wages higher than in Europe. Demand for scarce labor would inevitably lead to high wages. "So vast is the Territory of North-America, that it will require many Ages to settle it fully," Franklin argued. "Till it is fully settled, Labour will never be cheap here, where no Man continues long a Labourer for others, but gets a Plantation of his own, no Man continues long a Journeyman to a Trade, but goes among those new Settlers, and sets up for himself."[112]

Unbeknownst to Benjamin Franklin as he celebrated the health and longevity of the colonists and predicted limitless population increase, the material conditions that he extolled as the basis of colonial success were silently vanishing. In part, this decrease was due to fundamental changes in agriculture that changed the nutritional status and healthfulness of eighteenth-century New England colonists. Further, with the ever-increasing population due to large family size and low infant and childhood mortality rates, the average size of farms was *declining*. Sons married and subdivided their parents' land among themselves or sold their inheritance to others. In a matter of three or four generations, from the mid-seventeenth century to the mid-eighteenth century, the original family farms became smaller, leaving less and less land for cattle or other grazing stock. By the late eighteenth century, the New England farm family found that their diet had changed substantially. Meat, once a staple, was less available. The presence of vegetables in the average diet relieved the constant threat of scurvy, and potatoes became the crop of choice. In New England, land was increasingly scarce and overplanted.[113]

As a result, many young people moved to land farther west and spawned a geometrically expanding network of villages and towns. If Franklin envisioned and new migrants desired unlimited access to western lands, however, their objectives were soon stymied by the British Proclamation of 1763, which prohibited colonization of lands beyond the Appalachian Mountains. Following the French and Indian War in the 1760s, the British sought to limit tensions with Native Americans by imposing these boundaries.

Franklin's imagined world of an ever-expanding population of independent well-paid laborers with the possibility of unlimited access to land was slowly vanishing in the East. As a result, many of the children of the troubled countryside were moving to Boston and other small port cities. Populations that measured in the low thousands during the Revolution mushroomed in the early 1800s. Until early in the eighteenth century, commercial life had centered on relatively limited trade up and down the coast, and infectious diseases, while serious, were rarely threats beyond the borders of the towns in which they appeared. But with increased economic development and commerce over the 1700s, sailors and those who worked on the docks were now increasingly exposed to the mosquitoes, rats, and other vectors of disease that accompanied the indigo, rice, and tobacco of the southern slave economy. People too—sailors, passengers, stowaways, and slaves—moved disease up and down the coast in boats that traveled along rivers or on post roads along the coastline.

Yellow fever, first confined primarily to the rice-cultivating regions of the Carolinas, now emerged, beginning in the late 1600s with more regularity in northern port cities such as Boston (1693), New York (1702), and Philadelphia (1741). Such seemingly isolated epidemics spread with the flourishing commercial economy that linked together distant ports, peoples, and insect vectors. This development foreshadowed the types of death that would transform the American experience in the nineteenth century as mosquitoes that carried yellow fever and malaria moved up and down the coast and along inland trade routes. The demographic explosion of the previous three generations fed political and social tensions in the older New England towns, while smallpox and other epidemics struck various commercial hubs, increasing instability and anxiety in the decades preceding the Revolutionary War.

In 1721, the Boston physician Zabdiel Boylston recalled that he had narrowly escaped with his life during a smallpox epidemic nineteen years before, in 1702. But the smallpox epidemic of 1721 then raging, he wrote, was vastly more terrifying in a growing port city of nearly ten thousand people. It infected approximately half the population, killing nearly one of every seven of those infected. Boylston wrote a long treatise to George I's first wife, Queen Sophia, whose father had died of smallpox, in hopes of gaining her support for inoculation, a new technology that entailed the use of pus drawn from the smallpox sores of those already infected.[114] Placing a poultice of this material on a wound of a healthy person appeared to provide protection from the disease. Boylston and the Puritan preacher Cotton Mather had learned about the success of inoculation in the largely Muslim eastern Mediterranean and northern Africa from one of Boylston's slaves, Onesimus. Between the outbreak in April 1721 and February of the next year, Boylston experimented by inoculating his slave Jack, Jack's young sons, Jackey and Thomas, and scores of other Boston residents, Black, white, and Indian, wealthy and poor, young and old. Nearly all whom he treated survived what was sometimes a grueling course of treatment but at least generally less gruesome than the experience of those who contracted smallpox "the natural way." The uninoculated suffered "Purple Spots, the bloody and parchment Pox, Hemorrhages of Blood at the Mouth, Nose, Fundament, and Privities; Ravings and Deliriums; Convulsions, and Other Fits; violent inflammations and Swellings in the Eyes and Throat; so that they cannot see, or scarcely breathe, or swallow any thing, to keep them from starving." He described some victims of the "Pox" "as black as the

Stock, others as white as a Sheet" with their "Skin stripping off and their Flesh raw, like Creatures flea'd." The terror this disease wrought was overwhelming. "Some have a burning, others a smarting Pain, as if in the Fire, or scalded with boiling Water; Some have insatiable Thirst, others greedy Appetites; and will crave Food when dying. Some have been fill'd with loathsome Ulcers; others have had deep, and fistulous Ulcers in their Bodies." While many died, those who survived were forever marked by the physical scarring and the debilities that left some as "Cripples, others Idiots, and many-blind all their Days."[115]

Smallpox impacted many others besides its victims and survivors. As Boylston put it, "Parents [were] left Childless, Children without Parents, and sometimes Parents and Children's being both carried off, and many families broken up by the destruction the Small-Pox made in the natural way." Fear swept through the city, for "no one knew who were or who were not infected."[116]

Boylston and Mather met strong resistance to their inoculation efforts from a community that saw the suffering as a divine intervention, a judgment that had been justly imposed by God and therefore must not be questioned or contradicted. Boylston countered that, if such were the case, God would not have provided the means by which to prevent this suffering. What he interpreted as a largely isolated event had shown that "Providence has wisely and mercifully order'd it, that once only, in our Lives, we shall be distressed by it; & has now, in greater Goodness, discovered to us a Way or Method how to moderate that Distemper, & to render the Small-Pox, inoculated, no further dangerous than a common intermittent Fever, under the prudent use of its specific Bark."

The eventual acceptance of inoculation (the insertion of the pus of smallpox victims into the healthy subject) helped many people but did not stop the decline in health status, first among Bostonians and then later among other New Englanders, from the mid-eighteenth to early nineteenth centuries. In Boston, the center of growing coastal and international trade, thirty-seven of every thousand residents were dying by the middle years of the eighteenth century, just slightly below the rate in England at the time. But in farming communities just 10 to 20 miles away, the estimated death rates were only about twenty per thousand.[117] Laurel Thatcher Ulrich documents that in rural Hallowell, Maine, in 1787, the death rate was also half that of Boston and Salem. Similarly, maternal mortality rates were lower in rural New England than in its urbanizing areas, and extraordinarily lower than the mortality rate in London during the same period.[118]

By the decades during and immediately following the Revolution, the seemingly salubrious environment of New England farm life had changed, as had the predominant reasons for death and disease throughout the region. By the end of the eighteenth century, observers, including Thomas Jefferson, Secretary of War Henry Knox, physician Benjamin Rush, and many others, had already noted the changing patterns of disease in the new nation and the broad national epidemics that seemed more common. Jefferson wrote in 1793 of "a contagious and mortal fever which has arisen here, and is driving us all away. It is called a yellow fever, but is like nothing known or read of by the Physicians."[119]

Noah Webster, who today is remembered as the compiler of the first American dictionary, reacted to the changing world around him by compiling an idiosyncratic list of various geological, astronomical, astrological, and physical events that he believed to be linked to the changing health of Americans in the years just after the yellow fever epidemic of the 1790s. Webster acknowledged the growing ties between and commonalities among the older European empires and the newly emerging nation. Unlike earlier outbreaks of smallpox, diphtheria, and yellow fever, which were generally local in character, the yellow fever and other epidemics of the 1790s were more widespread, affecting communities along the coast and inland as well. Their intensity and rapid spread from one community to another marked new phenomena in a country that as recently as the 1750s still imagined itself as exceptionally healthy. Yellow fever had been the first truly national epidemic and as such represented a new chapter in both public health and economic history, for its spread was traceable in no small part to a commercial world of greater and more far-reaching contact among people than had been true of the rural, isolated communities of the early 1700s.

The shift was not lost on Webster. In 1789, a drought and accompanying diseases had produced near famine in Vermont, where "people were reduced to the necessity of feeding on tadpoles," he reported. None actually "starved to death but a few died of the flux." He wondered at the changes the country was now experiencing. "In old settlements, there was food enough for man, but the failure of a surplus in this country, is a rare event." While cattle "perished in considerable numbers . . . [i]t is certain that a similar scarcity had not been experienced in America for many years."[120]

Epidemics seemed to appear more and more frequently, Webster noted. "Two ladies who left Boston with me on the second of November [1789], before the disease [perhaps influenza] had appeared in their family . . . were seized with it in Hartford, at the same time it became epidemic in Boston," he related. Soon, it "pervaded the wilderness and seized the Indians—it spread over the ocean and attacked seamen a hundred leagues from land and . . . appeared in the West Indies nearly at the time it did in the northern states. It overspread America, from the 15th to the 45th parallel . . . in about 6 or 8 weeks." The American experience with disease was indeed changing as commercial development and involvement with international trade and the slave trade made the safety afforded by a vast ocean and limited interactions much less secure. Webster again:

> The scarlet fever re-appeared in December [1789], and became epidemic; often blending itself with the influenza. It exhibited one predominant feature of the whole series of succeeding epidemics, a prevalence of bilious matter, which was often discharged by purging and vomiting. This disease continued to prevail in Philadelphia, and if my information is correct, in some parts of New-Jersey, till the spring of 1790. The measles occurred in some cases, but was not epidemic. It is remarkable that the scarlatina anginosa was contemporary in Edinburgh with the epidemic measles in America in 1789, and nearly so, with the death of the haddock on the coast of Norway. It will be observed that the scarlet fever, tho epidemic in Philadelphia, did not spread over the country in 1790. It was little known in the northern states, till two years after.[121]

The last decade of the century appeared ominous in Webster's eyes. "In August 1793 commenced in Philadelphia that dreadful pestilence which alarmed the United States, and spread terror and dismay over that city," he recounted. "The spring diseases, which ushered in this malady, were influenza, scarlatina and mild bilious remittents. . . . About the 12th of September, fell a meteor between the city and the hospital,"

auguring a terrible toll from this latest epidemic. "The number of victims to this disease [probably yellow fever] was 4040." "A controversy
arose among the physicians in Philadelphia, relative to the origin of the
plague, one party tracing the disease, as they supposed, to infected vessels from the West-Indies," but Webster still hoped the true cause was
much more local. "Garbage, to the amount of a car load perhaps," had
been dumped on the dock and the "hot sun had rendered the putrefa-
cation of this mass of filth extremely rapid [and] the stench became
intolerable." Rotting fish, clams, oysters, and the general filth of the area
had obviously, to Webster's way of thinking, created the "miasmas," the
vapors and smells that were associated in the early to mid-nineteenth
century with the cause and transmission of various diseases. The growth
of towns, the crowding of people together, and the destruction of the
environment in which the poor lived augured the worst of times ahead.
In New Haven, "a great number of sick in a narrow close built street,
may render the air of it infectious, but a few diseased persons in the wide
streets of New-Haven could not produce this effect." In the face of such
disintegration of the environment, it was impossible "that the human
race should escape the calamity of epidemic disease."[122] For Webster,
infections were a minor element in the creation of epidemics. Far more
important were the pollution due to decomposing organic matter and
meteorological and other natural events.[123]

The changing disease experience during the colonial and post-
Revolutionary period was intimately tied to the human-constructed
conditions of what some have called the Age of Discovery, or the Age
of Mercantilism, and others have dubbed the Age of War Capitalism.[124]
Colonialism had created new conditions in the Americas, debilitating
Native American populations, introducing yellow fever, malaria, and
human carnage with its dependence on the slave trade, and altering the
health experience of residents of New England and the Potomac region
alike. The worlds that the colonial settlers had created led to specific
diseases and death and frightening new forms of disease transmission—
epidemic, national in scope, and devastating in effect—that had not
previously been encountered in the North American colonies, where
previous epidemics had been local affairs.

CHAPTER TWO

Life and Death in Antebellum America

Just as social, economic, and demographic events during the colonial era shaped the prevalence of disease and different rates of early death, so too did social transformations and shifting conditions of life between the Revolutionary and Civil wars deeply affect the ways Americans lived and died in the first half of the nineteenth century.

During the late eighteenth and early nineteenth centuries, the emergence of the industrial state, built around the factory, brought about a revolutionary change in production that, in the words of the historian Joshua Freeman, "ushered in a new world" of factories, forms of exploitation, and diseases.[1] This growing commercial economy, built around the ports of the East Coast and developing centers of inland trade, combined with the dramatically increasing population and the concomitant growth in urban populations to create conditions that were detrimental to health. The declining sanitary conditions of the expanding cities, a lack of pure water or sewerage systems, and an unstable and increasingly unregulated food supply resulted in increased incidences of disease and death that affected people of diverse classes, races, religions, and ethnicities differently.[2] Generally, the worst effects were felt by those in bondage. At the same time, the rapid expansion of a southern plantation system built around cotton and planters' omnivorous demand for slave labor and more land resulted in an increasing gap in wealth between those who did the work and those who profited from their labor. It also meant a deteriorating health picture for most Americans, the enslaved most dramatically but the free alike.

By the outbreak of the Civil War in 1861, the exceptional health of white northerners experienced during the colonial period was in decline as measured by life expectancy, a decline that would continue into the twentieth century.[3] The historical demographer David Hacker estimates that on average American "white male life expectancy at age 20 was approximately six years lower at mid-century than it was in the late eighteenth century."[4] The early factory system alone, however, did not account for the subsequent decline in health in the North. In addition, national epidemics like cholera and yellow fever linked to the creation of a national commercial economy transformed the health of the nation. And not surprisingly, in the South, the plantation economy ravaged the lives of slaves and even affected the health of owners.

NEW ENGLAND AND THE MID-ATLANTIC AT THE DAWN OF THE FACTORY SYSTEM

As outlined earlier, in colonial Boston and other small port cities where populations measured only in the low thousands by the time of the Revolution, commercial life had centered around relatively limited trade with Britain and the West Indies. Yet people in these port cities were exposed to the mosquitoes, rats, and other vectors of disease that came with the indigo, rice, tobacco, sugar, or other agricultural staples produced in southern plantations and Caribbean slave economies. People too—sailors, passengers, stowaways, and slaves—spread contagious disease up and down the coast in boats or in horse-drawn wagons on the post roads along the coast or in the interior. While the estimated annual death rates in farming communities just 10 to 20 miles away from Boston were about 20 per 1,000 in the middle years of the eighteenth century, in Boston, the center of growing coastal and international trade, 37 per 1,000 residents died, a death rate just slightly below that of England. At the same time, the scattered, isolated epidemics of yellow fever,[5] smallpox, and diphtheria that had previously affected mainly people in the South and in Boston, New York, and Philadelphia began to affect people living far from these cities in western New York,

Ohio, and rural Pennsylvania, and even among native populations in Arkansas and elsewhere. And so, by the early post-Revolution decades, the seemingly salubrious environment of New England and mid-Atlantic farm life had changed, as had the reasons for death and disease throughout the new nation. The living standards of many Americans declined as a result of such changes as smaller family plots and more crowded housing in cities and towns. This crowding in turn led to more widespread epidemics, which, combined with unhealthful working conditions at home and in new factories, resulted in shorter life spans, and even a decrease in the average height and nutritional status of residents of the northern states.[6]

The changes in agriculture in the late eighteenth and early nineteenth centuries had slowly eroded the economic base of the New England farm, driving children to seek out new farmland further west or families to move to places where they could either ply a trade or gain employment in the new industries springing up. The textile mills built in the 1820s and 1830s along the Housatonic, Quinebaug, Shetucket, Merrimack, Nashua, Cocheco, Saco, Androscoggin, Kennebec, and Winooski rivers, named after peoples long since displaced, profited from the problems of the rural world. The workers who moved from farms provided the labor for the textile factories in the capitalists' new company towns. There they wove the cotton purchased from southern slave-labor plantations, much as the British were doing in Manchester and Leeds.

About one-quarter of the cotton grown in the South was sent north to feed the rapidly growing textile industry in New England. Traders and merchants like Francis Cabot Lowell began to build their own mills along the numerous waterways of Massachusetts, Rhode Island, New Hampshire, and Vermont. The river waters turned the looms, spinning wheels, and gins that produced yarn and finished goods for the growing American markets. The factory system displaced the "outwork" systems of home production that had previously dominated textile production. Unlike the British mills that, after the mid-1820s, ran off coal-fired steam power, the early American textile factories still were sited where river water flowed with enough force to drive the machinery, making it essential for factory owners to attract laborers to previously unpopulated rural areas. Drawing on a labor force of young women from struggling farms throughout New England, the early factory owners in effect conducted a giant experiment in developing a particularly American industrial system. The mill towns of Lowell, Lawrence, Waltham, and Fall River marketed themselves as a new type of community in which young women would not be exploited but could earn a livelihood while having a time-limited cultural experience unavailable to them in the isolated farms and villages from which they came. Under strict moral supervision, it was promised, they would live in dormitories where they would be provided with food, shelter, and culture in exchange for paid work at the looms. After some years of this work, the women were still expected to return home and get married, thus reaffirming the traditional gender norms of the new industrial order.[7]

The country, as Franklin had defined it in 1750 and as Thomas Jefferson had reiterated, was to be built around the unlimited availability of land to the west and a labor force always able to take advantage of it. Franklin believed that urban workers, if unhappy with wages offered by employers, would always be able to move to the expansive western reserves, where they could get land to farm and thereby become their own masters. He hypothesized that to keep workers in the emerging textile towns, employers would have to treat workers decently and pay them adequately, thus avoiding the worst inequalities and tensions of a class-riven European society.

The paradox of the nascent expansion of industrial capitalism around the world was that it was creating enormous wealth while also creating extraordinary human suffering. The experience of England could have served as a lesson. As the factory replaced the home-based craft systems of production, the relative autonomy, sometimes the self-respect, and the health of large numbers of laborers disappeared. The great historian of British industrial capitalism, E. P. Thompson, quoted one observer who captured even as late as 1887 the dramatic effects of industrialism in England: "It is truly lamentable to behold so many thousands of men who formerly earned 20 to 30 shillings per week, now compelled to live upon 3s, 4s, or even less."[8] And in Britain, along with the development of the factories went the Enclosure Acts, which prevented agrarian peoples from tilling common lands and thus impoverished small farmers, destroying their ability to feed their families. These laws, in turn, forced many in rural communities to move to the towns where the textile mills, coal mines, and other industrial enterprises were in search of a ready and dependent labor supply. This crowding of peoples resulted in the creation of truly filthy environments. In England, the "dark satanic mills," which William Blake ruminated on in his 1808 poem "And Did Those Feet in Ancient Time" and later immortalized in the hymn "Jerusalem," occupied early-nineteenth-century British thinkers, politicians, and artists.

The British had initially constructed their textile mills along rivers so they could be powered by water, but in short order they shifted to steam, powered by coal, because the best stretches of rivers for powering machinery were rarely near population centers. Thus, as would later happen in the United States, they had to provide housing and other amenities to attract their workforce. By shifting to steam, factories could be sited where a workforce already existed and there was no need to provide housing. It was immediately apparent, however, that this shift from water power to coal-powered steam would have a major effect on health. One magistrate noted that "children employed in Cotton Factories . . . are generally puny and squalid, especially those who work in Mills where Steam Engines are used; but in Establishments where the Machinery be worked by Water Wheels, the Climate of the Rooms is more wholesome, and the Appearance of the children better."[9] The historian Andreas Malm quotes a poet who in 1848 described the damage that textile factories run by steam had on the workers: "Contending hard against mechanic power, / From early morn till midnight's last hour, / In heated atmosphere of smoke and fire, / He slaves for life to gain a scanty hire." As Malm explains, the triumph of coal-fired steam textile plants meant that a "considerable segment of the British working class would then have experienced the coming of the fossil economy as a palpable deterioration of the immediate environment" as manifested in "excessive heat, heightened concentration of carbon dioxide, air pollution by smoke and the risk of sudden explosive disasters."[10]

Noting the growing pollution in cities, along with declines in earning power and the living conditions of working peoples, numerous English and European authors, politicians, social reformers, health officials, and artisans responded. Charles Dickens provided a running commentary for the British reading public on the horrors of the workhouses, child labor, and urban living conditions; the social reformer Edwin Chadwick documented the impact of the mills on the health of city residents; groups of workers known as Luddites rebelled against the harsh conditions of the new factories through petitions, protests, and sometimes sabotage. All, from Tory and Whig politicians through political philosophers such as Jeremy Bentham and John Stuart Mill, debated the significance of and justifications for building empires of power looms, cotton gins, and steam- and water-powered factories where owners garnered huge profits while a labor force gathered from the countryside lived and died in often horrendous conditions.

The health of the worker became a poignant symbol of the excesses of capitalism. As Friedrich Engels, himself a factory owner's son, wrote in his classic 1845 book, *The Condition of the Working Class in England*, it was "self-evident that a social class which live under the conditions that we have described and is so poorly supplied with the most indispensable necessities of existence can enjoy neither good health nor a normal expectation of life." Not only were the factory towns destroying lives, but even the concentration of people there was altering the environment as "the carbon dioxide gas produced by people breathing [in close quarters] and fires burning fails to rise from the streets," leading to a lack of oxygen, "mental torpor and low physical vitality," Engels wrote.

> The way in which the vast mass of the poor are treated in modern society is truly scandalous. They are herded into great cities. . . . They are housed in the worst ventilated districts. . . . They are deprived of all means of keeping clean. They are deprived of water because this is only brought to their houses if someone is prepared to defray the costs of laying pipes. River water is so dirty as to be useless for cleansing purposes. The poor are forced to throw into the streets all their sweepings, garbage, dirty water, and frequently even disgusting filth and excrement.[11]

Engels painted an even bleaker view of what befell a worker in the new factories. For Engels, not yet at work with Karl Marx on *The Communist Manifesto*, the foundational document of communism, the industrial factory owner who allowed terrible conditions to continue was little different from a common murderer who lacked conscience and principles. He began his chapter on the impact of the factory system on laborers by writing, "If one individual inflicts a bodily injury upon another which leads to the death of the person attacked we call it manslaughter. . . . If the attacker knows beforehand that the blow will be fatal we call it murder." Engels maintained that the principles and laws that governed civil society should also govern industrialists who knowingly put their workforce in harm's way. "Murder has also been committed if society places hundreds of workers in such a position that they inevitably come to premature and unnatural deaths." And that was indeed what was occurring, he said: "English society has created for the workers an environment in which they cannot remain healthy or enjoy a normal expectation of life."[12]

Some Europeans held out hope that the American industrial experiment would not go the way of Britain's and that workers might be treated fairly. In fact, industrializing Massachusetts during the early 1800s seemed to confirm the exceptional nature of the American industrial model, albeit in ways that Franklin had not foreseen seventy years before. Rather than the availability of a vast countryside being a natural brake on the possibility of exploitation (since, he assumed, workers would for many decades to come have cheap land available to them), the factories now might be a means of improving life for the sons and daughters who would no longer inherit the subdivided lands that had become overcrowded in the Northeast. In the early nineteenth century, factory towns like Lowell, Massachusetts, built around the textile mills along the waterways of New England, appeared to be exemplars of a modern, responsible, and humane American industrial system, one that stood in direct contrast to the satanic mills of Manchester, Leeds, and other British and European industrial centers. Early visitors and propaganda focused on Lowell, Lawrence, and Fall River as models of responsible industrial capitalism, highlighting their efforts to integrate work in the factory with housing, moral supervision, and the cultural improvement of the women who were its primary workforce.[13]

Charles Dickens was one European who saw in the American example of the first decades of the nineteenth century the possibility of a more humane industrial system. In 1842, he included a stop in Lowell on his visit to the United States.[14] After his return to England, he began his observations of Lowell, which he described as a "large, populous, thriving place," with a backhanded compliment. "It was a very dirty winter's day, and nothing in the whole town looked old to me, except the mud," he said. Despite the dismal weather, "The 'Bakery,' 'Grocery,' and 'Book-bindery,' and another kind of store" looked as if they had "started in business yesterday." Even "the very [Merrimac] river that moves the machinery in the mills (for they are all worked by water power), seems to acquire a new character from the fresh buildings of bright red brick and painted wood."[15] Dickens was particularly impressed by the "woolen factory, a carpet factory, and a cotton factory," which he contrasted with the Manchester textile mills. Of special interest were the young girls in the workforce, "all well dressed, but not to my thinking above their condition." They not only were dressed neatly, he went on, but they showed "extreme cleanliness. They had serviceable bonnets, good warm cloaks, and shawls; and were not above clogs and pattens." It appeared that the seeming self-respect and intelligence of the workers were reinforced and encouraged by the factory management and organization. "There were places in the mill in which they could deposit these things without injury; and there were conveniences for washing. They were healthy in appearance, many of them remarkably so, and had the manners and deportment of young women: not of degraded brutes of burden."[16] Dickens expected a dispirited workforce and scenes like those in Manchester and other English mill towns. Yet, in Lowell, the mills he observed were remarkably clean and tidy. "The rooms in which they worked, were as well ordered as themselves. In the windows of some, there were green plants, which were trained to shade the glass; in all, there was as much fresh air, cleanliness, and comfort, as the nature of the occupation would possibly admit of." The young women who worked there appeared healthy and happy. "Out of so large a number of females, many of whom were only then just verging upon womanhood, it may be reasonably supposed that some were delicate and fragile in appearance: no doubt there were." But he was at a loss to find them. "I solemnly declare, that from all the crowd I saw in the different factories that day, I cannot recall or separate one young face that gave me a painful impression; not one young girl whom, assuming it to be a matter of necessity that she should gain her daily bread by the labour of her hands, I would have removed from those works if I had had the power."[17]

Not only was the factory apparently built with their needs in mind, but the entire town seemed organized to accommodate these young women. "They reside in various boarding-houses near at hand," controlled by the mill owners, Dickens noted. And "the owners of the mills are particularly careful to allow no persons to enter upon the possession of these houses, whose characters have not undergone the most searching and thorough inquiry. Any complaint that is made against them, by the boarders, or by anyone else, is fully investigated; and if good ground of complaint be shown to exist against them, they are removed, and their occupation is handed over to some more deserving person." He was particularly impressed by the few children who were employed in the plant, another contrast with the mills of Manchester, where children from the local orphanage were regularly "apprenticed" to work in the mills. In Lowell, the state, it seemed, had worked hand in hand with the paternalistic mill owners to establish laws that "forbid their working more than nine months in the year and require that they be educated during the other three." He noted in particular that "there are schools in Lowell; and there are churches and chapels of various persuasions, in which the young women may observe that form of worship in which they have been educated." Perhaps of greatest fascination was that the houses where the young women lived included pianos and books. It appeared that all the women were encouraged to read and improve themselves, even to write poetry and stories that were published in a magazine called the *Lowell Offering*, which Dickens described as a "repository of original articles, written exclusively by females actively employed in the mills . . . whereof I brought away from Lowell four hundred good solid pages, which I have read from beginning to end." To Dickens, this was a truly enlightened new world in which an industrial revolution did not necessarily entail degrading and ultimately destroying the very people who powered it.

Even the hospital in Lowell stood in direct contrast to the pesthouses he saw in England: "At some distance from the factories, and on the highest and pleasantest ground in the neighborhood, stands their hospital, or boarding-house for the sick: it is the best house in those parts, and was built by an eminent merchant for his own residence. . . . It is not parceled out into wards, but is divided into convenient chambers, each of which has all the comforts of a very comfortable home. The principal medical attendant resides under the same roof; and were the patients members of his own family, they could not be better cared for, or attended with greater gentleness and consideration."[18]

Dickens was overcome by what he saw in Lowell, and he tried to get his English upper- and middle-class readers to reconsider their own preconceptions of English working people, their habits and their moral failings, which, he argued, were rooted in class prejudices and privileges, not their essential character. "The large class of readers, startled by these facts, will exclaim, . . . 'How very preposterous!' On my deferentially inquiring why, they will answer, 'These things are above their station.' In reply to that objection, I would beg to ask what their station is." There was no contradiction between humane treatment, self-improvement, self-respect, and industrial production, he insisted. "They *do* work," he explained. "They labour in these mills, upon an average, twelve hours a day, which is unquestionably work, and pretty tight work too." To those who believed that cultural attainment, education, and the arts were "above their station," he asked, "Are we quite sure that we in England have not formed our ideas of the 'station' of working people, from accustoming ourselves to the contemplation of that class as they are, and not as they might be? I think that if we examine our own feelings, we shall find that the pianos, and the circulating libraries, and even the *Lowell Offering*, startle us by their novelty, and not by their bearing upon any abstract question of right or wrong." "For myself, I know no station in which, the occupation of to-day cheerfully done and the occupation of to-morrow cheerfully looked to, any one of these pursuits is not most humanising and laudable."[19]

Dickens, writing in 1842, was not alone in extolling the unusual industrial progress of the country. Lowell's image was nurtured by the owners themselves, who constantly welcomed visitors from afar to marvel at, and write about, the system they had constructed. In 1834, two years before he would be killed at the Alamo, Davy Crockett, frontiersman and U.S. Representative from Texas, toured Lowell and met with the owners. He too marveled at the extraordinary experiment. "I never witnessed such a combination of industry, and perhaps never will again," he told readers of his book *Tour to the North and Down East*. He noted the healthfulness of the "mile of gals" who did most of the work, the seeming good cheer and generosity of the owners, and the general industriousness and productive capacity of the looms, the spinning wheels, and the processing of cloth. "I saw the whole process, from the time they put in the raw material [cotton from Mississippi] until it came out completely finished."[20] After interrogating "a few women workers and town residents," he concluded that the majority of them "enjoy better health than before being employed in the mills." Even the men benefited, he claimed: of males, "one-half derive the same advantage."[21]

As late as the eve of the Civil War, the British novelist Anthony Trollope was equally impressed. In 1861, like Dickens and Crockett before him, he toured the country and made a special visit to Lowell, where he observed an industrial city very unlike Manchester. To him, Lowell was "the realization of a commercial Utopia"; it was "to New England what Manchester is to us," he noted. "It is the largest and most prosperous cotton-manufacturing town in the States." As with Dickens, the character of the people, the wholesomeness of their environment, and virtually every other aspect of the quality of life in the town were a contrast to Manchester back home. "That which most surprises an English visitor on going through the mills at Lowell is the personal appearance of the men and women who work at them," Trollope observed. "They are not only better dressed, cleaner, and better mounted in every respect than the girls employed at manufactories in England, but they are so infinitely superior as to make a stranger immediately perceive that some very strong cause must have created the difference." In the shops in New England, those behind counters "are neat, well dressed, careful, especially about their hair, composed in their manner, and sometimes a little supercilious in the propriety of their demeanour," characteristics that he certainly didn't associate with the factory workers of England. But, to his surprise, "it is exactly the same class of young women [as one finds in the shops in England] that one sees in the factories at Lowell. They are not sallow, nor dirty, nor ragged, nor rough. They have about them no signs of want, or of low culture." He wondered whether "superior wages" could account for the profound difference between Lowell and the Manchester women who worked as spinners and weavers, but he quickly rejected that notion because Lowell's wages were only slightly higher than Manchester's. Rather, the difference was in the accommodations that the factory owners provided their workers. "If wages at Manchester were raised to the Lowell standard," he argued, "the Manchester women would not be clothed, fed, cared for, and educated like the Lowell women." It was a difference in operating philosophy that explained it, he decided. "The fact is, that the workmen and the workwomen at Lowell are "not exposed to the chances of an open labour market." "They are taken in, as it were," into a "philanthropical manufacturing college" and treated as if they were "girls and lads at a great seminary," not demeaned "as hands by whose industry profit is to be made out of capital."[22]

Contemporaries suggested that Francis Cabot Lowell's experience on an 1810–1812 trip to Europe, on which he observed the Manchester mills, sensitized him to both their financial benefits and the toll they might take on the lives of their workers, and he determined to organize the company town he was developing differently. Trollope, seeking to explain the origins of the Lowell project to his British readers, quoted a contemporary "hand-book" detailing the factory owner's thinking: Lowell had observed the effect of Manchester on "the character of the people," and he, along with his partners, "looked for a remedy for these defects. They thought that education and good morals would even enhance the profit, and that they could compete with Great Britain by introducing a more cultivated class of operatives."[23]

Though the Lowell mills presented the tantalizing possibility of a capitalist enterprise ostensibly free of the extremes of exploitation, concerns expressed only a few years after the Lowell mills began production lingered. "I am of opinion," Alexis de Tocqueville observed in his chapter on early U.S. industry in *Democracy in America* in 1840, "that the manufacturing aristocracy which is growing up under our eyes [in Europe] is one of the harshest which ever existed in the world." He forewarned that "the friends of democracy should keep their eyes anxiously fixed" on this class of industrialists, "for if ever a permanent inequality of conditions and aristocracy again penetrate into the world, it may be predicted that" an industrial aristocracy would arise. And for that, Manchester, not Lowell, might prove the model.[24] Others saw the extraordinary experiment in paternalist manufacturing and the favorable comparisons with the European industrial system as simply a product of the relatively limited number of mills and the infancy of American manufacturing when compared to the British and European examples.

It seemed evident to Europeans such as Dickens and Trollope, who were witnessing the dehumanizing life of workers in Manchester, Leeds, Lancaster, and the coal towns of Wales, that the conditions in American textile towns were much better. But this was not necessarily the view of the women and other workers who made up the bulk of Lowell's and Waltham's workforce. Only a few years after Lowell's founding in 1826, women drawn to the mills from the countryside by the appeal of an apparently wholesome alternative to the struggling New England family began to object to the dormitories in which they were required to sleep two to a bed and, as time passed, to pay cuts, increased cost of room and board, speed-ups, and the greater work required of spinners and weavers, as they were now assigned two, even three, high-speed machines to watch over.[25]

A young woman operative from Manchester, New Hampshire, observed in 1846 that the textile mills had changed only a couple of decades after their founding: "those [workers] who are shut up within the 'Prison walls of a Factory'" were "continually inhaling cotton-dust, lamp smoke, and away from wholesome, pure air." And a sympathetic overseer wrote to the *Voice of Industry*, one of the leading newspapers published by workers in Lowell in the 1840s, that he had seen "girls faint in the morning, in consequence of the air being so impure in the mill. This is quite a common thing. Especially when girls have worked in the factory for considerable length of time." Weavers may have been particularly susceptible to respiratory problems because they had to suck the thread through their shuttles. "These 'kiss-of-death' shuttles forced workers to constantly ingest lint, sizing, and dyes from the thread. Since shuttles passed throughout the mill, there was also the risk of transmitting communicable diseases, such as tuberculosis."[26] "A young girl could leave her homestead for a factory town a plump, rosy-cheeked, strong, and laughing girl, and in one year comes back to them—better clad, t'is true, and with refined manners, and money for the discharge of their little debts, and for the supply of their wants,—but alas, how changed!" returning home often "weary" and having "los[t] my health."[27]

By the mid-1830s, short-lived strikes at Lowell alerted the public to the fact that all was not well in the mills, and by 1836 between 1,500 and 2,000 workers walked off the job, at some mills for weeks. In other mill towns as well—Pawtucket, Rhode Island; and Waltham, Massachusetts, for example—smaller job actions reflected a growing tension, undercutting the view of Lowell as representing a different kind of American capitalism than that experienced in the Old World. By the 1840s, mill workers typically labored from between 11.5 and 13.5 hours a day.[28]

The enormous financial success of Massachusetts's first mills along the Merrimac, Charles, Blackstone, and Taunton rivers in the eastern part of the state, and then farther west along the Connecticut River in Holyoke and the Housatonic in Pittsfield, spurred competition that even the prosperous, enlightened capitalists in Lowell couldn't withstand. In the coming years, factory conditions became even worse in the New England mills. By the outbreak of the Civil War, there were reports of working and living conditions that were as bad as the earlier conditions in Britain that Edwin Chadwick, Charles Dickens, and other European observers had decried. Now, as coal replaced water power as the source of energy in many factories, filth and poor-quality air and water became commonplace in the once-salubrious towns. By midcentury, every indicator of health, including life span, disease rates, and infant mortality, worsened in the worlds that the new industrialists created.

THE DECLINE OF HEALTH IN THE INDUSTRIALIZING NORTH

What effect did the developing American factory system and other changes in American society have on the health of the population? There was no national registry of diseases, nor were local and state data uniformly collected. The nomenclature of even the most devastating diseases like consumption and cholera had not been standardized. But what was undoubtedly accurate was the widespread belief among contemporaries that the remarkable experience of the first generations of New Englanders had changed and generally for the worse, reaching its nadir in the middle decades of the nineteenth century. And what was true in New England became true of the country as a whole.

In 1790 the total population of the country was 3,929,000, and by 1850 it had grown to 23,261,000.[29] But by 1850, the average life expectancy for whites had declined from over 70 years for New Englanders in the seventeenth century to 39.5 years, and for Blacks, both slave and free, the average age at death was staggeringly low, a mere 23 years. While high infant mortality, increased exposure to infectious diseases, high maternal deaths and poor nutrition, and lack of pure water and adequate sewerage, among a host of other environmental insults, affected the life spans of both whites and Blacks, the heaviest burden was borne by African Americans. For example, in 1850 the Black infant mortality rate was 340 deaths per 1,000 live births, and for whites it was 216 deaths per 1,000 live births, a difference of 57 percent.[30]

During the early 1800s, numerous signs of a coming health crisis emerged. Declining life spans, greater morbidity, and growing infant mortality became evident. Disease, once confined to periodic local epidemics of smallpox, had become an everyday reality for many northerners. Ben Mutschler details in *The Province of Affliction* the experience of Elizabeth Drinker of the growing port city of Philadelphia in 1777 as she watched her young son Henry die of "the bloody flux," long a concern of West Indian sugar planters whose slaves were regularly struck down by it. Her son had been plagued by recurrent bouts of "mucous-laden stools," but the long worms that accompanied his bowel movements had worried her that this time the outcome would not be happy. She had lost three children, one in infancy, before this. By the time of the Revolution, Mutschler reports, "a staggering range of afflictions" plagued northerners, leading local assemblies to establish some of the early public social welfare services aimed at housing, supporting, and even treating the sick. New York City established its almshouse in 1736, and private merchants and philanthropists established early charity hospitals starting with Pennsylvania General (1751), New York Hospital (1771), and Massachusetts General (1811). Diarrheal diseases in infancy, chronic and acute infections, and dietary insufficiencies during development from childhood through adolescence were noted with increasing frequency in the letters, writings, and reflections of men and women in the Revolutionary and early republic years.[31]

By the middle decades of the nineteenth century, a decline in health was noted by both statisticians and writers. In 1855, Catharine Beecher, sister of Harriet Beecher Stowe, author of *Uncle Tom's Cabin*, and Henry Ward Beecher, abolitionist and head of Plymouth Church in Brooklyn, wrote *Letters to the People on Health and Happiness*, a 200-page effort to "prove that the American people are pursuing a course, in their own habits and practices, which is destroying health and happiness to an extent that is perfectly appalling."[32]

Catharine Beecher nostalgically recalled that when she was younger, living in the rural communities of East Hampton, Long Island, New York, and Litchfield, Connecticut, "almost all [children] had rosy cheeks, and looked full of health and spirits." But this had changed. "Now, both in city and country, a great portion of them either have sallow or pale complexions, or look delicate or partially misformed."[33] "When I was young," she remembered, "I did not know of any sickly children." But now "I rarely find a school-room full of such rosy-cheeked, strong, fine-looking children as I used to see thirty years ago."[34] Beecher claimed that she was not alone in this observation. "Among all classes of our land," she maintained, "we are constantly hearing of the superior health and activity of our ancestors. Their physical health and strength, and their power of labor and endurance, was altogether beyond anything witnessed in the present generation."[35] By midcentury Beecher and the descendants of the older Protestant elites in the northeastern states were seeing the effects of the transformed commercial, social, and economic landscape reflected in the health conditions of New England's women and children.

Beecher believed that middle- and upper-class women and their children were particularly affected by an overall decline in health. That decline had dire implications for the future of the country, she argued. "In this nation, it is rare to see a married woman of thirty or forty, especially in the more wealthy classes, who retains the fulness of person and freshness of complexion that mark good health," she maintained. Beecher saw an unfolding spiral of disease, enfeeblement, and disability. "The more parents become unhealthy," she claimed, "the more feeble children will be born, and when these feeble children grow up and become parents, they will have still more puny and degenerate offspring."[36] In a recurring theme of her book, Beecher argued that "American women every year become more and more nervous, sickly, and miserable, while they are bringing into existence a feeble, delicate, or deformed offspring."[37]

Paralleling the broad agricultural and social transformations that were taking place as cities grew, commercial life expanded, and industries drew more young women from the countryside to the growing factory towns that were shaping their health experience. Beecher, however, laid the blame on women and on "the majority of parents in this nation [who were] systematically educating the rising generation to be feeble, deformed, homely, sickly, and miserable."[38] Beecher was quite specific about what she believed parents were doing wrong. "Children are allowed so many hours in wrong positions, either while reading or writing, as to bring on deformity." She also criticized parents for allowing children to "sleep on high pillows," a practice that also induced deformity. The contemporary diet of "butter, molasses, and sugar heaped on to hot cakes," as well as a diet rich in "meats, gravies, and fatty cooking" and the widespread availability of "candies and confectionaries . . . are all so many sources of debilitation, disease, and death to the young." The new diet of New Englanders was destroying the health of their children, she insisted. Beecher also worried that parents had too readily adapted to the products of the growing international trade: "Children are allowed tea and coffee [much of which was also dependent on colonial exploitation], which stimulate the nerves and brain," she complained, arguing that "the heat of these drinks tends to debilitate the stomach."[39] Not only were children being deformed, but it appeared to her that if "a plan for *destroying female health* . . . were drawn up, it would be exactly the course which is now pursued by a large portion of this nation, especially in the more wealthy classes."[40]

Beecher's perceptions were undoubtedly shaped by class and ethnic prejudices as well as by her distaste for crass commercialism and a typical prejudice of the elderly that the next generation wasn't living up to their standards. While she did offer suggestions for reform, she did not challenge the emerging economic and social relations. Instead, Beecher's prescriptions centered on educating the public on how various environmental factors might affect the physiology of the child and adult and on ways to alter habits, nutrition, housing, and working conditions to lessen disease and stunted growth. Buildings in urban areas, for example, should be built to maximize the amount of outside air in rooms and hallways. "The collecting of large numbers of humans in one building, to spend both day and night, always involves the gradual dilapidation of constitution to all," she commented. The rapidly expanding number of prisons, asylums, and other institutions, along with a rapidly growing immigrant population, many of whom now lived in crowded boardinghouses and tenements in the slums of the growing cities, augured a bleak future. In the 1820s and 1830s, some 222,000 Irish immigrants had come to the United States, whereas in the 1840s and 1850s, as Beecher was writing, almost 1,700,000 arrived. Similarly, in the 1820s and 1830s, 135,000 German immigrants had arrived, while in the 1840s and 1850s, about 1,290,000 came through the various ports on the East Coast.[41]

Another Beecher concern was the growing factory system, the "manufactories and shops of labor" where "thousands of the young congregate to labor in poisonous air, till their constitutions are undermined, and then return home to remain invalids for life."[42] Even "school-rooms and lodging houses are equally unprovided with *proper* ventilation. . . . The young inmates have their brain and nervous system on a constant drain by intellectual activity and moral responsibility." After a time, "we hear that fevers and various diseases sweep off young inmates by death" and their "friends are all wondering what *can* be the reason there is so much sickness there!"[43]

Rising infant mortality rates and declining life spans and, by the 1850s, yellow fever, malaria, and cholera, along with various other diarrheal diseases and fevers, plagued rural and urban populations in the North and South alike. "Common rumor has stigmatized Memphis as the graveyard of children," complained one author in the *American Journal of the Medical Sciences* in 1853. "The mortuary records of 1852 show the deaths among this interesting class of our population, of five years of age and under, to be 263; which number is a large fraction over one-third of all the deaths among our citizens for the year!"[44]

In general, the first half of the nineteenth century saw the paradox of a dramatic growth in the new nation's overall wealth and productivity at the same time that many people's health and well-being were being undermined.[45] According to some historical demographers, "White male life expectancy at age 20 was approximately six years lower at mid-century than it was in the late eighteenth century."[46] The medical historian Richard Shryock wrote that "in New York City, for example, the gross mortality rate for 1810 was reported as 1 death for every 46.5 persons; by 1859 this had risen to 1 for every 27!"[47] Growing economic and social inequalities in wealth and disparities in access to fresh foods, good housing, and sanitation contributed greatly to growing differences in life expectancy and experience with illness.

A concrete indication of the changing health status of early republic Americans was a decline in their average height. When Benjamin Franklin, in 1750, was delivering his optimistic assessment of the demographic experience in the New World, colonists averaged 7 centimeters (2.75 inches) taller than their English brethren. In fact, at the time of the Revolution, the average height of men has been estimated to be 5 feet,

8 inches, and by the Civil War it had declined by 2 to 3 inches. Other research indicates that white women in the nineteenth century were consistently two-thirds of an inch taller than African American women, undoubtedly due to nutritional and other environmental, economic, and social factors.[48] According to Dora Costa, this difference between white and Black women and the shrinking of Americans in general in the first half of the century were hardly surprising; as she points out, it has long been recognized that "large height differentials between social classes" are not uncommon and are linked to nutritional, housing, disease, and other socioeconomic differences. According to the medical records of army recruits during the Civil War, those born in 1840 were, on average, half an inch shorter than those born a decade earlier, and those born at the outbreak of the Civil War were 1 inch shorter than their 1830 cohort.[49] While historians argue over the causes—from differences between urban and rural populations, immigrant status, work, and wealth to ostensible genetic differences between nationalities and geographic regions, as well as limitations of the data—most agree with Dora Costa that "cohorts born from the early 1700s to those born in 1830 achieved a gradual increase in average stature of approximately one centimeter (.4 inches). Average heights fell by approximately four centimeters (1.57 inches) in the ensuing half century, reaching a trough among births in the 1880s."[50]

Interestingly, some historical demographic research indicates that height was in part a function of freedom. Free Blacks in Virginia, even in the midst of the slave South, were relatively tall until the mid-nineteenth century. Despite the harsh, repressive environment in which the small group of freemen lived between 1780 and 1830, they were nearly as tall as their white counterparts. While their farms were smaller than those owned by local whites and therefore were able to grow less and sustain fewer livestock, some historians suggest that outside income from their labor enabled them to supplement their family's caloric intake and hence provide their children with nearly as good nutrition as whites received and that this nutrition was reflected in their relative heights. By contrast, their enslaved counterparts ate diets that were restricted by masters to occasional rations of meat and reliance on a few staple vegetables, primarily corn.[51] However bad was the declining health status of northern white populations, the conditions for enslaved African Americans were substantially worse.

While the growing industrial economy was having a profound impact on health in the North, the world of the South was in many ways quite different. While yellow fever epidemics had occasionally broken out in Boston (1693), New York (1702), and Philadelphia (1741) before the Revolution, they were already permanent features of the southern health experience, affecting African Americans and whites alike. Brought over from Africa by the slave trade, two mosquito-borne diseases found fertile ground in which to propagate and spread, first in the swampy lowlands of the rice and indigo regions of the Carolinas and later in the sugar fields of Louisiana, where enslaved Blacks were particularly vulnerable. They spread along the Mississippi between Baton Rouge and New Orleans and the Delta. By the middle of the nineteenth century, epidemics of yellow fever and malaria plagued the South and along the Mississippi River further north as trade between the cotton South and the northern industrial and farming states expanded.

For enslaved African Americans, poor nutrition, poor housing, and overwork created an especially vulnerable population whose life spans were shortened and whose general health was always threatened, and not just by infectious diseases. The experience with disease was directly linked to the coercion of the slave system. In his definitive history of cotton in the creation of modern industrial capitalist states, Sven Beckert details the ways in which British, French, and Dutch merchant and military powers inserted themselves into distant societies, creating systems of exploitation, termed by Beckert "war capitalism," that ranged from control over the politics, social organization, and economics of a society to the abduction, enslavement, and forced movement of peoples across continents and oceans to do the work essential for the expansion of empires.[52] Sugar from the Caribbean; cotton from India, Brazil, Egypt, Turkey, and finally the American South; dyes and spices from Asia— all depended on creating a hierarchy of power and codified rights that gave control over body and soul to Europeans and white Americans and denied it to people of color elsewhere in the world.[53] Along with sheer military and economic power came the establishment of legal and social norms that condoned and encouraged slavery. Pseudoscientific rationales provided patinas of legitimacy for the raw exploitation of slaves by slavers, proto-police slave catchers, slave patrollers, and bounty hunters in the United States.[54]

Industrialization, first in Britain and later in the United States, and most importantly of textiles, led to an enormous increase in the demand for cotton. In the South, a further expulsion of native peoples to the west was stimulated by plantation owners' desire to expand their cotton production. The exploding demand overseas for cotton and the declining importance of tobacco as the primary cash crop in the South led plantation owners to overplant and exhaust their lands in Georgia and the Carolinas and to move the center of cotton production westward to Mississippi, Alabama, and Texas. To support that land-consuming system of cotton production, the South developed a labor scheme characterized by a rapacious demand for exploitation of human bodies rarely seen in world history. The production of cotton, the agricultural product central to Britain's textile-based Industrial Revolution, provides a glimpse of how radically work was transformed, how the plantation system and slavery were integrated into this transformation, and how human suffering and concomitant diseases were central to it.

The antebellum period was one of extraordinary growth in the demand for American cotton. The production of cotton in the United States grew from 750,000 bales in 1830 to 2.85 million bales in 1850.[55] It accounted for 77 percent of the cotton used in the British textile industry, 90 percent of the cotton used in France, up to 92 percent of the 102 million pounds spun in the German Zollverein (which included greater Germany, Prussia, and parts of Austria), and the vast majority of the cloth spun in Russia, as well as nearly all the cotton destined for the textile mills of Massachusetts, Rhode Island, and New Hampshire.[56] In 1850, less than 14 percent of U.S. cotton production was for the domestic market.[57] Intricate international businesses grew up to facilitate the transportation of cotton from the field to the trading houses, to the ships, and to the mills where it was ginned, spun into yarn, and then made into cloth. Banks and lending houses financed middlemen to distribute the cotton to domestic and overseas markets as finished products. In the United States, Beckert argues, planters hung on news of price changes on the Liverpool market; slight variations in price would determine whether plantation owners would buy more slaves or sell them downriver, push western expansion for new lands, or borrow from banks.[58] The abolition of the slave trade in 1808 led to the forced migration of slaves from the older tobacco regions of Virginia and the eastern seaboard to the new giant plantations in the Deep South and westward.[59] From 1800 to 1860, between 800,000 and 1 million African Americans were forcibly moved from the Upper South to the Lower South, in what the historian Edward Baptist identifies as among the largest forced migrations in world history.[60] By the start of the Civil War, three-quarters of the world's cotton was grown in the American South.[61]

By the early decades of the nineteenth century, the enslaved population represented a considerable percentage of the nation's "capital," that is, "property"—which included land, machinery, buildings, inventories, and, in this case, human beings. In 1774, the monetary value of slaves as a percentage of total wealth in the South was about one-third, while in the country as a whole it was less than 20 percent.[62] But by 1860 the monetary value of slaves as a proportion of the South's total wealth approached 50 percent. For the country as a whole, though, despite the rapid growth of the industrial economy in the North, the percentage of national wealth in that year represented by enslaved persons was still approximately 20 percent. In 1860, the value of slaves was $3.059 trillion of a $16 trillion national economy.[63] By the Civil War, ownership of other human beings, according to the historian David Blight, was the "largest single financial asset in the entire U.S. economy, worth more than all manufacturing and railroads combined."[64] Whippings, terror, backbreaking labor, poor nutrition, and early death were the prices paid by the enslaved to ensure the fortunes of planters, textile factory owners, and bankers.[65] Growing wealth in the form of "human capital," as economists would have it, depended on the creation of a system in which disease would thrive. Some would benefit while others would die. See figure 2.1.

The expanding slave-based cotton economy was supplemented by rapid growth in the South's slave-based sugar production. In 1795 the first U.S. sugar plantation was opened in Louisiana, and by 1850 Louisiana's planters were producing 25 percent of the world's cane sugar supply. The number of enslaved workers in sugar quadrupled between 1830 and 1850, reaching 125,000.[66] Working on sugar plantations was "exhausting work" throughout the year, as the historian Michael Tadman

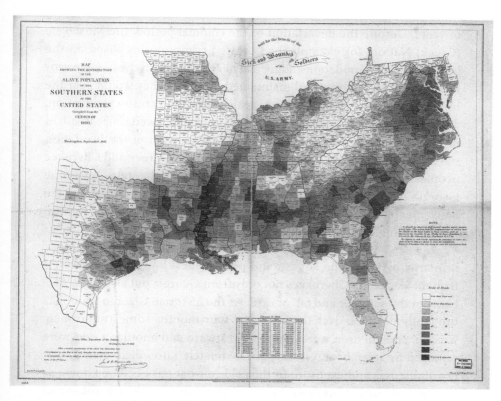

FIGURE 2.1 Distribution of slaves in the U.S. South in 1860. Edwin Hergesheimer, *Map Showing the Distribution of the Slave Population of the Southern States of the United States, compiled from the Census of 1860* (Washington, DC: Henry S. Graham, 1861). Courtesy of the Library of Congress, Geography and Map Division.

notes, but the "grinding season" from October to January "was by far the cruelest time for sugar workers." At that time, "cane cutting and hauling had to be synchronized so that grinding and boiling at the sugar mill could go around the clock. Unlike cotton the sugar crop would not keep." Tadman argues that on the U.S. sugar plantations, like those of the Caribbean, deaths exceeded births, and as a result of the horrendous conditions "slaves working on sugar plantations were, compared with other working-age slaves in the United States, far less able to resist the common and life-threatening diseases of dirt and poverty."[67]

By the first years of the nineteenth century, native peoples in the American Southeast had maintained their communities for hundreds of years. Despite the devastation of the colonial period, the Muscogee (Creek) Nation, for example, had created communities based on the belief that accommodation and formal negotiation with the U.S. government would be honored and maintained. But soon they would bear the brunt of the demand for land for greater sugar and cotton production, as Georgian plantation owners and their backers viewed those that had not been driven out as an obstacle to the expansion of the plantation slave system. As late as 1825, there were still 10,000 Creek and Cherokee peoples in Georgia, and they occupied 25 percent of the state. But as one Georgia politician opined, foreshadowing their forced migration, the native people were "simply occupants—tenants at will," and the rightful owners of the land were "the White people of Georgia."[68]

In 1836 some 1,600 Creeks were forcibly removed from Georgia, primarily by boat. The largest, and perhaps best-known, forced resettlement was of the Cherokees not only from Georgia but also from Alabama in the summer and fall of 1838. As the historian Claudio Saunt has brilliantly detailed, over the course of four months some 11,000 men, women, and children were marched westward and another 3,000 were removed by steamboat. Overall, approximately 1,000 died from a variety of diseases and exposure to the cold in what has become known as the "trail of tears."[69] But expulsions were not limited to the Cherokee and Creek tribes. In 1831, 4,000 Choctaw people were forcibly moved from Mississippi to the West, and 398 Senecas and Delaware peoples were expelled from Ohio in that same year.

Thus Indigenous peoples whose ancestors had lived in Florida, Georgia, Alabama, Mississippi, and other areas east of the Mississippi River for centuries were expelled, primarily but not exclusively to allow for the expansion of cotton production based on slave labor. They were forced to live in designated "Indian lands," what is now modern-day Oklahoma. By 1850, approximately 236,000 enslaved people were working the lands that had previously been inhabited by native people.[70]

Not only were plantations and slave labor emerging as the heart of the South's production of raw materials essential to textile manufacturing overseas, but that system shaped much of northern life as well. The building of a stable supply chain of cotton for both New England's and Great Britain's textile industries required a political and economic system that provided a legal and regulatory framework to support it and the infrastructure necessary to carry it out. The building of roads, canals, ports, and railroads essential to facilitating transportation of the raw materials grown in the South to the mills in New England and Manchester certainly supported the system of slavery. In addition, an acknowledgment of slavery itself was written into the U.S. Constitution. Article 1, Section 2, Clause 3 included the "three-fifths" clause, which provided that enslaved Africans would be counted as three-fifths of a person for tax, census, and apportionment of representation in the House of Representatives, despite their lack of citizenship or the right to vote.[71] Then Article IV, Section 2, Clause 3 required that slaves who escaped to another state had to be returned to their owners upon the latter's request.[72] In subsequent years many other federal laws were passed that sanctified and strengthened the institution of slavery. Further customs and laws were developed in the slave states that virtually freed plantation owners from restraints on their behavior by allowing whippings, child labor, and even murder and rape. The point was to increase the production of cotton and other cash crops; subordinating the enslaved who were deemed unruly or unproductive was part of that purpose. Though southerners in Congress and in public discourse proclaimed that what happened on the plantation was a private affair, northern abolitionists, escaped slaves, and free people of color made clear that because the slave system was an abomination that affected all of American society, it had to be confronted publicly. As debates in Congress indicated and slave narratives documented, slavery in the United States was not only cruel and inhumane but was also deadly— leading to high maternal and infant mortality, nutritional deficiencies, and even specific dread diseases.

Historians agree that capitalism was critical to the way that economic, political, and social systems developed in the North and the South of the United States and elsewhere.[73] As James Oakes summarizes, "Capitalism, not slavery, was the truly revolutionary force. . . . As it spanned the globe, capitalism drove indigenous peoples from their lands, [and] put slaves to work on plantations in the Americas."[74] If the industrial workers and farmers in the U.S. North were experiencing some decline in their health status, enslaved people in the U.S. South also found their lives shortened and health destroyed as slavery expanded to new areas further west and south.

SOUTHERN WHITES AND FREE BLACKS

The plantation system and its relationship to industrial capitalism created disparities between and among the South's different populations. Broadly speaking, the free white population in the South was essentially composed of three groups: planters and their overseers, whose slaves produced cotton throughout the South, tobacco in Virginia and North Carolina, and sugar in Louisiana; yeomen, some of whom owned slaves and produced, for example, hemp in Kentucky and wheat in Maryland; and poor subsistence farmers living on the worst land, especially inland in mountainous terrain.

Most of the population of free Blacks lived on farms, but others were artisans in, for example, Charleston, Baltimore, and the District of Columbia. In 1860 there were 262,000 Black freemen in the South, the vast majority of whom (216,000) lived along the southeastern seaboard. An additional 219,000 free Blacks lived in the northern states, more than half of whom lived in New York, New Jersey, and Pennsylvania. According to some sources, among the free Black population who lived in cities, mortality rates varied by region, with Blacks having a worse experience in northern cities because of inadequate housing and heat during the winter months.[75] The historian Christian Warren quotes one report from Philadelphia describing free Blacks "dying from exposure" because they lived in "'cold and exposed rooms and garrets . . . without any comforts, save the bare floor, with the cold penetrating between the boards,' or 'in cold, wet and damp cellars.'"[76] A study of free Blacks in four cities—two northern and two southern—suggests, however, that mortality gradually improved in some cities in the decades leading up to the Civil War.[77]

Before the Civil War, plantation owners made up over two-thirds of millionaires in the United States despite their small number.[78] Southern yeoman white farmers, however, were only half as wealthy as their northern brethren, and inequality in the South between rich and poor whites was extreme. Among whites in the South, the historian James Oakes writes, "the extreme levels of inequality [were equivalent to those] prevalent in England and France." Oakes concludes that there was "no doubt that slavery made the slave owners rich but [it] also made the South poor." Since most land produced products for export, there was less fertile land available for varied diets that included protein, fruits, and vegetables.[79] In the midcentury South, both Black and white poor were plagued by various nutritional and environmental diseases, including hookworm and pellagra, that directly reflected the dietary and social conditions under which they lived.

INADEQUATE DIETS AND HEALTH CONSEQUENCES

Access to nutritious food is a good barometer for evaluating not only the fundamental social justice of a society but also the extent to which basic sustenance is denied and susceptibility to illness increased. Control of food was especially important in the slave economy. As Walter Johnson explains in his book *River of Dark Dreams*, determining the quality, amounts, and types of food granted slaves was as much about a larger social calculus of control and plantation hierarchy as it was about calibrations of food economy. Slave owners calculated how much and what types of foodstuffs were necessary to keep slaves in their most productive years capable of doing the work. "Meat is generally not fed to the laborers in this part of the state," Johnson quotes one planter who lived along the Mississippi. This was both an economic determination and a means of maintaining social hierarchy and control. "By regulating the food that passed the lips of their slaves," Johnson notes, "planters materially affirmed and naturalized [their] version of social order."[80]

Johnson argues that decisions about the makeup of the slave diet in cotton-growing regions were in part a product of the unique demands of the cotton economy. Planters devoted so much of their land to growing cotton, the "white gold," that the amount of land left for food production was severely limited. Beef took up too much profitable land for grazing, and pigs running through cotton fields were a danger to the cotton crop. Planters reserved the prime meats for themselves. The land available to the enslaved for their own plots was quite limited, as were the amounts of food distributed to the slaves, and even the amount of manure that could be used as fertilizer was limited. "The entire economy was devoted to agriculture, yet it could not feed itself." As a result, the lower South "imported most of [its] wheat, corn, beef, and pork . . . from the Midwest and the Ohio Valley," Johnson tells us. *The American Cotton Planter*, a publication out of Montgomery, Alabama, was "*devoted to*

Improved Plantation Economy, Manufactures, and the Mechanic Arts."
First published as a monthly in 1853, its inaugural issue editorialized on
the paradox of the world's richest agricultural region having to import
its food. The journal noted that Alabama, Mississippi, and Texas "produce too *little grain . . . too little bacon,* too *few mules,* and *no wool,"*
making the region dependent on northern and western imports. It was
a "system . . . that must be changed, else the cotton States are to become
to the grain and [live]stock States what Ireland and Irish farmers are to
England and her Lords—'hewers of wood and drawers of water'!" An
"insidious effect . . . of this disastrous policy," a problem both in the
long run and the short, was "sapping the cotton States of the immense
sums of gold produced annually from our cotton fields—expended for
[imported] grain, meat and negro cloth."[81] "Why," the *Planter* asked, do
"our planters persist in paying out the substance of their fields and labor
for grain, bacon, mules, etc., which they may and can produce to better
advantage to themselves and country?"[82]

Some historians have argued with this analysis of the plantation's
dependence on imports, saying that, for much of the year before harvesting the cotton crop, plantations had a "surplus" of slave labor
available to grow corn and other vegetation, thereby providing the
nutritional necessities, independent of northern wheat, meat, and other
essential food products. In fact, the economic historian Robert Gallman
has argued that the cost of transporting foodstuffs from northern and
western regions was prohibitive; given the availability of "very valuable
surplus labor and relatively cheap land," planters "could grow corn without reducing cotton capacity." Since the harvesting season of cotton was
so short, for much of the year the planter could depend on using a surplus of workers to farm.[83]

While it may have been possible for plantation owners to produce
healthy food as well as cotton, the fact remains that the quality and
nutritional value of the food given to the enslaved were always poor.
Emancipated slaves remembered that they "never had meat of any kind"
and that their "allowance of food was one peck of corn a week to each
full-grown slave."[84] Irrespective of the amount of grains and hogs produced in the cotton-growing South, it is incontestable that planters controlled and distributed food to enslaved families at their whim.[85] The
historian Eugene Genovese, in his first book, *The Political Economy of*

Slavery, explains the bare diet that plantation slaves lived on: "The diet to which the slaves were subjected must be judged immensely damaging, despite assurances from contemporaries and later historians that the slaves were well fed," he begins. "The slave usually got enough to eat, but the starchy high-energy diet of cornmeal, pork, and molasses produced specific hungers, dangerous deficiencies, and . . . unidentified forms of malnutrition." Slaves received "occasional additions of sweet potatoes or beans," but they "could do little to supplement the narrow diet."[86] When allowed, they tried to add to their rations by sowing their own gardens, but as Genovese points out, that land "was generally the poorest available, and the quality of foodstuffs consequently suffered."[87]

What enslaved were fed, according to Genovese, was spurred by economic considerations, although the lines between economic self-interest and cruelty were often blurred: whipping and the control of diet were both tools in a system geared to maximizing production, which in the eyes of its adherents legitimated human cruelty as a necessary evil. Some "planters did try to provide vegetables and fruits, but not much land could be spared from the staples, and output remained minimal." Planters obviously could have devoted more land to fruits and vegetables, and their decision not to had a direct impact on the caloric, vitamin, and protein intake of slaves. Because the pork provided to slaves was mostly fat, it was low in protein, while "cereals in general and corn in particular cannot provide adequate protein[,] [which] greatly reduces the ability of an organism to resist infectious diseases."[88]

There may have often been a good *quantity* of food available. But it is clear from medical historians that the quality of food was deficient because it led to such diseases as pellagra (now understood as a deficiency in niacin and vitamin B3, which can ultimately lead to death), rickets (a vitamin D deficiency that causes softening of the bones that results in bowed legs), and scurvy (caused by a lack of vitamin C and resulting in open sores and poorly healing wounds). These are all diseases of inadequate nutrition. Pellagra's symptoms included severe diarrhea, a skin rash (sometimes referred to as a "butterfly caste" across the face), dementia and other neurological problems, and ultimately death. While pellagra was also present among poor whites, about half of the cases were among African Americans, even through the Depression of the 1930s.[89] Poor general health was undoubtedly also linked to the lack of variety in the slave diet. Enslaved men and women were given a mush of rice in the South Carolina lowlands and corn and some pork in much of the cotton regions. Historians have euphemistically called this paucity of protein a "monotonous diet."[90]

Nineteenth-century personal narratives and later historical analyses confirm that no matter what quantity of food was provided, adequate nutrition was certainly lacking, leading to high infant mortality rates and, in those infants that survived, stunted growth; in addition, women were in heightened danger of miscarriage and stillborn births. In *Twelve Years a Slave*, written in 1853, Solomon Northrup recalled his life on a farm in northern Louisiana: "All that is allowed is corn and bacon, which is given out at the corncrib and smokehouse every Sunday morning. Each [person] receives, as his weekly allowance, three and a half pounds of bacon, and corn enough to make a peck of meal." Slaves were not "ever likely to suffer from the gout, superinduced by excessive high living."[91]

In *Fifty Years in Chains, or, The Life of an American Slave* (1859), Charles Ball told the story of his enslavement in Maryland, South Carolina, and Georgia. Raised on a tobacco plantation in Maryland, he was forced to walk for a month from there to Columbia, South Carolina, where he was sold to a cotton plantation owner in Georgia. He remembers how little food his family was given, both on the plantation and on the journey, and how, before he was taken to be sold farther south, his mother "divided the scanty pittance of food [salt fish and cornbread], allowed her by her mistress between [his] brothers and sisters . . . and gone supperless to bed herself."[92]

Food, or its absence, was a constant reminder of power and control and the harsh life slaves endured. "As I was always very obedient, and ready to execute all his orders, I did not receive much whipping, but suffered greatly for want of sufficient and proper food. My master allowed his slaves a peck of corn, each, per week, throughout the year," Ball recalled. In December, when hogs were slaughtered, various grades of pork might be available—intestines, snouts, feet—those parts that were rejected by the masters or not valuable in any market. Other times of year, "we had meat once a week, unless bacon became scarce, which very often happened, in which case we had no meat at all." His diet as a child was supplemented by an "abundance of fish in the spring, and as long as the fishing season continued. After that period, each slave received, in addition to his allowance of corn, one salt herring every day."[93] Occasionally, his father would visit from another plantation and bring "apples, melons, sweet potatoes, or, if he could procure nothing else, a little parched corn, which tasted better in our cabin, because he had brought it."[94]

A study of the skeletal remains of one group of children, young adults, women, and men from a gravesite designated for slaves in North Carolina gives vivid evidence of the impact of slavery on the health of a community in the antebellum years. The anthropologist Patricia Lambert shows that evidence of "dental caries, antemortem tooth loss, enamel hypoplasia [a defect of the enamel that only occurs while teeth are still developing], porotic hyperostosis [a pathological condition that affects bones of the cranial vault], periosteal lesions [lesions involving the outer layer of the bones], lytic lesions [destruction of an area of bone due to a disease process, such as cancer] and stature" points to severe and prolonged vitamin and other dietary insufficiency and indicates that infants and children were the most negatively affected segment of the enslaved African American population.[95] Forensic analysis of seventeen enslaved people buried on a North Carolina estate from the 1830s through the 1850s suggests that among Black children the death rate was twice as high as that of white children at the time.[96]

Richard Steckel, a medical historian whose work has focused on pediatrics and child health, concluded that the health of enslaved children "was comparable to that in the poorest populations ever studied," a remarkable indictment of the savagery of slavery in the United States.[97] He notes that slaves were fed differently at different periods of their lives according to the owners' need for labor. Slave children, whose stomachs demanded nutritious foods but whose hands were generally unprofitable until age five, when they might be sent into the fields to pick cotton, were a financial burden for a slave owner. As a result, as statistical measures of development have indicated, their growth was stunted when compared to white children of the same age.[98] Comparisons of the average heights of children, Steckel documents, "show that slave children were among the smallest ever measured."[99] Upon reaching an age at which their labor could be productive, Steckel argues, young slaves received more nutritious and plentiful allotments of food and then gained some of the stature that other children their age had attained earlier.[100] Among the enslaved population, Steckel attributes the "high incidence of stillbirths during the late Autumn and the concentration of neonatal deaths in February to April . . . [to] acute nutritional deprivation during the late winter and early spring." Not only were women forced into the fields soon after giving birth, but pregnant women as well were forced to work "during peak seasons in the demand for labor."[101] Steckel estimates that 30 percent of enslaved infants died within weeks of their birth, most during the "peak season" after their mothers had been forced to work the fields. Another 20 percent died between ages one and four.[102]

Other evidence reinforces the impact of poor food on the health and well-being of African Americans in the antebellum period. One study of "the effect of geography and vitamin D on African American stature" used prison records to document that "nineteenth century African-American [heights] were consistently shorter than those of whites."[103] Other studies document deficiencies of calcium caused by a lack of milk, a nutrient reserved for white children, particularly during winters when supplies were short; others detail vitamin A deficiencies that led to poor eyesight and anemia due to an absence of iron in the diet.[104]

Ultimately, despite decades of research on the plantation diet, we are still left with Genovese's observation of more than sixty years ago: "There is nothing surprising in the slave's appearance of good health: his diet was well suited to guarantee the appearance of good health and to provide the fuel to keep him going in the fields, but it was not sufficient to ensure either sound bodies or the stamina needed for sustained labor." Those whose value to the plantation economy was limited—children, the elderly, the injured or disabled, women—were expendable.[105]

Diet was but one factor in why the enslaved population had a greater death rate than whites and why they suffered with greater frequencies from the array of horrendous diseases and other afflictions that were ever-present threats for mid-nineteenth-century Americans. Kenneth Stampp wrote more than sixty years ago that "to owners of river-bottom plantations in Alabama and Mississippi reports of 'a great deal of sickness among negroes' were distressingly familiar." The epidemics of cholera (the most significant ones were in 1832, 1849, and 1866), especially in the large plantations of the Deep South, seem to have affected the slave population more severely than the planters and their families. "In each of the great epidemics," Stampp commented, "cholera which struck its victims with terrifying suddenness and ran its course with dramatic speed, was fatal to thousands of slaves and reduced some of their owners to financial ruin."[106] The death could be a horrible one. If a person ingests the bacterium *V. cholerae*, the historian Claudio Saunt notes, it will make its way to the small intestine, "where it produces a toxin that the body flushes out with watery vomit and a voluminous and distinctive rice-water diarrhea." Because of the diarrhea and vomiting, sufferers become severely dehydrated. As a result, "blood pressure collapses, eyes recede in the skull, skin becomes shriveled and pallid and victims go into shock." Approximately half of those so affected die, "some within a few hours after the onset of symptoms."[107]

Even more prevalent were a wide range of diseases that attacked the slaves annually: "During the summer months," Stampp notes, "'bowel complaints,' or the 'bloody flux' (usually some form of dysentery or diarrhea), [was indicative of] the debilitating effects and mortality of malaria. During the winter months, pleurisy and pneumonia cut down the poorly clad and improperly housed field hands who were too much exposed during cold or wet weather." Stampp quotes a Louisiana physician that pneumonia was "one of the most formidable complaints, more fatal than any other." In addition, sore throats, colds, thrush, measles, mumps, influenza, whooping cough, dengue, scrofula, scarlet fever, rheumatism, typhoid, typhus, smallpox, diphtheria, dropsy, and tuberculosis were identified by doctors in the South as frequent causes of disease among the slave population. Hookworm, an intestinal parasite that is closely linked to poor sanitation, outhouses, and lack of shoes, affected many slaves; "Cachexia Africana," or dirt eating, was explained by slave owners as a "habit" but was undoubtedly due to dietary deficiencies. Numerous mental disorders, including depression, were regularly reported as diseases of slavery.[108]

The grueling work on the plantation took a particular toll on enslaved women. Stampp reported that "painful or irregular menses, suppurative infections of the generative tract, and prolapses uteri were extremely common; sterility, spontaneous abortions, stillbirths, and death in childbirth occurred two or three times as frequently among slave women as among white."[109] When enslaved women or men became ill, he also noted, rarely was a doctor called. Richard Shryock observed many decades ago, as other historians have since, that "considerations of economy" dictated that slaves were generally in poor health, receiving little or no medical attention.[110] Some planters were willing to call in doctors when slave women were not conceiving because that problem would limit the likely number of surviving children available for the plantation's workforce in coming years. One "country practitioner" reported on "Sterility Among the Negroes" in the *New Orleans Medical News and Hospital Gazette*, saying that "barrenness is more common among negro women than whites" and noting that some believed "the women have knowledge of an art or herb by which conception may be prevented or abort procured."[111] When someone became critically ill and was sent to a hospital, the conditions were horrible. Stampp quotes Fanny Kemble, an English visitor to a Georgia plantation in 1838–1839, who describes the scene at a hospital that slaves were sent to: "The floors were 'merely the hard damp earth itself,' most of the windows were unglazed, the rooms were dirty and malodorous, and the inmates 'lay prostrate on the floor, without bed, mattress, or pillow, buried in tattered and filthy blankets. Sick and well alike were 'literally encrusted with dirt,' and infested with 'swarms of fleas.'"[112]

The greater incidence of disease among slaves could be traced not only to their diet, their work, and the callousness of so many slave owners, but also to inadequate provision of other necessities of life, such as clothing and housing. Like the food provided to slave men, women, and children, clothing and shelter, to the extent provided, were meant simply to allow slaves to survive at a minimum level so that they could continue to work. The refusal of most masters to provide adequate clothing to the slaves, as Stampp observed, "during the winters . . . caused real discomfort and posed a serious threat to health." Most of the slaves "lacked sufficient clothing to keep warm when the temperature dropped below freezing. Many of them went barefoot even in winter weather, or wore out their shoes before spring; hence they often limped about on frostbitten feet."[113] Frederick Douglass described how, when he was a child, he "was kept almost in a state of nudity; no shoes, no stockings, no jacket, no trousers; nothing but coarse sack-cloth or tow-linen, made into a sort of shirt, reaching down to my knees, This I wore night and day, changing it once a week."[114]

The housing was typically so inadequate that even southern doctors at the time commented on it. As Stampp recounts, "'One of the most prolific sources of disease among negroes,' wrote an Alabama physician, 'is the condition of their houses. . . . Small, low, tight and filthy; their houses can be but laboratories of disease. According to a Mississippian, 'Planters do not always reflect that there is more sickness, and consequently greater loss of life from the decaying logs of negro houses, open floors, leaky roofs, and crowded rooms than all other causes combined.'"[115]

Evidence abounds that slaves who were considered unproductive were often discarded. They were often sold "downriver" (that is, to the Lower South, where larger cotton plantations were established as the fertility of land in the Upper South—Virginia, Maryland, and North Carolina—declined from overcultivation), and they were sold for lower prices than for those in their prime or whose bodies were whole. And then, in a further twist to the inherent cruelty of a system that so valued profit over the lives of others, there were the unproductive enslaved women who were offered to doctors to experiment on—as exemplified by the stories of enslaved women with prolapsed uteruses who were "donated" by local plantation owners to Marion Sims for his infamous human experiments.[116] More common, so common that it happened over and over again and to family after family, was the routine cruelty inherent in buying and selling human beings as if they were any other commodity, in the forced separation of families, of children being sold, of wives being taken, and of escapees having to leave their loved ones without a word lest their escape be discovered by the wailing of their children or wife. Psychic and physical stress went hand in hand. Some lost all hope, as well one might, but many others resisted when they could and never gave up on the idea of freedom. As Louis Hughes put it in his memoir *Thirty Years a Slave*, the new freedmen exulted at the arrival of Union troops, whom they viewed as true liberators, and thousands among them "in search of the freedom of which they had so long dreamed, flocked into the city of refuge [Memphis], some having walked hundreds of miles."[117]

While the plantation system devastated the health of slaves in the South, the emergence of a commercial economy built around rice, cotton, and sugar promoted the spread of another deadly disease, yellow fever, among Blacks and whites. In the decades between the Revolution and the Civil War, the growth of trade both within and outside the original colonies made epidemic diseases endemic to all sections of the United States, but especially in the South. Yellow fever was a constant threat to both Black and white throughout the South by the early nineteenth century. By midcentury, the disease threat seems to have intensified, according to the historian Margaret Humphreys. "In each year in the two decades before the Civil War, there was at least one major yellow fever epidemic in some southern maritime city. New Orleans, Mobile, Pensacola, Savanah, Charleston, and Norfolk were ravaged with varying frequency during these twenty years."[118] One southern doctor, Josiah Clark Nott, claimed that yellow fever was "confined predominantly" to what he called the "unwashed democracy." This perception, according to Humphreys, was a common one, leading, for example, to "the Irish slums [being] burned by an angry mob that blamed [Norfolk's] yellow fever epidemic on the condition of 'the dirty Irish.'"[119] The president of Louisiana's State Board of Health, E. H. Barton, measured the impact of filthy living habits by the prevalence of yellow fever in certain areas of New Orleans. He insisted that the worst aspects of yellow fever could be explained as the result of living conditions in both Black and white areas of the city, conditions that the Sanitary Commission of New Orleans described as "disgusting and revolting beyond all expression. . . . Filth of every character crowded the streets, gutters, pavements, and even the houses," conditions which were often ascribed by the elites as products of the "depraved" cultures of the Black and white poor.[120]

Yellow fever's symptoms were particularly fearsome. One Memphis resident described the experiences of "Lucille," who, according to Humphreys, was probably the resident's niece. "The poor girl's screams might be heard for half a square and at times I had to exert my utmost strength to hold her in bed. Jaundice was marked, the skin being a bright yellow hue: tongue and lips dark, cracked and blood oozing from the mouth and nose." But that was not the worst of her symptoms: "the most terrible and terrifying feature was the 'black vomit' which I had never before witnessed. By Tuesday evening it was as black as ink and would be ejected with terriffic [sic] force." The resident said that he had his "face and hands spattered but had to stand by and hold her."[121]

The incidence of yellow fever was tied to the transformation of the southern economy, as the historian Urmi Engineer Willoughby has detailed in *Yellow Fever, Race, and Ecology in Nineteenth-Century New Orleans*. Willoughby explains the underlying political economy of the disease in this way: "Ecological conditions produced by colonialism and imperial expansion resulted in the escalation of epidemic yellow fever (and other diseases) across the Atlantic. . . . In the nineteenth century, epidemic yellow fever emerged in the Americas and Africa as an unforeseen consequence of colonial expansion and maritime trade, and the disease became prevalent with the rise of plantation slavery, sugar production, and urban growth in swamps and prairies."[122] The "process of sugar production and the establishment of large scale sugar plantations" in the Caribbean, Brazil, and Louisiana, she notes, "facilitated the propagation of yellow fever in several ways." Sugar plantations could only be established by destroying forests and thus the habitats of the birds and bats that feasted on mosquitoes; that, in turn, allowed mass mosquito propagation in these areas. Sugar plantations depended on transatlantic commerce and were typically built close to ports and canals, most specifically New Orleans, where riverboats were then used to transport sugar and other goods throughout the South and into the northern cities. In the process, the boats became a natural means of transporting the disease-bearing mosquito *A. aegypti* to new and formerly untouched areas of the country. In addition, the plantations used a variety of storage containers, especially clay pots "to clarify crystalized sugar," that made attractive fertile breeding environments for *A. aegypti*.[123] These decisions to build economies around sugar and cotton literally built a world that killed no small number of its people.

The development of an industrial and commercial economy in the years between the Revolutionary and Civil wars led to severely negative effects on the U.S. population in both the North and the South. In the North, the growing market economy transformed rural life and affected the health of many classes, including the women and children who worked in the mills and even the middle-class women and northern merchants and financiers. In the South, slaveholders created a system that fostered new patterns of suffering, manifested in disease and death. By midcentury, it was clear that a peculiar kind of American capitalism based on slavery had created a new world that enriched some lives at the expense of the vast majority of the population. Waves of epidemic diseases now swept through the growing commercial centers, threatening Black and white, rich and poor, alike, although disproportionately African Americans and the poor. Once relatively local affairs, epidemics became national in scope. Human suffering of all kinds became a lodestone on the neck of the new nation.

CHAPTER THREE

"The Surging Tide of Business . . . Yielding Up the Bones of the Dead"

Overwork, Poor Nutrition, Unhygienic Homes, and a Hazardous Workplace

"Filth of every kind [was] thrown into the streets, covering their surface, filling the gutters, obstructing the sewer culverts, and sending forth perennial emanations which must generate pestiferous diseases."

CITIZENS' ASSOCIATION, *REPORT . . . UPON THE SANITARY CONDITION OF THE CITY* (1865)

As this book argues, the causes of ill-health lie in the creation of worlds that promote the conditions for disease, disability, and death. In the late nineteenth and early twentieth centuries, America was a world of industrial capitalism that featured the growth of the iron and steel, coal, metal-mining, oil, and textile industries. The dramatic transformation of the American economy in the decades following the Civil War required enormous infrastructure investment to support the growing industries across the nation. Government and private investment went into building a railroad system and an infrastructure of roads and ports that could efficiently transport goods from the Atlantic to the Pacific and to Europe. Similar transportation links were built between the northern industrial centers and port cities and the southern cotton fields. Cities like Pittsburgh, Cleveland, and Youngstown—all near the coalfields of the Appalachian region—exploded in population and became centers for the production of the steel, iron, and rubber that would be used to manufacture the railroad track, engines, and cars that would tie the nation together. Detroit, whose population grew from 9,000 to 116,000 between 1840 and 1880, was first the center of foundries producing stoves and other cast iron products and then, by the early twentieth century, a center of Ford, General Motors, and other firms of the new automobile industry. Chicago, in the pre–Civil War period not much more than a fort and trading center, grew to become the second-largest city in the nation based on its slaughterhouses and food-processing industries. Its population grew from about 4,000 people in 1840 to over 1.5 million people by 1900, only six decades later. Smaller cities built around industries that serviced the emerging giant industrial and consumer firms expanded throughout the Midwest and western states. Dayton and Akron, Ohio; Flint and Battle Creek, Michigan; Charleston, West Virginia; and Indianapolis, Indiana, for example, produced the batteries, bicycles, chemicals, paints, canned goods, processed foods, and packaging that were essential to the growing consumer economy.

To these transformed cities came masses of people looking for work in the factories and wharves. White people came from the rural Midwest, African Americans from the South, and immigrants from Germany and Ireland and then from Italy and eastern Europe. What they found, however, was that these industrial cities, given the overcrowding and greed of industrialists and landlords, were practically unlivable. The streets were filthy. Horse manure, animal waste, and refuse of all kinds accumulated there. Backyard privies were rarely emptied, leaving visual, ambulatory, and olfactory reminders of the physical deterioration of the city. The waste from tanneries, breweries, slaughterhouses, and other manufacturing and processing factories now drew armies of rats, mice, lice, pigeons, and other vermin that feasted on, among other things, the discarded feed from the huge number of horses that were used to transport goods and help lift the granite at building sites. In addition, thousands of horses, goats, and pigs died in the streets (the 130,000 or more horses in 1870 Manhattan were literally worked to death with a life expectancy of less than three years).[1] The glue factories to which the dead carcasses were hauled produced enormous waste and acrid odors. The tons of organic mash, the "swill" that flowed from the breweries, were used to feed the diseased and undernourished cows that produced the adulterated milk that was fed to poor working-class children. The blood and entrails of cows, pigs, goats, and lambs were dumped in overflowing bins in the slaughter-house districts. The city was transformed. Once economically diverse communities of artisans and shopkeepers living above their places of work became class-defined neighborhoods; the wealthy lived in one section of the city, where street cleaning and fresh produce were available, while workers, migrants, and immigrants crowded together into slums that were antithetical to good health.[2]

With this new social and industrial reality came substantial changes to the health of the nation. Factory accidents resulted in broken bones and lost limbs and lives. Industries structured work in ways that were harmful to workers—with long hours and unsafe conditions. Infectious diseases became epidemic. As in the past, many explained ill-health as due to the personal failings of individuals who were seen as morally suspect. But with the massive immigration that began in the middle decades of the century, elites no longer saw disease as rooted in the habits or beliefs of individuals, but rather as the characteristic of entire immigrant groups or classes. Older native English Protestants blamed Irish, Jewish, Italian, and other immigrants—those who were most affected by the changing urban environment—for the deteriorating conditions of cities and of people's health. But the situation in the nineteenth-century industrial centers led some to challenge that view. It became apparent that it was not solely individuals or groups who were responsible for disease and death—it was the world built around these industries that created the conditions in which accidents would occur and diseases would become widespread. Urban life was untenable.

Three illustrations show the contemporary understanding of disease. Figure 3.1, a scene of a street in an Irish neighborhood, leaves it ambiguous who are the "microbes" that chose this liquor-laden squalor as their "home." Figures 3.2 and 3.3, however, specifically identify the new Irish and Jewish immigrants, the likely victims of midcentury epidemics, as themselves the "microbes" responsible for the "cholera scare." Not even new, seemingly "scientific," bacteriological understandings of the cause of disease could neutralize the nativism and hatred of foreigners that marked so much of American culture. Racist and anti-immigrant theories were simply incorporated into the new bacteriological explanations of disease.

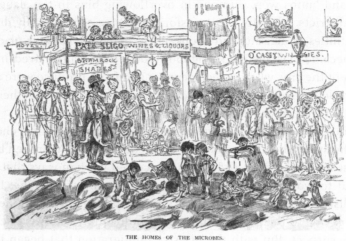

THE STREETS OF NEW YORK.—No. XXIV.

THE HOMES OF THE MICROBES.

FIGURE 3.1 "The Streets of New York—No. XXIV: The Homes of the Microbes," *Puck* (vol. 17, no. 421), April 1, 1885, 74. HathiTrust.

A CHANCE FOR THE CHOLERA.

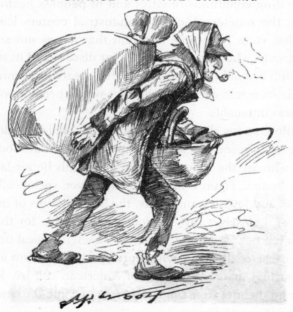

ONE OF NEW YORK'S "MICROBES."

FIGURE 3.2 "A Chance for Cholera," *Puck* (vol. 16, no. 415), February 18, 1885, 387. HathiTrust.

THE CHOLERA SCARE.

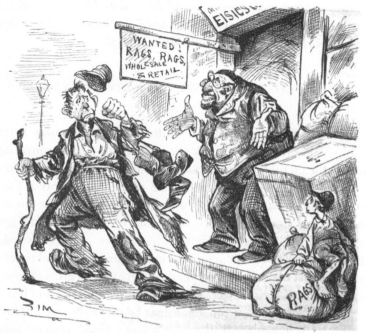

ANCIENT DEALER IN RAGS (*to Casual Tramp*).—" Hi, dere! you! Shoost you shtop—I puy you for dose Æchyptian raegs—fife cents a bound, ain'd it ?"

FIGURE 3.3 "The Cholera Scare," *Puck* (vol. 16, no. 395), October 1, 1884, 75. HathiTrust.

In this chapter we look at the impact of a changing nineteenth-century industrial, urban world on the lives and health of Americans. With the growth of industry and the crowding of people into cities, industrial accidents multiplied and infectious disease became rampant. In addition, work-related stress led to ill-health and early death. In contrast to much of the colonial era, when epidemics were of relatively limited duration and geographic spread, now poor nutrition, tuberculosis, diarrheal diseases of infancy, fevers, typhoid, typhus, cholera, and smallpox became ever-present threats to workers, their families, and the poor. As the demographer Dora Costa writes, "A white American ten-year-old boy born in the early 1880s . . . had witnessed three major cholera epidemics, widespread malaria in the Midwest, [and] the rise of typhoid fever as newly constructed sewers poured their contents into the rivers and lakes from which towns drew their drinking water." Babies would drink adulterated milk "from cows fed on distillery wastes."[3] The world of industry and commerce was clearly killing people.

THE IMPACT OF THE GROWING FACTORY SYSTEM ON HEALTH

The growth of the factory system shifted production away from the shop and the home, where work was under the direct control of the artisan, to the factory, where managers could more easily oversee work routines and the speed at which their employees labored. Further, many workers were increasingly dependent on wages for their live-lihood and for housing, where landlords took greater and greater percentages of their income for rent in smaller, more crowded, and less healthy housing that generally lacked water spigots and toilets. No longer could people live on the food they were able to grow themselves. Wages now were needed to pay for virtually every necessity of life: milk, bread, meat, and clothes from a garment factory rather than from the home loom.[4] Without a job that paid a wage, abject poverty loomed. And poverty bred disease.

Newly built factories produced new dangers to health for larger and larger numbers of workers. Steam and electricity fed the power looms, steel rolling mills, lathes, saws, high-speed drills, and presses that too often led to limbs being mangled, fingers being cut off, or eyes being poked out. Further, the use of new chemicals and materials in the oil industry, blast furnaces, tanning, hat-making, and match-making industry introduced new diseases that had previously been unknown. In South Carolina's textile plants, for example, asbestos fibers filled the air workers breathed, creating a new disease that would later be named asbestosis. In Cleveland's paint-manufacturing industry, workers suffered from lead poisoning, and in the Danbury, Connecticut, haber-dashery industry, men and women alike came down with symptoms of mercury poisoning.

Following the Civil War, the full impact of these social and economic changes on the health status of the population was becoming apparent. Episodic epidemic diseases regularly rampaged through the growing industrial and commercial cities, life spans declined, infant mortality increased, and the appearance of an often-sickly population fed a sense of disorder (including violent strikes and riots) and decline that civic leaders believed had to be addressed. The disparity in income between the rich and the poor increased dramatically, as did the gap in length and quality of life.[5] In fact, the long decline that marked American's health during the industrialization and urbanization of the nineteenth century continued until 1920. As noted earlier, the demographer and economic historian Dora Costa's discussion of a ten-year-old boy tells this story in stark form: "A white American ten-year-old boy born in the early 1880s could expect to live to age 48 and to grow to 169 cm [5 feet, 6.5 inches], a short, stunted life compared to his counterparts born at the time of the American Revolution," who could, on average, expect to live to 57 years and grow to a height of 174 centimeters,(5 feet, 8.5 inches).[6] African American babies, if surviving infancy, born in 1900 could expect to die in their early to mid-thirties.[7]

One of the most obvious changes for native-born Americans in the post–Civil War years was the dissolution of the previous generations' faith in the superiority of American cities, housing, and workplaces compared to Europe's. Observers from all walks of life had begun to notice that "protections" such as guaranteed housing and clean and orderly factories for working people, previously a point of pride for textile manufacturers in Lowell and other Massachusetts mill towns, had disappeared. The operatives in these Massachusetts factories "labor more hours per day than do the operatives in like pursuits in Great Britain," concluded the Massachusetts Bureau of Statistics of Labor's report of 1873. The report went on to note the increasing disparities in wealth and well-being between social classes: "I think it cannot be denied that society is becoming sorted into classes, more clearly divided, and each knowing and caring less about the other than ever before."[8] Even in Lowell, which had forfeited its place to Fall River as the largest textile town, the Ten Hour League, a group devoted to lowering the length of the working day, had gained a foothold, and the boarding system, the heart of the paternalist cotton textile towns, had lost its appeal, with many of the "factory girls" now abandoning the company-controlled homes for more private and cheaper, if more crowded, boarding rooms farther from the mills.

For some, especially among longtime, native-born residents, the decline in the conditions of American life was attributed to the growing number of immigrants who were bringing disease and foreign habits with them from Germany (over 700,000 in the 1870s), Ireland (over 400,000 in the 1870s), and other locales, an immigration that totaled over 2.7 million people for the decade.[9] One patrician, appealing for charitable support for a new children's hospital, walked around "the dirty narrow sidewalks" of Boston in the 1870s, "remembering a time when I could walk whither I would" with little worry or concern. But now what he saw were "streets where poverty in its worst estate stared at me on every side." He saw "a row of tenement houses, several stories high, each story of which opened on a balcony . . . thronged with men, women and children, from every window and door. . . . Men whose brutal faces made me shiver, women from whom every grace of womanhood had departed." More "pitiful than all" were the children whose "poor, wan faces [were] so pinched and pale with want and sickness."[10] The extent of poverty and deterioration in the urban environment reinforced a view among the native-born that drunkenness, depravity, and generally loose morals among the newcomers led to disease and underscored the need for establishments such as the new children's hospital. In Lowell alone, according to the state's labor bureau, there were "586 licensed rum shops . . . and the most pervasive vice is drunkenness," representing over 70 percent of the 3,025 arrests in 1872.[11]

EFFORTS AT REFORM

Growing recognition of the poor pay and unhealthy conditions in which working people lived and died spurred a dramatic growth in labor unrest in the post–Civil War decades. These reforms underscore the important role that reform efforts played in reducing disease and death. Old artisans' guilds joined with, or at least identified with, newer industrial associations such as the Knights of Labor, founded in 1869, an organization of skilled and unskilled workers who pressed for the ending of child labor, greater safety conditions in factories, payments for accidents that occurred on the job, and equal pay for men and women. The organization grew from a few thousand members in the years immediately after the Civil War to nearly 700,000 members by the 1880s. Railroad workers who faced the constant threat of accidents costing them life or limb brought the nation to a near standstill in 1877 and 1886 when companies cut their wages. Massive strikes shut down coal mines in Illinois, Ohio, and West Virginia, among other states. In the 1870s, the Molly McGuires, a secret society of primarily Irish immigrant miners in the eastern Pennsylvania coalfields, resorted to violent attacks on landlords and mining companies in an attempt to win better living conditions, improved working conditions in the mines, and higher wages. In the 1880s, labor radicals marched and demonstrated in Chicago's Haymarket Square to achieve an eight-hour day. In early 1894, the American Railway Union, led by Eugene V. Debs, struck against the Pullman factory in Chicago leading to the calling out of government troops. This strike led to a national shutdown of the railroad system in the spring and summer of that year in an effort to achieve wage increases and lower rents in Pullman, the company town where the sleeper cars were built. All of these actions and much more augured a chaotic and dangerous threat to industrial capitalism, or so it appeared to many.

While many cities shared the disastrous health effects of industrialism, differing economies, ethnic and racial makeups, and political realities led to differing responses to disease. Massachusetts was the home of the first American factories and the first state department of health, and the *Springfield Republican* acknowledged the dramatic changes that had overtaken Massachusetts cities and industrial towns in the few decades since Davy Crockett, Charles Dickens, Anthony Trollope and Alexis de Tocqueville had lauded the Lowell experiment. "The struggle between capital and labor" was "growing bitter," the paper reported by 1873, with strikes and walkouts by laborers stunned by the speed at which their lives, skills, and even their home lives were being destroyed by an industrial system that left many plagued by illness and desperate poverty.[12]

Skilled craft unions as well pressed governments to intervene in the disintegrating work conditions in the new factories. Under pressure from groups such as the Knights of St. Crispin, a union of shoemakers with forty thousand members in Massachusetts alone, and despite opposition from employers (and some labor unions that distrusted the state to represent their interests), the state of Massachusetts in 1869 organized a Bureau of Statistics of Labor, the first in the nation, to help define the problems that plagued the growing population of wage earners flooding into already crowded cities. With little power other than to report to the legislature the conditions of working people throughout the state, the bureau's inspectors produced extraordinary portraits of the desperate conditions that then existed among broad swaths of the state's working class, both in the factory and in the home.[13] Their reports threw "increasing light on the relations between labor and capital" in order, as one letter said, "to secure the highest degree of a true Christian civilization."[14] "The rich and the poor we shall always have," one reader wrote to the bureau's inspectors, "but this [fact] is not inconsistent with a social equalization that will secure to honest industry . . . respect, especially . . . self-respect, and prevent extreme wealth terrorizing over the toiler, or looking down on him with contempt."[15] As a result of their investigations, the commissioners recommended limiting work time to no more than ten hours per day or sixty hours per week, no employment of children under thirteen years of age, and no employment of those aged thirteen to fifteen unless they had completed elementary school.[16]

In 1870, Massachusetts's newly established departments of labor began inspections of factories and working-class homes in Lowell and other mill towns. In 1875, Massachusetts government inspectors presented a detailed report on both the deteriorating working conditions within the mills and the quality of life to which workers and their families were being reduced.[17] In every factory-dominated community in the state, workers and their families were paying a terrible price for industrial progress. In Holyoke, for example, where the Hadley Textile Mills and Parsons paper mills lined the Connecticut River along with the canal system that powered them, in workers' homes the "sanitary arrangements . . . are very imperfect"; "slops" were "allowed to run wherever they can make their way." "Portions of yards are covered with filth and green slime," the inspectors reported, while tenement houses where hundreds of people lived had "neither air nor light" and "no windows and no means of ventilation." The inspectors concluded that "it was no wonder that the death rate . . . was greater in Holyoke than in any large town . . . excepting Fall River," which not coincidentally also housed giant textile factories.[18] In Newburyport, the Massachusetts port and mill town, conditions were not any better.[19]

By the 1870s, any illusion of equality in wealth between working people and those profiting from their labor was all but gone. In Rhode Island, the top 1 percent of the population owned 47 percent of all property in 1870, while in Connecticut and Massachusetts, the top percentile owned 41 and 35 percent, respectively. In the same decade, in the country as a whole the top 1 percent owned 27.9 percent of all property.[20] Such a skewed distribution meant that in Massachusetts "the majority" of "workingmen in this Commonwealth do not support their families by their individual earnings alone," while the "earnings contributed by wives . . . is so small that they would save more by staying at home," reported the state's labor inspectors. Families "are forced to depend, upon their children for from *one-quarter to one-third* of the entire family earnings" and those "under 15 years of age supply, by their labor, from *one-eighth to one-sixth* of the total family earnings." Child labor, then, was critical to the survival of the family: "Without children's assistance . . . the majority of families would be in poverty or debt."[21] See figure 3.4.

No. 164.	LABORER, IN IRON-WORKS.			*Irish.*
EARNINGS of father, ...				$490
son, aged 14, ...				270
				$760

CONDITION.—Family numbers 8, parents and 6 children from nine months to fourteen years of age. Have a tenement of 4 rooms, situated in a disagreeable neighborhood, in an over-crowded block, to which belong only two privies for about fifty people. When this place was visited the vault had overflowed in the yard and run a considerable distance; the sink-water was also running in the same place, and created a stench that was really frightful. How people can live, or why they are allowed to live, in such places, is beyond comprehension. The house inside, partaking of the character of the surroundings, was badly furnished and dirty, and a disgrace to Worcester.

FOOD.—*Breakfast.* Bread, butter, corned meat or salt fish, potatoes and coffee.
  Dinner. Meat, potatoes, sometimes vegetables, bread.
  Supper. Bread, butter, warmed potatoes and tea.

COST OF LIVING, ...				$716
Rent, . . . $120 00	Fish, ... $14 20	Dry goods, . . $13 00		
Fuel, . . . 23 00	Milk, ... 17 25	Sundries, . . . 47 04		
Groceries, . . 370 61	Boots and shoes, . 16 35			
Meat, . . . 49 75	Clothing, . . . 44 80			

FIGURE 3.4 "Laborer, in Iron-Works" (1875). Figure shows that the $760 combined yearly income (the equivalent of about $21,000 in 2023) of an Irish ironworker and his fourteen-year-old son was used to support a family of eight in 1875 in Worcester, Massachusetts. Massachusetts Bureau of Statistics of Labor, *Sixth Annual Report* (Boston: Wright and Potter, March 1875), 275.

The health of young women and children took on special significance for the Massachusetts inspectors as an indicator of the moral and social, not to say physical, decline produced by industrialization as it was then practiced in the state. The labor inspectors in Massachusetts conducted a special survey asking owners of textile mills whether there were "any diseases which you have noticed as being particularly prevalent amongst" the workers and whether there were any manufacturing processes that were "specially injurious to women and children." The growing concern was whether the now-maturing textile industry was transforming the commonwealth's cities into the same hell holes as those of Europe, from which the American nation had thought itself immune.[22]

Long hours of work in unhealthy conditions could lead, the inspectors said, to "loss of vital force, time and money," growing debt, and "bodily and mental distress sometimes tending to intemperance and crime." The effect on women included "lessened probabilities of maternity or vigorous offspring, with possible resultant loss of social and domestic happiness, and even a worse train of sequelae, including secondary disease and death." Would the new factory system produce future generations of "non-vigorous and non-productive offspring," as well as sterile women and enfeebled workers, and would a shrinking "productive" labor force create greater dependence and a lack of healthy people "required to care for the sick"?[23] The new routines, the inspectors reported, were creating real problems for women in the workplace: "Profuse, difficult, deficient or retarded menstruation, . . . chlorosis [anemia], anasarca [swelling of the whole body] and edema of feet, pains of back and limbs, nervous headaches, hacking coughs, by-and-by tubercular symptoms, and more or less early decline" was "the usual list and order of complaints."[24] "Amongst the women of factory operatives, much more than among the general population," the inspectors remarked, there were "derangements of the digestive organs . . . e.g., pyrosis [heartburn], constipation, vertigo, and headache." The factory routine demanded "a neglect of the calls of nature through the early hours of work, the short intervals at meals, the eating and drinking of easily prepared foods, as bread, tea and coffee, and the neglect of meat and fresh-cooked vegetables," which, in turn, led to *other deranged states of a still worse character . . . e.g., leucorrhoea* [vaginal discharges], *and too frequent and profuse menstruation* [italics in original]. Cases also of displacement, flexions, and versions [*sic*] of the uterus, arising from the constant standing, and the increased heat of and confinement in the mill."[25]

Working conditions were part of a larger threat to "the individual, and the community alike," argued the factory inspectors. Workers, both male and female, young and old, were now working "in occupations which cannot be undertaken without injury." Young women "of tender years" were in special danger because the conditions in the factories were "radically unfavorable to health." "The disregard (even in defiance of statute) which our managers of industries exhibit for the cardinal principles of continued prosperity and individual happiness" was embodied in "summoning these girls to a long day of labor and requiring their unremitting attention to it."[26]

What, specifically, were the causes of the deaths, diseases, miscarriages, poor reproductive outcomes, and poor general health of the young women working in the mills, in the eyes of the Massachusetts factory inspectors? First was "severe overwork"; then came "severe overwork coupled with innutrition [*sic*] and non-hygienic surroundings"; and lastly came exposure in the workplace to hazardous conditions, such as inhalation of cotton dust, that resulted in other diseases, specifically phthisis or consumption; these lung complaints were later identified as silicosis, brown lung, and tuberculosis.[27]

The deteriorating conditions in the once-exalted textile mills were just part of a much broader concern over deteriorating conditions for the growing industrial workforce in Massachusetts and elsewhere in the nation. Foundries were established in states across the country where iron would be molded to make casings for everything from locomotive engines to potbellied wood-burning stoves, tools, farm equipment, and soon the cast iron siding of office buildings in New York, Boston, Philadelphia, and the other growing commercial cities of the East Coast as well as Chicago. In the new foundries and many other large factories, owners introduced new machinery and broke down the work process into tasks that depended less on the knowledge and expertise of the skilled worker and increasingly on the brute energy of the semiskilled and unskilled, who lacked authority over the work process, speed, and conditions that their skilled colleagues had once largely controlled.[28]

Much like the reformers in Massachusetts, reformers across the country were eager to ameliorate the worst excesses of the new industrial and urban worlds. Some reformers focused on ways to improve the social conditions that gave rise to discord, disease, and violence, while others sought ways to control or repress the populations that appeared to threaten the social order; still others were beginning to challenge capitalism's legitimacy. Organized charities, once the province of paternalistic women's groups or local elite leaders attempting to meet their moral and religious obligations to care for those less fortunate, understood the social importance of their traditional charitable missions and recast them in political terms. Many believed, along with the patrician seeking funds for Boston's new children's hospital, that "there is a practical side of this charity which may commend itself to thoughtful men. In it I see one clew [*sic*] to the future settlement of several of the questions of the hour, such as communism, socialism and the reconciliation of labor to capital."[29]

The ill-health of these and other workers was not simply the result of their jobs, many observers realized, but also the result of the housing and sanitary conditions in which many of these workers and their families were forced to live. The Massachusetts bureau inspectors made no fine distinction between the environments of the factory and the home. They were particularly outraged by the housing in which the poor were forced to live. In purple prose, the labor inspectors detailed one group of especially foul tenements in Boston: "beastly abominations, these pestilential stench-holes, reeking with frowzy fluids, and bestenching [*sic*] the atmosphere with their malarious effluvia, these fertile nurseries of disease and death, and skulking haunts of villainy and crime, are still permitted to remain in their unmitigated defilement."[30] Landlords were not required to provide the most basic amenities to their tenants, and (in this case) the city of Boston ignored the conditions that so many workers were forced to endure. "Boston, the Athens of America; the home . . . of culture and refinement, of high art and pure morals," the labor inspectors sarcastically noted in their 1875 report, "still indulges all this violation of sanitary statute, this squalor of filth, this physical debasement and depravity." "Who, we ask, are the owners of these courts of death to the body and ruin of the soul?" Who were the men, they asked rhetorically, with perhaps the Lowells and Lawrences in mind, "who buy fame and town names" by renting to "the hapless tenants of these fouled-aired pest holes, with their dingy ceiling, their dark grimy window, their murky and stench atmosphere"?[31]

The impact of such conditions on tenants was impossible to ignore. "A laborer in a stone yard" who lived in Boston with his wife and five children in two rooms, one 15 feet by 10 feet and the other 8 feet by 6 feet, was sick with cellulitis—St. Anthony's fire, as it was called—and a three-week-old child was also ill, lying on the floor. Three other children were caring for the fourth, also sick. The mother, unable to leave the apartment out of fear for the children, told the inspector that "they lived most wretchedly from Christmas to March," when the ports were often closed because of ice and when unemployment soared. The family, she reported, "subsisted principally on bread and crackers." The inspectors visited home after home only to report similar indignities, hunger, suffering, and illness: "sharp misery had worn them to the bone," in "this miserable, worn-out, dirty, dilapidated rookery, with its moldy and dingy walls, in summer swarming with multitudinous vermin, in winter cold and cheerless as an iceberg, and at all seasons begrimed with filth, unfit for even hens or pigs; the chimneys moaning in the winds, with cracked and asthmatic voice, and wheezing out to the rotten roof the dolorous dirge of age and decay."[32]

Conditions of life for the masses of urban workers—dockworkers, stone masons, common laborers, junk dealers, washerwomen, garment workers, unemployed or disabled, and their families—were the same in Boston's North End and along the port: Stone's Yard, Young's Court, Johnson's Block, Cove Place, Kingston's Court, and other places had cramped, airless, heatless, tenement rooms, papered with newsprint, furnished with a couple of rickety chairs, a washtub in a "living room," and a bed generally without sheets and often without a blanket, or water with overflowing privies in backyards that were used for human and other waste produced in the cramped homes. Almost without exception, every household surveyed by the bureau had at least one person, whether husband, wife, or child, who was ill from a poorly defined disease or disabled by an industrial accident.[33]

The report was scathing about the hypocrisy of a state that would allow these obscenities to exist while punishing the poor themselves if they turned to crime to feed themselves and their families. "Does not everybody know that if one of the penniless starvelings found therein, were, in desperation of hunger, to steal a baker's false-weighted loaf, or under the impulse of poverty to filch a dollar from the counter of a bank . . . or, were he shivering with nakedness and cold, to pilfer a yard of cloth from a mill whose scot-free official had swindled it of millions,— does not everybody know that the sheriff, the court and the prison, would victimize him with pitiless speed and certainty?"[34]

Particularly galling was that the entire system supported the "miserly landlord" who was allowed "to slay his fleeced tenants, to poison the air they must breathe, to taint the neighborhood with the foul stench of deep stratas [sic] of filth, that breed dirt, flies, fleas, lice, and all the verminous curses that plagued the Pharaoh, to grind the face of the poor on the roughest grindstone" and to remain "as safe, as unmolested, and unchastised, as the frauds of the cheating baker, the . . . banking robber, or the . . . peculating official!"[35]

The worsening conditions on the job and in the home were both seen by the Massachusetts inspectors as symptoms of a capitalist system run amok.[36] Trade and commerce were at the root of the disaster overtaking Boston; trade and commerce "elbowed out of place" everyone, "like Death": "The very temples of God retire before the surging tide of business, the sepulchers beneath them yielding up the bones of the dead, who, when living, chanted his praises and uttered their prayers within their consecrated walls."[37]

In response to these voluminous Massachusetts government reports, along with a number of well-publicized industrial catastrophes such as the collapse of a textile mill in Lawrence, the state passed the 1877 Factory Act, the first in the nation to require factory inspections for structural as well as health and safety violations. The inspectors were asked to investigate the state of factory equipment, watching for faulty or worn-out belting, gears, and drums and identifying poorly guarded machinery that could maim the worker. Ventilation and cleanliness were also their focus. In addition, the legislation addressed safety and health conditions in public buildings such as schools, theaters, and churches where the public generally assembled.[38]

Massachusetts was not alone in experiencing dramatic changes and growth in the middle and latter part of the nineteenth century as the nation's developing commercial and industrial economy encouraged the growth of urban centers and transformed the lives of its citizens. Millions of people were drawn from the American countryside as well as Europe to the older cities along the East Coast and newer cities in the Midwest. During the course of the nineteenth century, older cities such as Philadelphia, Boston, and New York grew exponentially in population, while numerous towns of between 10,000 and 50,000 people in 1800 saw their populations increase into the hundreds of thousands by the end of the nineteenth century. In New York, the extraordinary growth of the Irish immigrant population following the potato famines of the 1840s and the poverty and ill-health that they faced eventually forced the city to recognize the need to organize, as part of a general reform effort, what would become a world-famous department of health. In Philadelphia and Baltimore, commercial ports with large numbers of African Americans and immigrants also faced outbreaks of epidemic disease that spurred the development of active health departments. While all had their individual histories, all were faced by disparities in wealth and a growing desperation of the poor that forced elites to engage in dramatic efforts to control what appeared to be health conditions that could exacerbate social disruptions.

NEW YORK AS EMBLEMATIC OF SOCIAL CHANGE AND DISEASE IN THE LATE NINETEENTH CENTURY

New York's demographic and physical transformation was particularly hard to miss as an English-speaking, largely Protestant community became, by the 1880s, home to hundreds of thousands of desperately poor Catholic immigrants from Ireland and Italy and Jews from central and eastern Europe. Along with these changes went a profound reorganization in work, neighborhood, housing, family, and transportation. As a result, New York's problems and reforms often led the way for other growing cities.

In 1800, New York City had a population of about 60,000, having nearly doubled in the previous decade. With the completion of the Erie Canal in 1825, it was linked to the emerging cities of the Midwest by the Hudson River and the Great Lakes, making it the largest port in the country. By the Civil War it had surpassed Philadelphia as the most populous U.S. city and its population had already grown exponentially to over 1 million. For many New Yorkers in the middle and late decades of the nineteenth century whose memories of the city stretched back a few decades, the changes in the city's population size and the social backgrounds of new immigrants were stunning. On the one hand, the city was obviously emerging as the nation's preeminent center of commerce, finance, industry, culture, and wealth. Opera houses, museums, theaters, amusement parks, and music halls all indicated the cultural dynamism of urban America. On the other hand, urban poverty, waves of illness, crowding, and the evident "foreignness" of so many appeared frightening. To older, largely Protestant New Yorkers, there seemed an obvious connection between "plagues and peoples." Especially to those in authority, the cause of the "plagues" was usually taken to be the people who came from elsewhere.

Just north of City Hall, at the northern edge of the old city's settlement, lay an area that had been, in the early nineteenth century, a freshwater pond known as the Collect. In 1800, it was the "largest pond on Manhattan Island," surrounded by groves, fields, and a "high hill rising abruptly from its sides," remembered the authors of a later report. Its waters had been of "great depth and of unusual purity," providing nearly ten thousand New Yorkers with fresh spring water. Yet, by the late 1830s, the Collect, at the edge of the notorious Five Points, had been filled in because the rising landlord class wanted the area for tenement housing. The Collect quickly became a dumping ground for dead horses, goats, pigs, and other animals and offal, giving the area "an insufferable stench." By the end of the Civil War, the area was covered with tenements "containing 4 to 8 families in as many rooms." The lodging houses of the area had "as many as thirty persons . . . packed into one small room," promoting, as in the case of one such house on Baxter Street, large and virulent outbreaks of fever.[39]

By 1870, the commercial avenues of the area were paved with cobblestones, which provided deep cracks in which refuse could collect and rot.[40] In winter, when the filth was frozen in place under ice and snow, accumulations of manure from the horses that traversed the area filled the streets along with the remains of dead pigs, horses, dogs, cats, and rats; household and vegetable refuse could reach depths of 3 feet or more. "Garbage boxes," rarely emptied, overflowed with offal, animal carcasses, and household waste; stagnant water collected in the carcasses of dead animals, and open sewer drains were generally clogged. "Filth of every kind [was] thrown into the streets, covering their surface, filling the gutters, obstructing the sewer culverts, and sending forth perennial emanations which must generate pestiferous diseases," reported the sanitary inspector William Thoms in 1865. "Drainage is generally imperfect, the courtyards being . . . below the level of the streets," and "everything is thrown into the street and gutters at all times of the day." Most of the population depended upon outdoor "water closets" and privies in the courtyards of the tenement buildings, unfortunately close to wells used for drinking.[41]

The public health historian John Duffy describes attempts to cajole private contractors to do the public service work of cleaning the streets. In general, contracts were awarded to the lowest bidder, but "not infrequently, the lowest bidder turned out to be someone with neither the equipment, the knowledge, nor the intention of living up to the terms of the contract," who then did the minimal amount of work in order to maximize his profit.[42] In wealthier neighborhoods and along the commercial avenues, street cleaning was done more regularly and by more responsible and better-paid contractors. (In 1895 the city established a Department of Sanitation under the leadership of Colonel George Waring, who had gained a national reputation following the Memphis yellow fever epidemic in 1878.) The fundamental structural changes that sanitarians suggested addressed some of the inequities in the conditions of the city but not others. People in poorer neighborhoods gained access to running water and indoor plumbing only when it became a legal responsibility of tenement landlords. Because owners had to pay to have the pipes delivering water from the Croton reservoir system connected to their building, there were huge disparities in access to freshwater. Access to the system of sewer pipes, which allowed for indoor plumbing and the elimination of the backyard privies, was set up in a similar way. Nevertheless, conditions were slowly improving, and death rates from cholera, typhoid, childhood dysentery, and "cholera infantum" were declining. New York's construction of clean-water reservoirs beyond the limits of the expanding city was an extraordinary accomplishment, more ambitious than the reservoir projects being built, and that would be built, in Boston, Philadelphia, and other cities across the country. This reservoir system achieved significant protections against the water-borne diseases like cholera, dysentery, and typhoid that coursed through nineteenth-century American cities. But even with such technological innovations, class still played a role. In Pittsburgh, for example, pipes in working-class neighborhoods were smaller than those in more affluent areas, and so the poor received less water than the wealthy. From the viewpoint of the city business community, the improvements in the aesthetics of city life were of no small importance as well.

In part, the astonishing crowding that characterized New York and other growing cities in the mid-nineteenth century was a product of the extraordinary growth of urban populations brought about by the expansion of the new commercial and industrial enterprises. Manufacturing plants, trading houses, shipping and finance, and new housing and transportation networks promised a new start for millions of destitute Europeans. In the New York of 1800, 60,000 people lived in an area of about 1.5 square miles, or approximately 39,000 people per square mile. By 1870, that density had grown to more than 85,500 in 1.5 square miles, or more than 57,000 per square mile, in a city that had expanded to an area of 25 square miles.[43]

The relatively class-free distribution of the city's population of the early nineteenth century crumbled under the weight of this exploding population and a growing class of absentee landlords. Their ability to manipulate rents and increase housing density took its toll on the health of New York's working-class and immigrant population. As the city's population increased and as more and more of its economic life centered on the downtown port and commercial districts, the older patterns of housing changed dramatically. Single-family homes, capable of sheltering an artisan, his family, and often a journeyman apprentice, were unaffordable as commercial enterprises competed for space and pushed out middle-class households. In the early nineteenth century an apprentice learning a trade in the workshop of a cobbler, for example, may very well have lived in the home of his master, and that home may very well have been above a workshop in an economically integrated, if ethnically or racially segregated, neighborhood. Now, successful shopkeepers moved from the commercial center to a cheaper neighborhood and middle-class entrepreneurs and their families traded up and moved from Lower Manhattan to the uptown refuges of Grammercy Park or Greenwich Village. This change left a housing market

dominated by absentee landlords who subdivided single-family housing and rented out cramped "apartments" to poverty-stricken families
or rooms, sometimes by the hour, to single men of little means. The
market for housing, as the historians Elizabeth Blackmar and Elizabeth
Cromley detail, led to the creation of an overpriced rental market for
those unable to afford single-family dwellings or those unable to move
a distance from the ports and the commercial neighborhoods where
they were employed.[44] See figure 3.5.

Elizabeth Cromley summarizes the process that transformed the
neighborhoods and living environment—and that, in the process, as we'll
see, determined the geographic pattern of infectious disease transmissions,

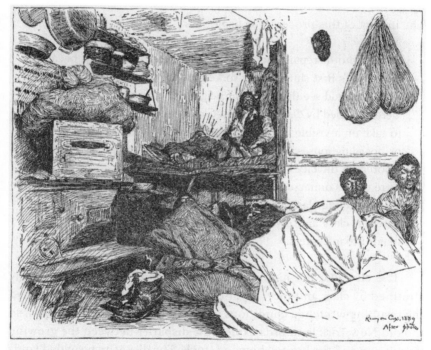

LODGERS IN A CROWDED BAYARD STREET TENEMENT—"FIVE CENTS A SPOT."

FIGURE 3.5 Jacob Riis, "Lodgers in a Crowded Bayard Street Tenement—'Five Cents
a Spot,'" *How the Other Half Lives* (1890). A room in a Lower East Side tenement
where renters supplemented their income by giving immigrant men a place to sleep
in lice-, mouse-, and rat-infested rooms for a few cents a stay.

particularly among the working class—during the decades between 1800 and 1870:

> As well-to-do families moved to improve their residential cir-
> cumstances, they left behind buildings that could be rented to
> people with fewer resources; the housing, in other words, "trickled
> down." Many poorer families could each rent a fraction of a former
> single-family house, creating an ad hoc multiple dwelling. Some of
> the houses that trickled down to low-income workers in the 1820s
> and 1830s were solid, well-built houses, but others were of cheaper
> wood-frame construction. The poorer the quality of the original
> house, of course, the less likely it could withstand heavy use by
> several families at once.[45]

The impact of this process was profound:

> Falling into disrepair, these ad hoc multifamily dwellings became
> New York's first slums. New Yorkers of the 1830s, looking around
> the city, could see that different neighborhoods and dwelling types
> were occupied by distinct classes. Class stratification was beginning
> to take on a visible form. The wage earners lived in rented rooms
> or boardinghouses; the merchants and artisans in private homes;
> laborers in the city's earliest tenements. Multifamily arrangements
> were often connected to deprivation, while a place in the respect-
> able, middling class was signified by a single-family house—a link
> between class and dwelling that is still in force today outside of
> major urban centers.[46]

The city, like the nation as a whole, was becoming increasingly stratified by class and race. As in Boston, where inspectors bemoaned the resulting wretched conditions in the city's poor neighborhoods, so too did New York landlords exploit the disparity between the growing population and the limited housing stock. The disparity provided land-lords with enormous profits while denying workers and their families wholesome living quarters.[47] See figure 3.6.

New York was, in 1865, still geographically identical with Manhattan Island, located between the Hudson and East rivers and bounded on the

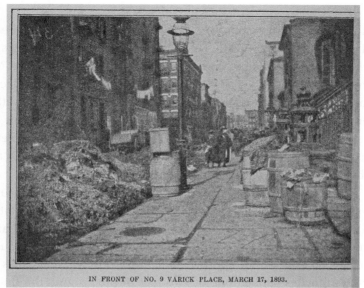

(A)

IN FRONT OF NO. 9 VARICK PLACE, MARCH 17, 1893.

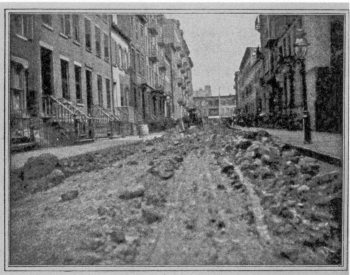

(B)

MORTON STREET, CORNER OF BEDFORD, LOOKING TOWARD BLEECKER STREET,
MARCH 17, 1893.

FIGURE 3.6 A Lower Manhattan street in the 1890s. Note on the left the piles of manure and other refuse piled in the street and the overflowing garbage bins on the right. Horse manure piles could make streets virtually impassable, and the jammed tenements fostered disease. *(A)* George E. Waring, "In Front of No. 9 Varick Place, March 17, 1893." *Street-Cleaning and the Disposal of a City's Wastes: Methods and Results and the Effect Upon Public Health* (New York: Doubleday & McClure, 1898). *(B)* George E. Waring, "Morton Street, Corner of Bedford, Looking Toward Bleeker Street, March 17, 1893," *Street-Cleaning and the Disposal of a City's Wastes: Methods and Results and the Effect Upon Public Health* (New York: Doubleday & McClure, 1898).

north by Westchester County and on the south by the sea. The island, far from being a level, neatly laid-out grid of rectangular blocks, was marked by hills and gullies, streams, marshlands, and meadows. Much of the original shoreline had been filled in over the preceding decades, yet areas along the rivers still had large pockets of swamp and wetlands where mosquitoes could multiply, leading to outbreaks of yellow fever and malaria. The densely populated area between Houston Street and Fourteenth Street and as far west as Tompkins Square, in what is today the heart of the East Village, was an uneven marshland.

The few amenities provided in the crowded tenements of the Lower East Side and the Five Points, the area north and east of City Hall, were generally inadequate, often becoming public health hazards themselves. Water closets were generally "covered and surrounded with filth, so as not to be approachable," while elsewhere latrines were "merely trenches sunken one or two feet in the ground, the fluids of which [were] in some instances allowed to run into the courts, stones and boards . . . provided to keep the feet out of filth." Half the houses in the Five Points had no sewers connected to them, making the stench that arose during the summer "absolutely unbearable and perilous." Twenty-nine brothels, 43 stables, and 406 "dram shops" added to the generalized decay of a district that seventy-five years earlier had boasted the purest water in the city.

In New York, efforts were under way to address the reasons for the increasingly evident high disease and death rates in the city and then to develop a plan for public and private action. These efforts would prove to be extremely significant in ameliorating the damage done by the creation of this huge industrial and commercial hub. The Citizens' Association, a voluntary group of city civic leaders, physicians, and politicians, in 1865 called upon New York's leading physicians to participate in a fact-gathering expedition. Valentine Mott, a pioneer of vascular surgery; Willard Parker, the first American to remove an appendix successfully; John Griscom, the author of the famous 1845 study, *Sanitary Conditions of [New York's] Laboring Population*; Stephen Smith, soon to head New York's new Metropolitan Board of Health and founder of the American Public Health Association; and other prominent physicians and civic leaders agreed to participate in a systematic inspection of the city's various sanitary districts, the boundaries of which were generally synonymous with those of city council members' political boundaries.[48] In 1865, the Citizens' Association issued its report on the "sanitary condition of the city." Dedicated to the benefit of "all classes in the city," the report provided more than 300 pages of detailed description of the city's physical, social, and moral characteristics. Coming at the end of a bloody war that had cleaved not only the nation but also communities of the city, the report reflected both the hopes and fears of the merchant leaders who had commissioned it.

Beginning with the observation that "pestilential diseases" laid bare "the impotence of the existing sanitary system," the physicians noted that outbreaks of disease paralyzed the commercial and political life of the community: "The people are panic-stricken [and] the interests of commerce suffer by the insensible and certain *loss of millions* [of dollars]." In a city of fewer than 1 million people, fully 7,000 to 10,000 lives could be saved, it was estimated, if proper sanitary practices could be instituted. It was clear that "the relation of the health and vigorous life of a people to the State, or to commercial prosperity, requires no discussion." Disease was from this perspective a commodity in the developing commercial capital whose cost could be measured in dollars and cents. An organized response to the high disease rates became, in this context, a political and social necessity.[49]

Most obvious to the various inspectors who wrote the district reports in the mid-1860s was the stench that characterized the city's various poor sections, of which Five Points was only one. In district after district, the inspectors detailed the smell of the "sewer gas" that escaped the inadequate sewerage system, the polluted water supply, the filthy streets, the overflowing garbage, the collapsing tenement houses, and other airless, overcrowded firetraps.

Inspector after inspector worried that the "miasmas"—vapors created by rotting foods, animal waste, and filth that lay in the streets and were believed to cause disease—threatened not only neighborhoods but the larger city as well. They feared that the "worthy" and the "unworthy," the "deserving" and "undeserving," the young and the old, and the rich and the poor were all susceptible to the fevers and plagues that were carried through the air. The report's introduction praised the work of the inspectors, who, "familiar with the haunts of fever and other pestilential diseases, . . . have fearlessly penetrated the dismal and unwholesome

quarters where infectious poisons and deadly maladies menace inhabitants and visitants, and from whence emanate the most dreaded diseases that find their way to the more favored districts of the city." In New
York, "disease, debasement, and pauperism . . . are found closely allied"
and "seriously endanger the sanitary safety of all other classes."[50]

The cholera epidemic of 1848, the growing population of poor Irish
following the potato famine in Ireland, the large immigration of Germans
beginning in the 1830s and 1840s, the deterioration of housing, and the
growing tenement neighborhoods—all appeared to contemporaries to
confirm the community's decay. By the time of the Civil War, the health
of New Yorkers and of residents of other large U.S. cities had declined.
Vital statistics gathered by the city showed that while 1 out of every
44 people died in 1863 in Boston and 1 out of 44 in Philadelphia, New
York's rate was 1 in 36. Even when compared with European centers
such as London and Liverpool, New York fared badly: in London and
Liverpool, death rates had hovered around 1 in 45.

Outbreaks of cholera and other epidemic diseases were the terrifying
symbols of the transformed social, economic, and health conditions
of the growing cities.[51] By the middle years of the century, epidemics of typhus (whose symptoms included a purple rash, high fever,
headaches, and often hallucinations), yellow fever, cholera, typhoid
(characterized by severe abdominal pain and high fever), and other
diseases swept through the tenements and slums of New York with
fearsome impact. In 1832, 3,500 deaths occurred during the previously
mentioned cholera epidemic; in 1847, almost 1,400 deaths resulted
from a typhus/typhoid epidemic; in 1849, over 5,000 New Yorkers died
during a cholera epidemic; in 1851, 1,100 New Yorkers died from a
typhoid/typhus epidemic; and in 1854, over 2,500 New Yorkers died in
another cholera epidemic. Near the end of the Civil War, in 1864–1865,
2,500 died in a typhus/typhoid epidemic, and in 1866, 1,100 New Yorkers would die in yet another cholera epidemic. Epidemics continued
in the following decades: smallpox claimed over 1,880 lives in 1872
and almost 1,900 lives in 1875. Diphtheria then claimed almost 4,900
children in 1881 and over 4,500 in 1887. The historical demographer
Gretchen Condran quotes the New York City Board of Health, explaining that those living near the ports on the Lower East Side and in
the "crowded and filthy dwellings, mostly ten[ement] housing of the

poorer classes; filthy streets, gutters and courts, obstructed and faulty house and privy sewerage, and a foul condition of privies" were especially vulnerable to the spread of disease.[52]

Some demographers argue that epidemics, while significant in specific years, were relatively minor contributors to overall death rates during the nineteenth century, especially when compared with the extraordinarily high rates of endemic tuberculosis and the excessive number of infant deaths. But the highly visible and often dramatic experience of seeing people actually dying in the streets had an enormous impact, affecting where and how the city developed. Mortality data specific to particular areas or groups were often referenced to cast blame for the disintegrating environment on immigrants or to spur efforts to reform and improve the city's sanitary condition.[53] By the middle decades of the nineteenth century, the toll of cholera and other epidemics in the United States had become undeniable. Cholera, typhoid, and yellow fever swept through cities along the East Coast and up and down the Mississippi River from New Orleans to Minneapolis. In years of cholera, smallpox, or other epidemics, uncounted thousands of infants and adults, Black and white, died in the rural South and Midwest.[54]

The 1863 draft riots were perhaps the most horrible race riots in New York City's history. Primarily Irish mobs roamed the city, ostensibly protesting the ability of rich men to buy themselves out of the military draft but also taking their anger out on an African American community they blamed for personal and social costs of the war against slavery. The rioters targeted African Americans, among the poorest people in the city, by burning the blocks in which they lived, lynching some who were caught outside, and even storming, sacking, and setting fire to the Colored Orphan Asylum, home to more than two hundred children. The brunt of the rioting was directed at African Americans, with whom the rioters were often competing for unskilled or semiskilled work. For the authors of the report, however, the causes were primarily the social conditions of the rioters, including poor housing and poverty, in addition to their pent-up anger at those who were able to buy their way out of the draft and therefore the Civil War. "The mobs that held fearful sway in our city during the memorable out-break of violence in the month of July, 1863, were gathered in the overcrowded and neglected quarters of the city," the committee report reminded readers.

The "closely-packed houses where the mobs originated seemed to be literally *hives of sickness and vice* [italics in original]." The report went on to point out sardonically, "It was wonderful to see, and difficult to believe, that so much misery, disease, and wretchedness can be huddled together and hidden by high walls, unvisited and unthought of, so near our own abodes." Morals and disease were inseparable to the inspectors, as "lewd but pale and sickly young women, scarcely decent in their ragged attire, were impudent and scattered everywhere in the crowd. But what numbers are made hideous by self-neglect and infirmity!"[55]

The riots seemed a fitting backdrop to help explain the suffering the inspectors were documenting. The report quoted a journalist who witnessed the "Draft Riots" of 1863: "To walk the streets as we walked them, in those hours of conflagration and riot, was like witnessing the day of judgement, with every wicked thing revealed, every sin and sorrow blazingly glared upon, every hidden abomination laid before hell's expectant fire." The city was in the midst of a moral reckoning, the journalist said, as "the elements of popular discord are gathered in those wretchedly-constructed tenant-houses, where poverty, disease, and crime find an abode. Here disease in its most loathsome form propagates itself and moral degradation."[56]

Published just two years after the attacks on Black residents of the city during the 1863 New York draft riots, the 1865 report made only six references to the Black population, and most of the authors blamed African Americans for aggravating the Irish working-class community. African Americans were described as "a poor, lazy class, gaining their livelihood by pursuits attended with as little work as possible." The inspectors did note that there were "exceptions," particularly the "washerwomen" who "work hard for all they have."[57]

Not all New York City inspectors who contributed to the 1865 report were equally inured to the suffering of the poor. Nor were they equally willing to focus on the ostensible "personal failings" of "Negroes" as the source of disease. In the Five Points section, for example, one physician reported that the previous year there had been over 200 cases of typhoid and typhus fever, along with 70 cases of dysentery and 50 cases of smallpox. One street in particular, Jersey Street, a "short and narrow lane running from Crosby to Mulberry Streets, but one block from Broadway," was "thickly inhabited by the poor, three-fourths of whom are negroes," and was the site of the first 40 or 50 cases of dysentery of whom 10 had died. It was the squalor of their conditions that accounted for the disease's deadly spread, one physician recognized, not the moral character of the residents: "The houses in this street are all old; many of them wooden, with brick fronts and stone foundations. The street is always filthy, and the effluvia arising therefrom are extremely offensive. The privies are generally full nearly to overflowing, and the yards are also in a dirty condition, heaps of refuse matter being allowed to remain and to accumulate continually in many of them. There is no sewer in this little street, though the streets at each end of it are sewered."[58]

Thirty-three thousand people lived in Five Points as a whole, but "there have been no improvements made in this district during my inspection," reported the sanitary inspector Nolan in 1865. He had not made any formal complaints, he said, because "the greater number of nuisances are permanent, and require legislative action for their removal."[59]

On the Lower East Side, around Grand Street, the inspectors noted that when the tide rose or there was a storm, the existing sewers vomited up their content onto the street and sidewalks. To remedy this problem, they suggested that a "tidal trap," or floodgate, that opened and shut "with the rising and falling of the tide" be installed to "prevent any reflow of sewage or water" whenever the tide was above the sewage pipe.[60] In contrast to those who saw their role as documenting the moral and social failings of the inhabitants, Nolan argued that "this district could be made a very healthy part of the city by removing the nuisances before mentioned; by keeping the streets, sewers, and privies clean, and free from filth and offal of every description. The removal of all rear tenant-houses is necessary, in order to secure free ventilation." The impact of the "overcrowding of people in tenant-houses and other buildings, as is the custom in this city, is very injurious; and thoroughly effective measures ought to be adopted to prevent it." Nolan went on: "There is no excuse for this oppression of the poor by landlords. It is a crime to crowd fifty or one hundred families into a building that has only ground and air-space for a fraction of such numbers. The privies should all be made to communicate with the sewers, and there should be such provisions and arrangements for the proper care of garbage, ashes, house-slops, &c, as would tend to insure domestic cleanliness and some degree of social refinement."[61]

THE ASIAN COMMUNITY ON THE WEST COAST

Racism directed at African Americans was a pernicious reality in every American city, but Asians felt its brunt as well, especially on the West Coast. Asian immigrants, who had long felt the pain and suffered the restrictions of prejudice and discrimination, experienced high rates of disease as well as a high degree of victimization. An examination of the experience on the West Coast, particularly in San Francisco, highlights the ways that racism contributed to poor health.

The conditions of life and work for the Asian community in San Francisco led to high rates of disease and death in the late nineteenth century. One immigrant newspaper editorialized in 1886 that "overcrowding both in the workshops and in the sleeping rooms" of homes resulted in "constant inhalation of bad air both day and night." As in other cities, these conditions encouraged the spread of a variety of diseases and left the community vulnerable, especially to high "mortality from consumption."[62] Tuberculosis rates in early-twentieth-century San Francisco, for example, were in the neighborhood of 203 per 100,000, nearly 30 percent higher than the average of the United States as a whole. The disproportionate burden of tuberculosis fell on the Chinese, Japanese, and African American populations of the city. The mortality rate of the white population was 173.94, while the Chinese rate was 621.9, the Japanese rate 228, and the African American rate 651.5 per 100,000. The Chinese and African American rates of disease were thus almost four times the rate for white San Franciscans.[63] Not only did Asian immigrants suffer disproportionately from disease, but the suffering they experienced was used to stigmatize them not as victims of crowding and disease but as perpetrators of the larger community's crises. As the historians Nayan Shah and Natalia Molina have detailed, Asian as well as Mexican immigrants in the nineteenth century and beyond were depicted as filthy and immoral vectors of smallpox, syphilis, and even bubonic plague; their communities were quarantined; and they were subjected to racist attacks and taunts.[64] After the smallpox outbreak of 1868, for example, one San Francisco health officer described the Chinese as "moral leper[s] in our community. . . . Their habits and manner of life [are] of such a character as to breed and engender disease wherever they reside."[65] In 1900, during an outbreak of bubonic plague in San Francisco, the city authorities imposed a quarantine on the Chinese quarter, which the Chinese community there denounced as a "blockade of Chinatown."[66] A few years later, the public health community identified fleas carried by rats as the bubonic plague vectors, yet racism continued to animate the public to use disease to stigmatize Asians as dangerous, dirty, and suspiciously different.[67]

The use of race and ethnicity as a rationale for exclusion has been deeply rooted in American public policy. The 1882 Chinese Exclusion Act prohibiting further immigration of all but a few Chinese laborers, for example, was enforced until World War II, when Congress repealed the act. Even so, incredibly low quotas remained as a result of the Immigration Act of 1924, which limited the number of Chinese allowed into the country to a mere 105 per year. The 1891 Immigration Act explicitly identified the presence of a "loathsome or dangerous contagious disease" as a basis for excluding an immigrant's entry. On its face, barring entry to the diseased was not particularly nefarious, but entry was selectively enforced, with the assumption often made that the Chinese, particularly men who came without papers and without contacts in America, were carrying a disease.[68]

RESPONSES TO THE SUFFERING OF THE POOR

As institutions developed to provide medical and other care, decisions continued to be made about who was worthy of what kind of care and of whether people had brought their conditions on themselves. Some were overtly hostile to charitable efforts to aid the poor and immigrants for fear that such aid discouraged initiative and a work ethic and encouraged "pauperism" and dependency. For others, the right approach was to make structural changes that would improve the conditions that caused disease, such as introducing water lines and sewer systems into poor neighborhoods.

Reformers such as the physician John Griscom in New York and Lemuel Shattuck in Boston surveyed their cities and found some of the same conditions that Edwin Chadwick, the author of Britain's *Report on the Sanitary Conditions of the Labouring Population*, identified across the ocean. Griscom and Shattuck were motivated in part by their own moral outrage at the apparent destruction of life in the cities that they had personally experienced from the time of their youth. Griscom wrote the *Sanitary Condition of the Laboring Population of New York* in 1845.[69] While social circumstances certainly influenced health, Griscom admitted, he still saw the habits of the poor—not the inequalities linked to the way urban commercial and industrial society was developing—as the root of the problem. In his view, improving social conditions would improve the character of the poor. Would not education, for example, instruct the poor to avoid filthy habits and therefore disease? "Teach them how to live, so as to avoid diseases and be more comfortable," Griscom lectured his medical colleagues in April 1845, "and then their school education will have a redoubled effect in mending their morals, and rendering them intelligent and happy. But without sound bodies, when surrounded with dirt, foul air, and all manner of filthy associations, it is vain to expect even the child of education to be better than his ignorant companions."[70]

Unlike in Britain, where disease was more often cast as a social problem whose reach might extend across social classes, in the United States, the source of disease was still popularly considered to be the behavior of certain individuals and groups, not so much the social environment. It was therefore deemed necessary to distinguish between the "worthy" and the "unworthy" poor. Physicians and other health personnel as well accepted the moral and social categories of worthy and unworthy as applicable to whole ethnic groups, races, or classes. A Brooklyn physician, H. N. Hoople, summarized the views of many in 1902: "The extremes [of wealth] should not be so marked in America as in foreign cities. But poor foreigners from the lowest dregs of European countries have poured into our cities bringing with them, of course, their debased standard of living, intelligence, morality, earnings, etc. They segregate, fail to assimilate and reproduce the foreign conditions under our very eyes."[71] Poor people of high moral character could be aided by the charitable "visitor" who would come to their houses and, albeit often condescendingly, provide guidance on how to remedy their ways and improve their conditions. Those who were "unworthy" would not benefit from such instruction and aid and were either ignored or sent to public hospitals, almshouses, or jail.

The stratified systems of health care the United States adopted were informed, in part, by this notion that poor health often signaled moral failing. Dwight L. Moody, perhaps America's most popular and influential revivalist preacher in the 1870s, spoke to hundreds of thousands in Chicago, Boston, Brooklyn, and New York, explaining to his largely middle-class audiences why there was such "great misery and suffering in the great city." It was, he argued, because "the sufferers have become lost from the Shepherd's care," not because millions escaping pogroms, poverty, and famine were being squeezed into the crowded tenements of America's cities.[72]

Throughout the mid- to late nineteenth century, there was not only the possibility but the reality that the poor could die in the streets, without care and without attention. Some among the healthy and better-off viewed such lack of attention as itself a kind of perverse motivation, one that would prompt the poor to reform their ways and thus improve society. Too much, or ill-conceived, state or private aid, in this view, would promote a "dependent" class and keep the poor from improving themselves. Others saw in unbridled poverty and suffering a threat to the larger society, because both the "deserving" and "undeserving" could themselves threaten stability in a rapidly changing urban order. Not only were the poor a potential source of violence and social disruption in the crowded commercial districts of the city, but they might also spread infectious diseases to those of their own station and those of higher classes as well.

As late as the 1880s and 1890s, hospitals in the United States were often undifferentiated welfare institutions that provided the poor and homeless with services that were only tangentially related to medical practice. For instance, women's and children's hospitals often sheltered unmarried pregnant women from social ostracism with a hospital stay that was often measured in months or even years. Some women were sheltered while nursing their own child or another child whose mother had died in childbirth or shortly after. Some orphaned children would spend years in foundling hospitals. Even what might today be considered a general hospital would likely house working-class patients who were temporarily unemployed, unable to continue working, or displaced from their homes by urban development or another form of social dislocation.[73]

By the late nineteenth century, it was seen as necessary to establish more clearly defined institutions to care for the poor. The question became how to care for the virtuous poor as well as the growing army of "unworthy," who would provide this care, and under what conditions.

After the Civil War, health care for the poor was provided through an evolving system of dispensaries and hospitals. Those deemed "worthy" by hospital superintendents appointed by Protestant elites would be admitted to private charity hospitals, and those deemed "unworthy" would be housed in public facilities. In larger cities such as New York, Boston, Philadelphia, and Chicago, local charity or community organizations offered care of the community. The origins of relatively small nongovernmental charity hospitals in the United States were intimately linked to the communities that sponsored them. Many featured a name that denoted the particular group they initially served: Jewish, Lutheran, Cabrini (Italian Catholic), and German (which changed its name to Lenox Hill during World War I) hospitals in New York City and Brooklyn, for example. Unlike the larger institutions and citywide organized charitable societies, these institutions were closely linked culturally, economically, and politically to the communities they served and therefore exhibited fewer of the condescending, victim-blaming attitudes of the larger facilities. In the late years of the century, the number of these hospitals, dispensaries, soup kitchens, and other services grew significantly to meet the obvious need of large numbers of homeless, unemployed, and sick people in diverse communities, especially during the severe economic depressions of 1873–1877 and 1893–1897.[74]

In smaller cities these residents ended up in almshouses or even jails, and in some cities public hospitals were outgrowths of both older institutions. The largest public hospital in New York, Bellevue, was a former almshouse, and Kings County Hospital in Brooklyn was initially an adjunct of the county prison. In Chicago, what was originally an almshouse was repurposed as an emergency hospital during the 1832 cholera epidemic, and by the turn of the century it became Cook County Hospital, then Chicago's sole public hospital.[75] Medical technologies and treatments for much of the nineteenth century consisted of a few medications such as opium and calomel. Surgical interventions in the generally unhygienic world of the nineteenth-century hospital were generally limited to amputations and interventions to address problems like prolapsed uteruses, complicated births, and, at the end of the century, appendicitis, often generally dangerous procedures. It is not clear that medical treatments were effective in any institution, but the cleanliness and attention that were provided to patients certainly were.

By and large, nurses, doctors, or aides paid more personal attention to the possible salvation of the "worthy" in charity hospitals than to the "unworthy" served in the public institutions. The situation for family members of artisans, the middle class, and the rich was different. They would be treated in private doctors' offices or at home by private physicians and nurses, some of whom might live in a spare room of wealthy households for the duration of a patient's illness.

Given the nativist tendencies among many charity spokesmen and spokeswomen, they were open to social Darwinist notions that were being popularized by industrialists like Andrew Carnegie, who sponsored a speaking tour by Herbert Spencer, the British sociologist who coined the phrase *survival of the fittest*. Spencer argued that those at the top of the social ladder had achieved their success through their own efforts, while those at the bottom lacked the will, character, and intelligence to succeed in a competitive world. It was concluded that there were now large numbers of poor who were incapable of escaping poverty because of "inherited" weaknesses, who were made dependent by diseases and disability, or who were in danger of becoming dependent on public or private charity because of character flaws, which would make them "professional paupers" who "plead destitution for purposes of dishonest gain."[76] Early in the twentieth century, active efforts to shape human biology took the form of eugenics, which promoted sterilization of the "unfit," hospitalization of the mentally "retarded," and selective marriage and procreation of those deemed to be most fit. Eugenics was not simply a conservative movement but was adopted some of the most progressive members of society.

By the end of the nineteenth century, academic sociologists, religious leaders, charity workers, and hospital trustees took up the task of identifying the "worthy." Some sought to develop absolute categories by which to evaluate the needs of the poor. Robert Hunter, for instance, a well-known Progressive, developed a system designed to consider all those factors that were useful for "philanthropy if any real progress is to be made in the treatment of pauperism."[77] In his table of "dependents and their treatment," he listed those who were "truly" dependent: the aged and children, the crippled, the blind, the deaf, and the insane. For this group he suggested that care in institutions or in the community should be provided as long as necessary. The second group were those "dependents capable of self-support," including "professional vagrants," beggars, and the "morally insane." For them, Hunter prescribed "industrial education, repression, confinement for [the] protection of society." The third group were those who were "temporary dependents likely to become chronic," which included "the sick" (especially convalescents), inebriates, and drug addicts. Their complete cure was required, after which all charity was to be terminated.[78]

In all of these various institutions, the social situation of the patient, rather than the medical capabilities of the institution, determined whether the patient should be placed in the hospital. Consider the superintendent's description of one group of patients who were deemed worthy to be admitted to Methodist Hospital in Brooklyn:

> Thirty-one of our patients were clerks. Most of them lived probably in a boarding house. They were young men, just beginning to make their way in life. They occupied a small cold hall bedroom perhaps. They could afford nothing better. . . . The life they lived was tolerable and even pleasant while health continued, but how dismal it became when broken in upon by illness. What a desolate room that is in which one of these young men lies sick. The landlady is kindly disposed, but what can she do? Her other rooms are all occupied, and there are no conveniences for warming this. . . . There creeps over the house also, quite possibly, a suspicion of typhoid fever, and all shun that room, and some talk of moving away. The young man soon sees that he is ruining his landlady's business. If he could only go to a good hospital, what a relief it would be to everybody concerned. He can go. He comes to ours, and without money and without price he is tenderly nursed back again to health. Can that young man ever forget such Christian kindness? On the contrary he will go forth from the hospital better fitted morally, as well as physically, to fight the great outside battle.[79]

The hospital provided this respectable young man not primarily medical treatment but an alternative to the boardinghouse. The nineteenth-century hospital saw its role as both a medical and a social institution.[80] In this instance, the clerk was one of the respectable, working poor in need of temporary aid.[81]

By the end of the nineteenth century, the charity hospital and dispensary system began to break down as increasing pressure to care for the expanding population of poor people stressed hospital finances. In addition, rising standards of cleanliness and the increased cost of maintaining nurses' and doctors' residences pressed administrators to attract classes of potentially "paying" patients who could afford private rooms and doctors. This development helped to support the hospital financially. As a result, the nature of these institutions changed from charity hospitals to what are now termed "voluntary" hospitals. There the middle class and wealthy paid for private rooms, improved food, nursing service, and more hotel-like amenities. Meanwhile, the working class—the "worthy" poor—were relegated to the hospital charity wards. For the "unworthy poor," public institutions continued to provide care. In smaller cities, the poor were cared for in county hospitals funded by local philanthropists. The structure of the health care system had thus fundamentally changed in the space of the few decades between the end of the Civil War and the turn of the century. But the fundamental division between those who could and those who could not afford care remained the same.

THE DEVELOPMENT OF PUBLIC HEALTH INSTITUTIONS

The poor health of so many in large cities also led to the development of public health institutions. In 1865, as we've seen, the Citizens' Association of New York issued its final report on the "sanitary condition of the city." Widely distributed in a variety of forms—book, booklets, and pamphlets—the report was used to pressure the city and the state to organize a permanent metropolitan board of health. Hamilton Fish, John Jacob Astor Jr., Robert Roosevelt, August Belmont, and other members of elite merchant society hoped that the city would embark on a reform effort to lift it from the depths of disorder and disease. Only a permanent organization with police powers, they argued, could possibly control the social forces of disorder fostered by the changing character of both the population and the commercial economy. In New York, but also across the country, this period of reform produced departments of sanitation, public health, and public works that improved the environments and health of millions of Americans. The investment in improving the city would be monumental. It is hard to imagine today what was involved in installing plumbing and sewerage lines and in building reservoirs tens of miles away and water tunnels and aqueducts to bring freshwater to virtually every tenement and middle-class home. The efforts of New York prove what can be done when the society decides to make the environment more healthful (see figure 3.7).

This 1865 report underscored the need for increased action, especially if New York wished to become a commercial center equal to London, Paris, or other centers of trade. The city faced a monumental task. It would need to better control the environment that fostered diseases and would need to provide a reliable source of pure water for more of the city's poor, a sewer system, and good transportation, as well as fresh produce and milk, better housing, and streets free of animal and human waste. To accomplish these objectives, New York realized it would need to establish a department that was focused on such structural changes. Even though this project would clearly involve a huge investment of public and private money, there was little public opposition. The city's newspapers rallied around this cause, overcoming concerns of primarily upstate legislators in Albany, the state capital, who were worried about costs.[82]

As a result, in 1866 the city created a permanent institution, the Metropolitan Board of Health, to regulate the conditions that caused disease. Previously, public health boards had been established on an ad hoc basis in response to specific epidemics or other health-related crises. Public health officials now set about inspecting butcher shops to ensure that they were selling good-quality meat, free of maggots or adulterants, and they closed (sometimes with guns drawn) the "swill milk" factories where cows were hung from the ceiling and fed on the slop that was discarded by the breweries that lined the industrial areas (figure 3.8).

Officials also contracted with private haulers to provide at least an irregular garbage collection and street-cleaning system under, first, the Metropolitan Board of Health in 1866, which became the Department of Health in 1870, and then within the latter's Bureau of Street Cleaning. Previously, decisions to clean streets and collect garbage had been left to the whims of the local ward boss, who typically organized such activities only after the winter thaw, after millions of pounds of horse

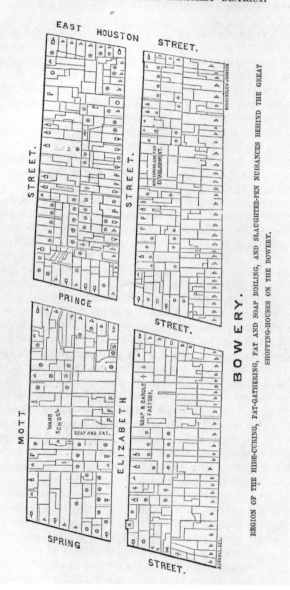

FIGURE 3.7 Street layout showing slaughter houses mixed in with people's residences on the Lower East Side, "Report 7th Sanitary District," in Citizens' Association of New York, Council of Hygiene and Public Health, *Report of the Council of Hygiene and Public Health of the Citizens' Association of New York Upon the Sanitary Condition of the City* (New York: D. Appleton, 1865), 88.

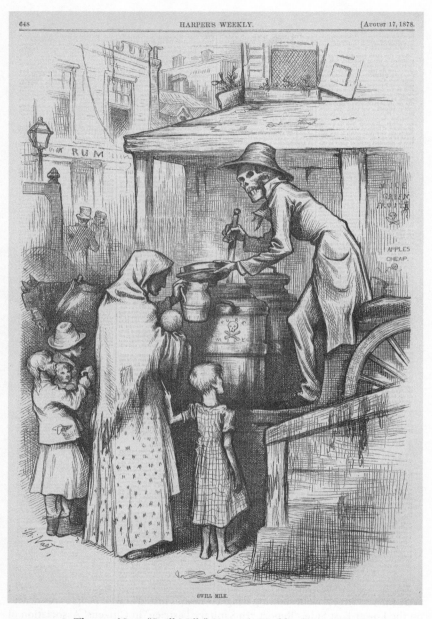

SWILL MILK.

FIGURE 3.8 Thomas Nast, "Swill Milk," *Harper's Weekly*, August 17, 1878.

manure, animal offal, garbage, and filth had accumulated. This cleanup was designed to allow for the freer flow of traffic in the emerging commercial city, to beautify it and to eliminate the stagnant pools of mosquito-breeding and polluted water and rotting organic matter that had fed disease-carrying rats, lice, and other vermin.

This effort was herculean. In short order, the department organized a Sanitary Bureau to regulate tenements and lodging houses, with divisions to address contagious diseases, sanitary inspections, plumbing and ventilation, and food inspection. It also organized a Bureau of Records to document births, deaths, and marriages in the city; a division of hospitals to provide care for strangers to the city and to "those suffering contagious diseases"; and a "Summer Corps" composed of forty-eight physicians whose "duty it is to visit each and every tenement-house, especially in the poorer or more crowded districts of the city, prescribe for the helpless sick, give needful advice, distribute rules for the care of infants, and search out and cause to be corrected all unsanitary conditions." Vaccination campaigns to prevent smallpox were organized through a "Permanent Inspectors of Vaccination" group that went from house to house, providing "free vaccination to all persons needing it," particularly children, who, under the sanitary regulations of the Board of Education, could not attend school without being vaccinated with the smallpox vaccine produced in the city's "Vaccine Laboratory."[83] Doctors were even sent back to the homes to ensure that the vaccination had been done properly.[84]

By 1873 the department had issued a number of important regulations for cleaning up the city. Regulations were passed mandating the "removal of manure" from the city's streets and from the more than six thousand stables around the city that housed the tens of thousands of horses that transported people, hauled goods, and hoisted building stone.[85] In addition, new fire safety codes augmented stricter enforcement of housing laws. Soon the newly organized Department of Health became a model for other cities throughout the nation, employing what were considered the latest advances in the bacteriology of the time.

These public health initiatives in New York and elsewhere made a tremendous difference in the lives of many, particularly by reducing the incidence of infectious disease. They even had an ameliorative effect on some of the vast inequalities in health. Even if the wealthy had sewer connections before the poor, eventually the poor got them as well. Similarly, water lines were gradually introduced to poor, working-class communities, and garbage collection became more systematic throughout the city.

While reforms like street cleaning, garbage removal, indoor plumbing, and the laying of sewer pipes and aqueducts were having some impact, differentials in the death rates of different classes and racial groups continued to be an issue. In 1894, the U.S. surgeon general John Billings issued a report on the health status of people in New York and Brooklyn detailing the various causes of death and disease and delineating the different experiences of both native- and foreign-born populations. The report documented that poor immigrants who lived in crowded tenements had far greater rates of death and disease than the middle and upper classes. It compared four different kinds of neighborhoods. "Group C" was composed of those city wards populated by immigrants living in crowded tenements on the Lower East Side. Group D referred to the districts of the middle and upper classes, "localities of high and good ground covered by the better class of residences." The difference in their disease experience was striking. Those living in crowded tenements were dying from scarlet fever, malaria, diphtheria, consumption, pneumonia, measles, stillbirths, and diseases of the liver at significantly higher rates than those living in more salubrious conditions. Also significantly higher were rates of typhoid fever, diarrheal diseases, whooping cough, heart disease, diseases of the nervous system, and diseases of the urinary organs and all other causes, which included accidents and injuries. Overall, the death rates per 100,000 people in the poorer districts were more than twice the rates for the wealthier areas.[86] See table 3.1.

The public health community was quick to trumpet the overall and dramatic success of the public health measures initiated in the second half of the nineteenth century. In 1913, the city's Department of Health reported that "the death rate from all causes reached the lowest level on record," a drop of 28 percent from the average of the previous fourteen years, "equivalent to a saving of 20,174 lives during the year 1912" alone. The report highlighted the dramatic impact that improved sanitary conditions had on the city's health. Children particularly had benefited

TABLE 3.1

Death rates per 100,000 of total population due to certain causes in four different groups of districts as reported in the 1890 census

Causes	Group A	Group B	Group C	Group D
All causes	2,825.49	3,313.95	4,191.58	1,864.34
Scarlet fever	22.38	41.41	28.70	8.99
Typhoid fever	12.43	21.50	35.88	22.12
Malarial fever	7.46	23.10	16.74	8.99
Diphtheria	79.58	101.15	93.28	55.99
Croup	46.01	42.21	55.01	16.59
Diarrheal diseases	293.45	399.01	398.23	159.08
Consumption	328.80	458.74	576.42	202.54
Pneumonia	381.11	363.97	548.91	219.13
Measles	21.76	22.30	88.50	2.07
Whooping cough	31.71	35.04	28.70	18.66
Cancer and tumor	44.76	52.56	63.38	68.43
Heart disease and dropsy	94.50	130.01	180.58	116.13
Childbirth and puerperal diseases	22.38	27.08	16.74	18.66
Diseases of the liver	25.49	39.03	47.84	20.05
Diseases of the nervous system	192.11	254.06	281.03	167.97
Diseases of the urinary organs	137.40	197.52	245.16	131.34
Old age	19.89	28.67	27.51	17.97
Stillbirths	257.39	258.04	309.73	176.96
All other causes	606.17	815.55	1148.05	431.34
Unknown	0.02	2.39	1.20	0.69

Source: John S. Billings, Bureau of the Census, *Vital Statistics of New York and Brooklyn Covering a Period of Six Years Ending May 31, 1890* (Washington, DC: Government Printing House, 1894), 66.

Note: This table shows the social and economic distinctions in death rates in four groups of districts in New York and Brooklyn in 1890. Group A are wards composed primarily of Russian and Polish Jews; Group B are "waterside districts with comparatively heavy death rates," most likely family of unskilled and semiskilled dockworkers; Group C includes wards in the southern districts of Manhattan with "heavy death rates"; Group D include "localities on high and good ground covered by the better class of residences."

from the improvements: the statisticians calculated that the mortality rates for children under five years of age had declined more than 33 percent over the previous fourteen years. The report noted that "the death rate of children under five years of age is considered by demographers as a most trustworthy index of the sanitary conditions prevalent in a community, and this excellent showing is due in great measure to the steps taken by the sanitary officials to minimize the mortality among children, especially from the infectious diseases of childhood, to wit, measles, scarlet fever, diphtheria and croup and diarrheal diseases." Dramatic declines in smallpox, scarlet fever, whooping cough, and pulmonary tuberculosis were also documented for the preceding decade.[87] The vast differences in health outcomes between rich and poor, Black and white, and immigrant and native-born were ameliorated.

Despite the improvements, however, the fundamental social inequalities that resulted in unequal disease burdens remained. Poor people and people of color continued to live shorter, harder, and more painful lives than those with wealth. While the 1865 report, for example, suggested significant programs for improving and creating an infrastructure, it did not agitate for more fundamental reforms to deal with the inequities of commercial relationships, rent laws, employment opportunities, or the industrial relations that had transformed urban life in the preceding half century. Landlords could still jam residents into airless, filthy tenements, and factory owners could still force unskilled laborers to accept an average daily wage in 1870 of $1.66 (the equivalent in today's prices of $36.86, or $3.70 an hour in a ten-hour day).[88]

SHIFTING PUBLIC HEALTH PERSPECTIVES

By the 1880s, the general understanding of the causes of disease was shifting in very big ways. The focus on filth and immorality as the cause of disease was slowly being supplemented and in some respects supplanted by a focus on disease as caused by specific pathogens associated with specific diseases. The discovery of the tuberculosis bacillus by Robert Koch and Louis Pasteur's work in the 1880s on rabies and the bacterial origins of yeast opened new vistas for those coming out of new programs in bacteriology and for those working in the laboratory. The medical community began to objectify the source of disease less as lifestyle and living conditions and more as germs. Laboratory science began to hold out the possibility that disease could be explained rationally through the discovery of specific microorganisms. For the practitioner, this meant that a detailed life history was no longer as essential for diagnosing disease. Medical practitioners continued to speak of the significance of taking the patient's "history," but now they focused less on environmental conditions like homelife, work history, personal habits, and morality. They increasingly focused on the disease history of patients and their family members. This trend became even more true in the years following Robert Koch's 1882 discovery of the tuberculosis bacillus.[89] Traditional sanitarians continued to focus on engineering and the provision of pure water and the extension of sewage lines to prevent cholera, typhoid, and other water-borne diseases, but new techniques for managing disease were developing. New campaigns to inoculate entire populations were used to limit the spread of smallpox, and laboratory analysis of milk and meat could stop the transmission of food-borne diseases.[90]

Bacteriologists and epidemiologists developed the ability to identify disease carriers with microscopes and laboratory technologies. Technical experts and trained professionals were seen to have the answers to disease. A whole new world of disease prevention appeared to be opening up. Some public health practitioners had faith in laboratories and medical practitioners. Other public health advocates and older sanitarians continued to emphasize the importance of improving the environmental conditions that allowed disease to fester. Milk stations, bathrooms, public laundries, the provision of pasteurized milk, the cleaning of streets, public baths and laundries, the provision of school lunches, vaccination campaigns, visiting nurses, and a host of other efforts by social reformers in settlement houses and philanthropic organizations ameliorated some of the worst aspects of urban life.[91]

THE GREAT WHITE PLAGUE: THE MANIFESTATION OF INEQUALITIES IN URBAN AMERICA

Tuberculosis was the biggest killer around the world in the nineteenth century. The prevention, diagnosis, and treatment of tuberculosis— consumption or phthisis—developed within two sometimes contradictory understandings of the disease. Public health practitioners saw consumption as a manifestation of social and economic conditions. Bacteriologists saw the disease as caused by a specific germ that might spread from person to person, depending upon specific conditions.

Physicians often used the two terms *consumption* and *phthisis* (Greek for "to waste away") interchangeably to identify what later would be called tuberculosis. Consumption was generally associated with lung diseases characterized by shortness of breath and symptoms such as coughing blood, wasting away, and fevers. It had been a scourge throughout recorded history, and through much of the nineteenth century it was often the leading cause of death in European and American societies. It is estimated that as many as one in every four to six deaths in those societies was due to consumption for much of the century.[92]

While the symptoms appeared in victims regardless of class or social strata, the disease took on different meanings for different classes and groups. As the microbiologist René Dubos and the biological researcher Jean Dubos have written, physicians, "faced with a confusing array of signs and symptoms, bearing no obvious relation to one another," saw these manifestations as "the expression of different maladies." In light of its prevalence even among the gentry, consumption was seen not as a disease of immorality or personal failing, but as a sign of frailty, even as a sign of true womanhood among the middle class. As one medical historian has summarized: "During the first part of nineteenth century, the [young, middle class] consumptive was presented as sensitive, morally refined, inwardly and outwardly, perhaps [a] precociously talented individual." The translucent flush of Victorian ladies suffering from this disease became a standard image in the nineteenth-century novel. During the latter part of the century, given its wide spread among the poor, the disease was "more likely to be associated with . . . lack of control, effeminacy, sensuality and moral depravity."[93]

For the working class and poor, consumption or phthisis was popularly linked to an ongoing moral and social environment that predisposed a victim to disease.[94] As the historian John Harley Warner explains, "Treatment was to be sensitively gauged not to a disease entity but to such distinctive features of the patient as age, gender, ethnicity, socioeconomic position, and moral status, and to attributes of place like climate, topography and population density."[95] Until the discovery of the germ as the source of disease, it was thought that a practitioner needed to know the life history of the patient to make an accurate diagnosis and plan of treatment. Ironically, none of the treatments—the rest cure, bloodletting, purges, cod liver oil, or vinegar massages—had a direct effect on the progress of the disease.

Many public health practitioners understood that the structural realities of poverty were the seedbed that allowed the bacteria to thrive. Practitioners such as Hermann Biggs in New York City and Charles Chapin in Rhode Island, among others, documented a variety of important sources for phthisis—dusty or unsanitary conditions in the home, crowding, impure air, and dust in the workplace. In New York City in 1879, Roger Tracy, the registrar of vital statistics, noted symptoms of the disease among workers in the metal trades. "The disease comes on very gradually . . . and its duration may be extended over four or five years." It "begins with the cough of irritation, dry and hacking at first, with very scanty expectoration, whitish and stringy in character. . . . The expectoration gradually increases in amount and becomes reddish, and soon after this tinge appears there may be haemoptysis," or coughing of blood from the lungs.[96] Consumption or phthisis could be of an acute nature and "prove fatal in a few weeks," or it might start with acute symptoms and evolve into a chronic condition. Its symptoms might appear slowly, gradually getting worse over many years. It could affect lungs, bones, the brain, and other organs of the body, although pulmonary consumption was the primary fear, as it signaled almost inevitable early death, with up to 80 percent mortality of those who became ill.[97]

Increasingly, consumption (or phthisis) came to be understood as tuberculosis, caused by a specific organism that trained experts, using culture dishes and microscopes, could identify. "Medical science claims that the presence of the tubercle bacillus in the lungs is the fundamental cause of phthisis, or consumption," a New Yorker wrote to *Scientific American* in 1904. Such a redefinition held out the possibility that an effective vaccine could be developed, thereby undercutting expensive efforts to make structural changes.[98]

With the revolution in bacteriology that followed the discoveries of Pasteur, Koch, and Joseph Lister, who pioneered the uses of carbolic acid and other sterile and antiseptic surgical techniques, a new faith in laboratory science emerged not only among physicians but also among public health workers. Bacteriology thus became an ideological marker, "sharply differentiating the 'old' public health, the province of untrained amateurs, from the 'new' public health, which belonged to scientifically trained professionals," points out Elizabeth Fee.[99] Members of both professions began to share a common faith in the significance of a disease-specific germ entity in creating consumption. Public health practitioners came to understand that the modes of transmission of the bacteria had to be clearly identified if an effective campaign to eliminate the sources of the disease was to be mounted. It was not enough to simply identify the cause of tuberculosis.

By the turn of the twentieth century, public health had begun to answer key questions that would lead practitioners to become "microbe hunters," trying to figure out where the germ could be found and how it was transmitted.[100] They asked and answered significant questions. Why were the poor so likely to be struck by tuberculosis? Because the hot, crowded dwellings in which they lived allowed the germ to propagate and to spread among a population weakened by inadequate nutrition and horrid living conditions. Why did children appear to be a high-risk group? Because tainted milk from tubercular cows poisoned children. How did individuals outside any particular risk group come down with the disease? Because they had a hereditary predisposition that left them vulnerable to infection. Why did workers have a higher rate of tuberculosis than farmers? Because close quarters combined with long hours and inadequate diet left them more susceptible.

In the view of the medical community, the slums of large cities were the "breeding grounds" for the tuberculosis bacilli. Tuberculosis came to be viewed, then, as a disease that could be transmitted to susceptible individuals by means of air impregnated with bacteria from dried sputum, breathing, and other sources. Dusting furniture could throw into the air the "dried sputum" of tuberculars. Crowded public spaces or unclean home conditions with moist, warm, and stagnant air were seen as the most likely conduits for the disease, a view still true today but one that has been supplemented by an understanding of the risks of weakened immune systems; another cause was certain high-risk areas such as mines or foundries where workers were exposed to silica, a dust that increased tuberculosis rates among exposed workers.[101]

It became clear that, while bacteriology held promise for specific cures and preventive vaccines, the development of disease prevention programs could result in more efficient uses of public health resources. "A careless or ignorant expectorating consumptive can eliminate and distribute seven billions of bacilli in twenty-four hours," warned a prominent surgeon, S. A. Knopf, in the journal *Charities* in 1901. Tuberculosis victims were encouraged to carry and use flasks to dispose of their spittle so that "it cannot dry and be blown about to be inhaled by others," the social work journal *Charities* declared[102]; in this way responsible "tuberculars" could stem the disease.

Focusing on the sources of specific infection rather than on the general sanitary conditions of the broader city had numerous attractions. One could stem infection without disrupting existing social relationships between tenant and landlord, employer and worker, and political leaders and voters. Health and wealth could both be attained, it seemed.[103] But, importantly, a diverse group of Progressive Era reformers, socialists included, continued to press the point that the inspectors from the Massachusetts Department of Labor and labor leaders had made during the strike of 1877 decades before: that disease could not be divorced from the terrible conditions of life and work and that health and social problems had to be addressed together. Reformers in Boston, New York, Chicago, and other cities established "settlement houses" that provided a range of social and public health services for the poor in low-income communities. For example, Henry Street Settlement on New York's Lower East Side sent visiting nurses into the homes of the poor and set up milk stations where residents could get unadulterated milk for their children, offered language instruction, and provided educational and some recreational programs for new immigrants and their children. Charity and settlement house workers, for example, documented that nearly one out of every four dwellings in New York City in 1890 experienced a death from tuberculosis. In the poorer neighborhoods, it was clear, the toll was much higher, leaving these communities devastated by the disease.[104] For these reformers, tuberculosis was as much a disease of poverty as of germs.[105] Certainly, this was reason to continue to improve the living conditions of the poor. Even as late as 1917, near the end of World War I, the power of the social definition of disease shaped public health studies. In that year, the Framingham Community Health and

Tuberculosis Demonstration Study began, the "crown jewel of Metropolitan Life Insurance Company's health projects." The study prioritized preventive services and community involvement in educational campaigns and public health initiatives. This approach, it was claimed, led to a decline of the tuberculosis rates in the city by 68 percent "compared with only 32% in the control towns" where these interventions were not employed.[106]

Notably, even the most progressive social reformers of the era focused on the problems of white immigrants, generally ignoring the growing African American presence in cities and the impact of segregation and discrimination during the Jim Crow era. As Samuel Roberts documents in his study of Baltimore, tuberculosis festered in the Black community while public health officials generally paid only passing notice. As late as 1920, the overall mortality rate for African Americans of all ages exceeded that of whites, with the differences for young adults being particularly striking: for ages twenty-five to thirty-four, the death rate for Blacks was 275 per 100,000, while for whites it was 120 per 100,000, less than half.[107]

Despite an increasing emphasis on germs as a source of disease, the Department of Health, and New York City as a whole, still understood that they needed to continue to face daunting environmental hazards. In 1912, the department issued an annual report that, in language as dispassionate as any, detailed the continuing environmental problems New Yorkers faced. The department recorded 343,000 complaints from citizens, inspectors, and officials about inadequate ventilation, leaking cesspools and water closets, unlicensed manure dumps, and animals kept without permits. The department also removed nearly half a million smaller animals such as pigs, hogs, calves, and sheep. Its meat inspection unit removed 5,669,470 pounds of spoiled poultry, fish, offal, pork, and beef and carted 1,946 cubic yards of night soil from the backyards and privies of the city's tenements.[108] And even as late as 1900, the city had to deal with 130,000 horses in Manhattan alone.[109]

The scope of the Health Department's activities had expanded enormously over the course of the previous half century as the city population expanded from 1,068,000 at the beginning of the Civil War to 4,230,000 in 1900, and the department's budget now amounted to nearly $1 million per year. Significantly, a "remarkable and continuous decrease in the death rate . . . accompanied the development . . . of public sanitation," the 1912 report began. In 1866, the year in which the department was organized, New York City's death rate was 36.31 per 1,000. The rate then declined decade after decade, and by 1910 it had recently fallen below 16 per 1,000. The department was justifiably proud: over the course of just forty-five years, there had been a decrease in the death rate of over 50 percent.[110] In 1870 the average length of life of an American was just over thirty-nine years; by 1910 it had increased to just over fifty-one years.[111]

By the early decades of the twentieth century, substantial changes had occurred both in the workplace and in the society at large. Fundamental reforms changed the lives of millions of people, both rich and poor, improving their health and offering eventual escape from the infectious diseases that ravaged nineteenth-century life. In the coming decades fewer children died in childbirth or infancy as pasteurization of milk and the provision of pure water limited the transmission of bacteria and cholera; young people could expect to grow taller and live longer lives as improved nutrition and the inspection of meats limited rickets and parasitic diseases like trichinosis; and everyone benefited from legislation requiring fresh air in every room of the growing tenement districts. Other reforms, such as street cleaning, indoor plumbing, and sewerage systems, augured even more broadly observable improvements in health. Electric street cars, subways systems, and automobiles replaced horse-drawn trolleys and brought an end to manure in the streets. Even the gradual elimination of the granaries needed to store feed for horses gave hope that the rodent population could be controlled.

The improvements in New York were monumental, and metropolitan areas throughout the nation also initiated reforms like those in New York. The older cities of the Northeast as well as the emerging cities across the country (Milwaukee, Chicago, St. Louis, Pittsburgh, San Francisco, and Atlanta, for example) developed sanitation and water distribution and sewerage systems. They established departments of public health that began to dramatically improve the worlds in which their citizens lived. Throughout the nation, life spans increased and infectious disease rates declined.

RACE, CLASS, AND DEATH IN PHILADELPHIA AND BALTIMORE

Despite all these advances, disease and death rates among African Americans continued to be higher than among whites. Thanks to the pioneering work of the great sociologist W. E. B. Du Bois, we have detailed data for the condition of African Americans in the city of Philadelphia, which at the end of the nineteenth century was home to over 1,200,000 people.[112] By examining race as well as class, Du Bois was able to document how racism affected people's health in a way that public health reformers in New York had not been acknowledging.[113] Published in 1896, Du Bois's book, *The Philadelphia Negro*, detailed the social, political, cultural, and health conditions of African Americans in a municipality that in the antebellum period had been a center of abolitionist activity, a terminus of the Underground Railroad, a base of operations for both Harriet Tubman and William Still, and after the Civil War continued to be a destination for African Americans. As a result of this migration, Philadelphia had a strong and vibrant African American middle class as well as a large number of recent Black migrants escaping horrible conditions in Maryland and farther south. The death rate between 1884 and 1890 for African Americans in one of Philadelphia's slums, the Fifth Ward, was 48.46 out of 1,000, but among African Americans in a middle-class ward, the Thirtieth, it was less than half of that, 21.74.[114] As Du Bois explains, "The influence of bad sanitary surroundings is strikingly illustrated in the enormous death rate of the Fifth Ward—the worst Negro slum in the city and the worst part of the city in respect to sanitation. On the other hand the low death rate of the Thirtieth Ward illustrates the importance of good houses and clean streets in a district where the better class of Negroes have recently migrated."[115] Again, the increased prevalence of disease and death could be traced to the nature of the world that Blacks were forced to live in.

The major disease conditions in 1890 that affected Philadelphia's Black population were consumption, neurological problems, and pneumonia, with the death rate from consumption at 426.50 out of 100,000, almost 50 percent higher than for whites.[116] Du Bois saw this rate as a result of the social conditions in which poorer African Americans were forced to live: "The strikingly excessive rate here is that of consumption, which is the most fatal disease for Negroes. Bad ventilation, lack of outdoor life for women and children, poor protection against dampness and cold are undoubtedly the chief causes of this excessive death rate."[117] Although the death rate for African Americans had been declining in the city since 1820, in 1884–1890 it was 38 percent higher than that of whites, and in 1891–1896 it was still almost 20 percent higher (indeed, in the Fifth Ward it was almost 50 percent higher).[118] The statistics that he uncovered, Du Bois wrote, "seem to adduce considerable proof that the Negro death rate is largely a matter of condition of living."[119]

Du Bois felt that racism contributed to the higher rates of mortality from consumption and other respiratory diseases. African Americans feared hospitals because of the treatment that they received there, what Dubois described as the "roughness or brusqueness of manner prevalent in many hospitals."[120] He went on: "The most difficult social problem in the matter of Negro health is the peculiar attitude of the nation toward the well-being of the race. There have, for instance, been few other cases in the history of civilized peoples where human suffering has been viewed with such peculiar indifference."[121] It was clear from the evidence Du Bois collected that the racism and poverty imposed on African American residents, who were denied equal employment opportunities and adequate, affordable housing, resulted in increased disease and death.

In Baltimore, conditions of housing, nutrition, and racism in the late nineteenth and early twentieth centuries paralleled those of Philadelphia and other cities. As the historian Samuel Roberts, in his study of race and disease in Baltimore, documents, there was a glaring difference in the life expectancies of "white" and "nonwhite" Americans living in Baltimore in the early decades of the twentieth century. In 1905, the life expectancies for whites there was 49.1 years, while for African Americans it was 31.3. In 1915, it was 55.1 for whites and 38.9 for nonwhites.[122] He quotes the account of George Edmund Haynes, the historian and cofounder of the Urban League, who saw "the connections between ghettoization and poor health" and described the conditions at the turn of the twentieth century in Black communities not only in Baltimore but also in New York, Philadelphia, Chicago, Washington, Louisville, Atlanta, and other cities: "Crowded into segregated districts; living in poor houses for the most part for which they pay high rentals; . . . walled in by inefficiency, lack of training and the chance to get the training; usually restricted from well-paid occupations by the prejudice of employers; with a small income and the resulting low standard of living, the wonder is not that Negroes have a uniformly higher death rate than whites in the cities and towns, but that the mortality is as small as it is and shows signs of decrease."[123] Haynes noted that in Atlanta in 1882–1885 the death rate per thousand population for African Americans was 37.96 while for whites it was half that, 18.22; in 1891–1905, the death rate declined slightly for whites to 18.03; for African Americans it declined more, to 32.76, but this was still close to double that of whites.[124]

THE POSSIBILITIES AND LIMITATIONS OF LATE NINETEENTH CENTURY REFORM

The targeted public health interventions of the late nineteenth century were extremely important in improving the overall health experience of Americans. Somewhat startling, however, was the emergence of changing patterns of death among city residents. By 1912 public health officials could see that an "enormous reduction in mortality [had] taken place in all age groups below forty-five, while there has [been] an actual increase in the mortality at all ages over forty-five." The infectious diseases of the nineteenth century such as smallpox, typhoid fever, diphtheria, and pulmonary tuberculosis appeared to be claiming fewer and fewer of the city's children and young adults. Structural improvements, widespread vaccination campaigns against smallpox, and effective antitoxins to combat diphtheria all contributed to a decline in infectious disease rates. What became apparent was that cancer, heart disease, and pneumonia were claiming larger and larger percentages of the elderly, however. "Without exception," the report pointed out, "the diseases in which a reduction of mortality has been effected belong to the class of infectious diseases, while of those diseases in which there has been increase in the mortality only one, pneumonia, belongs to that group." Public health officials claimed a major success against infectious diseases and recognized that as people were now living longer, the field "needed to focus on reducing mortality from the diseases of middle and old age."[125] They thus recognized that one impact of their reforms was that cancer and heart disease would now become more prominent as causes of death.[126]

But the different structural economic and social relationships between Blacks and whites, rich and poor, and immigrant and native-born all resulted in disproportionate risks of getting sick, being disabled, and dying early. The world of the poor continued to sicken them. Despite the important ameliorative actions promoted by people in public health and other reformers, the elite's control over the conditions of work and life still resulted in widespread suffering. What had not changed were the disparities in housing, work, and environment—between the rich and the poor; the working immigrant and native-born white; African Americans and whites; Native Americans, Mexican Americans, and Anglos; industrial workers and their managers; and landowners and sharecroppers. Housing reforms and indoor plumbing were not equally available to all people. The wealthy still lived "up on the hill" away from the blight that was destroying lives below; they still ate better food and had access to more fresh fruit, meat, and fresh air than those who did the work. Workers still took the dangerous jobs that caused them to lose an arm, a leg, and even a life, and in many cases these injuries could have been avoided if elementary safeguards had been put in place. Owners took no such risks and profited from the dangers their machinery, chemicals, and workplaces posed to the workers and their families. A great deal of work remained to be done. As diseases of middle and old age increased, people became exposed to new industrial toxins that exacerbated these trends as the twentieth century progressed. A developing consumer economy also exposed people to new hazards like tobacco products, ultraprocessed foods, and car exhaust, to name a few.

CHAPTER FOUR

Resetting the Ground Rules for Inequality

Labor, Law, and Health After the Civil War

"It may seem strange that any men should dare to ask a just God's assistance in wringing their bread from the sweat of other men's faces."
ABRAHAM LINCOLN, SECOND INAUGURAL ADDRESS, 1865

"We no longer own slaves; now we can rent them."
EDWARD R. MURROW, *HARVEST OF SHAME*, 1960

While the North was dealing with the world created by industrial capitalism, the South was creating a postslavery world. The victory in the Civil War was a win for the idea of freedom and basic equality in rights of citizenship for all, but in the succeeding decades new rationales were found in both the North and South for maintaining the inequalities in power and control, and thereby health, that elites deemed essential for sustaining a corporate capitalist economic system. Despite Lincoln's second inaugural address, in which he condemned slavery as an immoral system of exploitation in which owners wrenched "their bread from the sweat of other men's faces," there were those intent on maintaining a system of exploitation based on "free labor" that would profit a few while harming many. They turned to the law to support these efforts.

The use of the law in this endeavor was instrumental in maintaining the power of white planters over Black sharecroppers but also, more broadly, managers over employees.[1] The law as it developed was used to legitimate the right of masters and managers to maintain dangerous and unhealthy working conditions in both the North and the South. But it was not all one-sided. While the rights of employers and landowners typically predominated, the law would also be used, especially in the North, to reform working conditions and improve safety in industrial and agricultural workplaces. The struggle was not only over wages; perhaps more importantly, it was over the conditions of work that sickened and crippled vast numbers of railroad workers, miners, steelworkers, and others in developing factories throughout the nation. The fight over hours of work, for example, was largely based on the belief that exhausted workers were more prone to accidental dismemberment and death. These contests between owners and workers were certainly lopsided in owners' favor, sometimes devastatingly so, but they also sparked some major legislative changes. Workers' compensation systems spread throughout the industrial states, as did more regular factory inspections. Union efforts to limit hours of work and improve conditions within the plant met with some success.

"SOCIAL SYSTEMS . . . TO PERFORM THE DRUDGERY OF LIFE"

While the Civil War formally ended chattel slavery, the question of how then to reorganize work in the South and find "free" workers to replace slaves emerged as a major problem. The South needed "social systems . . . to perform the drudgery of life."[2] In the years following the Civil War, landowners, county and state governments, and local vigilante groups like the Ku Klux Klan found both illegal and legal ways to coerce newly freed people to remain on the land and continue to produce the cotton that for many decades had powered the southern economy. After a brief hiatus in white southern control over the political apparatus of the states of the former Confederacy during the Reconstruction era, planters and allied politicians put in place laws tying freedmen and freedwomen to the lands on which they had previously been enslaved. The basic tools for reimposing control have been well documented by others. Sharecropping, as well as the crop lien system, in which Black families farmed on planters' land in exchange for shares of the crop, put thousands of families in permanent debt to landowners, from whom they were forced to buy their seed and tools. The "Black Codes" instituted by state legislatures made it illegal to leave lands on which you owed money. The enactment of vagrancy laws threatened arrest for those who quit onerous jobs, resulting in imprisonment and long sentences during which prisoners were returned to work for planters until the debt was paid off and the prison sentence served. The use of eligibility restrictions, as well as terror, lynchings, and intimidation by sheriffs and the Ku Klux Klan, denied former slaves their basic rights, including the right to vote.[3]

Long-term hopes for a freer, safer, more healthful future for the formerly enslaved were also undermined by promises not kept: William Tecumseh Sherman's promise of 40 acres and a mule, for example, promised former slaves and their families the wherewithal essential for their future health, but it did not come to fruition.[4] Such a radical redistribution of land from defeated plantation owners to freedmen would have inevitably led to better health outcomes for the freedmen and their descendants, but the proposal was soon squelched by a Congress and a southern planter class that resisted such radical change. In the immediate aftermath of the Civil War, for example, Congress established the Freedmen's Bureau, one of whose mandates was to establish twelve hospitals which provided much needed medical care for some of the millions of newly emancipated. Yet, even this limited effort was quickly dismantled two years after the end of the war, in 1867. As the historian Eric Foner points out, the Freedmen's Bureau did not undertake efforts to "train Black physicians or medical assistants," nor did it undertake "a general program of health statistics." As a result, "its activities did little to alter the fact that control of medicine remained firmly in white hands."[5]

All of these events affected the health of the African American population. In the immediate aftermath of the Civil War, many freedpeople were on the move, both to find new opportunities and to escape a massive drought and subsequent famine, but this migration had some immediate health consequences. As the historian Jim Downs recounts, "The forced migration and independent movements of freedpeople that crisscrossed the South throughout 1866 and 1867 redoubled their vulnerability to sickness, suffering and diseases," including dysentery, smallpox, and cholera.[6] By the late nineteenth century, the grinding poverty and oppressive living conditions of the rural Black population had taken an increasing toll on their health and well-being; that, together with the imposition of Jim Crow segregation and the enactment in the

1890s of poll taxes, grandfather clauses, and other legislation designed to drastically restrict African American voting, led to the first great migration of African Americans to the North and the West between 1890 and World War I. However, there were periods of African American and interracial resistance to exploitative conditions in the post-Reconstruction era. Most prominently, Blacks and whites created farmers' alliances and the Populist Party in the South, both made up of farmers, tenants, and sharecroppers who sought to curb the power of the railroads, bankers, and newly formed large corporations. The era of Reconstruction and beyond did allow the vast majority of freedpeople to take some measure of control over their health and treatment; that in turn buttressed their political and personal agency, expressed, for example, through their demands for access to state health and welfare institutions.[7]

THE HEALTH OF INDUSTRIAL WAGEWORKERS

Throughout the nineteenth century, the number of wage laborers in America grew. Whereas in 1850 about 1,350,000 people worked as wage earners in manufacturing, transportation, and mining, by 1900 over 10,860,000 did so.[8] As a result, the fear of what came to be called "wage slavery" spread, energizing ongoing struggles between those who owned land and factories and those who did the work. Fundamental questions were raised at the time about the meaning of freedom and liberty. When was a worker truly free, and when was he or she being coerced through threats of violence, deprivation, or lost wages? What was the effect of such conditions on a worker's health and well-being? When, as a condition of being hired, was a worker's nominal acceptance of the dangers of a job—danger from accident or injury, from poisoning and disease—a reasonable outcome of the "free" negotiations between a worker and the employer? And when was it an outcome of the coercive power that employers had in their negotiation with workers?

Ironically, before the Civil War southern politicians self-servingly used the inequalities that marked the free labor market to justify slavery, their own main system of exploitation. In 1858, for example, James Henry Hammond, plantation owner, attorney, and senator from South

Carolina, rose on the Senate floor to deliver his influential defense of slavery by comparing the two means of keeping a workforce in line: chattel and wage slavery. "In all social systems there must be a class to do the menial duties, to perform the drudgery of life. . . . Such a class you must have, or you would not have that other class which leads [to] progress, civilization, and refinement," he began. "Your whole hireling class of manual laborers and 'operatives,' as you call them are essentially slaves." He went on to compare "our slaves" in the South, who were "hired for life and well compensated," to northern workers, who were "hired by the day, not cared for, and scantily compensated." Not only was the southern system more humane in Hammond's characterization, but it was also more efficient and more stable. He bragged that the southern system, based on race, completely denied political power to those it exploited, while the absence of racial difference between employer and worker in the North had led to laborers there gaining the vote and therefore the potential to overthrow the system. If the northern workers "knew the tremendous secret, that the ballot box is stronger than 'an army with banners,' and [they] could combine, where would you be?" he rhetorically asked the Senate. "Your society would be reconstructed, your government overthrown, your property divided . . . by the quiet process of the ballot-box," a critique that could just as easily apply in the South after Reconstruction, which was why southern Redeemers restricted the ballot to whites.[9]

It is an aspect of the American system of law that the legal system, backed up by force when needed, provided a stable basis for the continued inequalities of the workplace before, during, and following the Civil War. Particularly valuable as the basis of labor law was the continuing tradition of English and European feudal law by which the owner and worker, master and slave, and manager and laborer embodied the inequalities that were so fundamental to the American economic and social system. Many scholars have looked specifically at the basic concept of "free" labor, work done under a contract in which both parties enter into an agreement of sorts in which one's labor is offered in exchange for wages. Based on the ideology that the worker and owner entered as equals into this negotiation, this concept ignored the extreme power differentials between the two parties. Even today, the terms *master* and *servant* are used in labor law briefs and court decisions. These issues of "freedom" of contract and the assumed equality between owners and employees were laid out in two important court decisions in the nineteenth and early twentieth centuries, *Farwell v. Boston and Worcester Railroad Corp.* in 1842 and *Lochner v. New York* in 1905.

ASSUMING THE RISKS OF THE JOB: *FARWELL V. BOSTON AND WORCESTER RAILROAD CORP.*

An early effort to use the court system to legitimate the "free labor" form of exploitation and to justify the health consequences of such exploitation was the case of *Farwell v. Boston and Worcester Railroad Corp.* In October 1837, Nicholas Farwell, an engineer driving a passenger train between Boston and Worcester, was seriously injured when the engine passed over a rail switch that had not been properly placed. The derailment left Farwell, who earned the princely sum of $2 per day, without an arm and without his job.[10] Farwell sued the railroad, arguing that a fellow worker's carelessness and negligence had led to his injury and that the company bore responsibility to compensate him for the loss of the use of his arm.

In the nineteenth century, the nation's railroad system expanded dramatically from a total of 40 miles in 1830 to over 160,000 miles by 1890. Compared to the textile mills, coal mines, and other industrial enterprises that were mushrooming in antebellum America, the railways were a quite different industrial form. Rather than rooted in one spot, their tracks and other infrastructure reached deep into the American continent, and management of the tracks, schedules, and maintenance was at once a deeply complex, yet often very local, affair. Teams of workers, often miles away from the nearest town, were in constant danger as they operated massive steam-powered engines hauling tons of freight in the cars behind. Workers were also killed during track switching, derailments (as in Farwell's case), coupling and uncoupling of cars, and sometimes head-on collisions. Brakemen, those workers who applied the brakes when ordered by the conductor and who made sure the couplings between cars were functioning, were at special risk. Workers were also killed or maimed by boiler explosions in the shops where the engines were built. Railroad work was, next to mining, the most dangerous occupation for much of the century, responsible for thousands of injuries and hundreds of deaths every year. For example, between 1870 and 1900, 19,707 coal miners lost their lives in accidents, with almost 1,500 dying in 1900 alone, while over the same period, over 2,900 railroad workers perished, with 370 dying in 1898 alone.[11]

The legal issues in the *Farwell* case revolved around responsibility for the many inevitable accidents that occurred among railroad workers. Farwell's attorney argued that the contract to take a job implied that a safe environment would be maintained. In contrast, the railroad argued that, while Farwell himself might not have been responsible for the accident that claimed his arm, a fellow worker who was tasked with maintaining the switch in its appropriate position was responsible. Hence, it wasn't the company's fault; rather, it was the fault of the "fellow servant."[12]

In 1842, when the case was decided, the United States was still overwhelmingly a rural nation with a large number of "shopkeepers" and artisan workers, and much of the law ignored the industrial settings that were beginning to replace the homes and artisan-owned and -controlled shops. The Massachusetts supreme court found for the defendant, largely adopting the defense's argument that the corporation had contracted with workers for the skills necessary for carrying out the assigned tasks and had paid them a wage commensurate with these skills. The court held that Farwell's decision to take the job meant that he knowingly accepted the dangers that attended it as well. His willingness to assume the risks of the job was indicated not only by his having taken the job but also by his having accepted a higher-than-prevailing wage for his labor. Farwell and his "fellow servant" had been "selected" because of their skills, and therefore both were experts capable of controlling the worksite. While Farwell was obviously not at fault that the switch had been wrongly placed, it was another railroad worker, not the company, with whom he had a legitimate gripe.[13]

Chief Justice Lemuel Shaw, in his 1842 decision, recognized that the case involved "a principle of great importance" in the new nation because it raised a key question of accountability: Was there an "implied contract" for a safe environment for the worker with an employer whose money an employee received, or did responsibility for injury reside with "fellow servants," also individuals who presumably had the skills and knowledge necessary to protect themselves and their coworkers from the "perils incident to the service"? It was not a customer suing a business for an injury on its premises or for damage caused by its products, Shaw pointed out: here, two employees were hired and paid "for their respective services according to . . . the labor and skill required for their proper performance." While masters were generally held accountable for their servant's misdeeds, here the master was hiring the servant ostensibly *because* of that person's expertise, as acknowledged by the fact that the servant accepted the job and earned a higher-than-normal wage because of a presumed skill.

The supreme court in the *Farwell v. Boston and Worcester Railroad Corp.* ruling established two principles that would be used throughout the rest of the nineteenth century and into the beginning of the twentieth to deny redress to workers who were injured or poisoned on the job: first, that workers who took a job were freely entering a contract and thereby generally "assum[ed] its risks," and second, that injuries caused by the negligence of other workers, or "fellow servants," were not the corporation's fault. The development of an ostensibly free market of labor, in which there was an ostensible negotiation between the worker and the owner over the pay and conditions of employment, relieved the employer of any responsibility. It papered over the blatant inequalities of employer-employee relationships that drove the evolving industrial economy.[14]

Between the Civil War and World War I, the United States shifted from a largely agricultural society to the world's leading producer of coal, oil, steel, and railroad track, outstripping England, France, and Germany. Along with this expanding economic base came a transformation of the workforce. In 1870 there were over 6.8 million people who worked on farms and just over 6 million people who worked in nonfarm occupations. By the end of World War I, the farm labor force had grown to almost 11.5 million, whereas the nonfarm labor force had exploded to almost 31 million workers.[15] A largely agricultural, rural workforce, with a considerable number of autonomous skilled tradesmen and artisans in cities and towns, was turning increasingly into an urban workforce, often employed in factories whose management actively sought to undercut the autonomy of their employees. Manufacturing establishments were no longer under the control of a skilled worker or the artisan in his or her shop. Now, workers were more often unskilled or semiskilled and ignorant of the overall production process. The adoption of assembly lines, the division of work into simple repetitive tasks, speed-ups, increasing supervision of the work process, intensifying competitive pressures, and the exploitation of low-paid immigrant workers to undermine the native-born working population created a harsh and contentious environment. Workers were exposed to dangerous, largely unguarded machinery along with chemicals, dusts, heat, and fumes that caused a variety of diseases previously unknown and against which they had no ability to protect themselves.

LOCHNER V. NEW YORK: THE "RIGHT" TO WORK EIGHTEEN-HOUR DAYS

As a result, American workers in the post–Civil War period rose up to protest not just low wages but also unsafe and unhealthy working conditions, conditions that they could not ameliorate. Responding to these uprisings and to the development of labor organizations such as the Knights of Labor, the American Federation of Labor, and the Industrial Workers of the World, some state legislatures passed regulations that challenged the notion, established in the *Farwell* case, that individual workers were truly free to negotiate the terms of their employment and could therefore expect no protection from owners. For example, in the 1880s and 1890s a series of strikes took place in the bakeries of New York to protest the unhealthy conditions bakers endured during eighteen-hour workdays in hot, unventilated basements. In 1895 the New York State legislature responded by passing a law limiting bakery workers to no more than ten hours per day or sixty hours a week.[16]

In 1901, John Lochner, a bakery owner in upstate Oneida, was found in violation of this 1895 law. His employees successfully argued that they were required to work in the dark basement to make bread that would come out of the ovens in time for the morning rush. Lochner appealed his conviction with an argument that the state could not interfere with contracts "freely" entered into by his workers. The case eventually was heard by the U.S. Supreme Court.[17]

The Supreme Court took the opportunity to directly confront the question of whether state legislatures could regulate the hours and working conditions of workers in a "free labor" economy. The case, *Lochner v. New York* (1905), was decided in a 5–4 decision, with the Court determining that the state law protecting workers was unconstitutional because it interfered with the right of owners and workers to "purchase and sell labor."[18] Chattel slavery no longer existed, but the Court held that "free" laborers were "guaranteed" the "right" to work eighteen-hour days, and the state could not prevent them from doing so. In other words, because laborers made a contract with their owners, they forfeited any protection by the state. For industrial workers and their advocates, this "contract" was akin to what was now regularly called "wage slavery." Accidents on the job came to symbolize the huge costs borne by those employed in America's production system.[19]

In the post–Civil War era, the idea that managers and workers bargained equally with each other was a fiction but one that justified the new social order. An exception was made for working women. In the late nineteenth century, a number of states passed legislation limiting the hours that women could work in a day. For example, Ohio enacted a maximum ten-hour day for women in 1852. Minnesota, Massachusetts, and Illinois passed similar statutes after the Civil War. In 1885, Rhode Island passed a law limiting women's work to ten hours daily or sixty hours a week.[20] In 1896, the Pennsylvania superior court upheld a law limiting womens' work to twelve hours per day and a maximum of sixty hours per week. The common justification for these laws was laid out by the Pennsylvania superior court in 1896 and was based on a belief that women were a "weaker" sex and needed special protections: "Adult females are a class as distinct as minors, separated by natural conditions from all other laborers, and are so constituted as to be unable to endure physical exertion and exposure to the extent and degree that is not harmful to [male] workers." A second justification at the time was that women, as childbearers, were responsible for the future of the race and therefore constituted a special class that needed to be protected from the ravenous greed of their employers: "Surely an act which prevents the mothers of our race from being tempted to endanger their life and health by exhaustive employment can be condemned by none save those who expect to profit by it."[21]

The laws regulating the hours of work for women in the nineteenth century were the exception to the legal principles as laid out in *Lochner* that such laws were an "unnecessary and arbitrary interference with the right and liberty of the individual to contract in relation to labor."[22] As with *Farwell*, the courts reinforced the traditional master-servant relationship with new arguments not only rooted in feudal traditions but also now rendered in the language and ideology of individual freedom, the supposed equality between workers and managers to join in a mutually agreed-upon and freely established contractual relationship.

While legal scholars have struggled to impose logic on the Court's decision, at the time *Lochner* provided a usable fiction that legitimated the inequality intrinsic to master-servant—or, more politely, employer-laborer—relationships. Justice Rufus Peckham, writing for the majority in the 5–4 decision, claimed that the decision was a "victory" for workers because it upheld the employee's right "to earn the extra money which would arise from his working more than the prescribed time."[23]

In order to reach this conclusion, the Court made hair-splitting distinctions about the meaning of words. It said, in effect, that New York State's legislature did not mean what it wrote. The legislation had forbidden an owner to *require* a worker to labor more than ten hours. The Court interpreted this restriction as an unconstitutional impingement on the "right" of the worker to labor as long as they had contracted for. The New York State law was unconstitutional under the Fourteenth Amendment, which prohibited any state from making or enforcing "any law which shall abridge the privileges or immunities of citizens of the United States" and which also said that "any State [could not] deprive any person of life, liberty, or property, without due process of law." As this implication couldn't have been what the legislature intended, the Court maintained that it had really meant to use the term *permitted*, meaning that a worker could take on a long workday if he or she so chose. "There is nothing in any of the opinions delivered in this case," the Supreme Court argued, "which construes [that the legislature's regulation] in using the word 'required,' [w]as referring to any physical force being used to obtain the labor of an employee . . . [or] . . . that the statute was intended to meet a case of involuntary labor in any form." Hence, "there is no real distinction . . . between the words 'required' and 'permitted,'" because *required* meant being compelled through force: the Court thereby ignored other forms of coercion, such as the threat of being fired with no other means of support, as the Court's dissenters pointed out. Because laborers were "free" to quit, there was no reason to pass legislation to protect them.

The Court also rejected the argument that the state had a right to use its policing power to protect workers from threats to their health and welfare and that such threats were a legitimate basis for state intervention. A New York State appeals court had previously justified New York State's law in the *Lochner* case by arguing that the law could be sustained if the state was "able to say, from common knowledge that working in a bakery and candy factory was an unhealthy employment." The lower court had held that "the occupation of a baker or confectioner was unhealthy, and tended to result in diseases of the respiratory organs." Since this was the case, the state had the right to intervene and limit the hours and conditions of work, even if a worker "agreed" to stay on the job.[24]

The Supreme Court's majority rejected that argument. "There is . . . no reasonable foundation for holding this to be necessary or appropriate as a health law to safeguard the public or the health of the individuals who are following the trade of baker." Further, the diseases that the baker faced from an overheated, dusty atmosphere were no threat to the general public because the very conditions that made work so uncomfortable also provided protection to the general public. "Viewed in the light of a purely labor law, with no reference whatever to the question of health," the Supreme Court's majority said, "we think that [the condition of work in Lochner's bakery] involves neither the safety, the morals, nor the welfare of the public. . . . Clean and wholesome bread does not depend upon whether the baker works but ten hours per day or only sixty hours a week."[25]

THE SHIFTING CALCULUS OF INDUSTRIAL WORK AND HEALTH

By making *Lochner* a question of Fourteenth Amendment rights, the U.S. Supreme Court created a high bar before health would trump a worker's "power to contract . . . his own labor." And the Court decided that bakers had not jumped high enough: "We think that there can be no fair doubt that the trade of a baker [is] not an unhealthy one to that degree which would authorize the legislature to interfere with the right to labor . . . either as employer or employee." Statistics showed, the Court's majority wrote, that while "the trade of baker does not appear to be as healthy as some trades, [it] is vastly more healthy than still others." After all, "almost all occupations more or less affect the health," the Court admitted. But "some small amount of unhealthiness [cannot] warrant legislative interference with liberty."[26] If the negative impact on health were a reason to interfere with the work to be done, the Court predicted (or opined), the economy would come to a grinding halt: "No trade, no occupation, no mode of earning a living could escape this all-pervading power [to regulate]."[27] In the fictional world of the U.S. Supreme Court's majority, a laborer and an employer were on a level playing field, each able to negotiate the terms of their "free market" exchange of services, time, labor, *and health* for wages.[28]

Such a narrow interpretation of constitutional law ignored the transformation overtaking working conditions in the new industries of the nation. As Justice John Marshall Harlan argued in his dissent from the *Lochner* decision in 1905, "the police power of the State" had "doubtless been greatly expanded . . . during the past century owing to the enormous increase in the number of occupations which are danger- ous, or so far detrimental to the health of the employees as to demand special precautions for their well-being and protection." And while "the police power cannot be put forward as an excuse for oppressive and unjust legislation it may be resorted to for the purpose of preserving public health, safety or morals, or the abatement of public nuisance."[29]

The question was, how to decide when that power was oppressive and unjust? A series of Supreme Court decisions in the late nineteenth and early twentieth centuries sought to define this boundary. *Lochner v. New York*, *Holden v. Hardy*, and *Muller v. Oregon* were all cases brought to the Supreme Court in a brief period between 1898 and 1908. They addressed the question of how much was too much when it came to the sacrifice that miners, bakers, women, and children, among others—the workforce—would be forced to bear. In the case of *Lochner*, the health of the worker and his or her family were clearly to be sacrificed for the "good" of an economic system dependent on their coerced labor and should not be protected by the state: "It is unfortunately true that labor, even in any department, may possibly carry with it the seeds of unhealthiness. But are we all, on that account, at the mercy of legislative majorities? . . . No trade, no occupation, no mode of earning one's living, could escape this all-pervading power, and the acts of the legislature in limiting the hours of labor in all employments would be valid, although such limitation might seriously cripple the ability of the laborer to support himself and his family."[30] In his dissent, Justice Harlan, speaking for the four justices in the minority, pointed to the long list of court decisions that upheld the right of state legislatures to use their police and regulatory powers to protect "life, health, and property." Harlan was referring to the 1898 Supreme Court decision in *Holden v. Hardy* in which a Utah law limiting the hours of work of miners and smelters was upheld because of the highly injurious nature of the work. The Supreme Court was willing to acknowledge that there were exceptional circumstances in which work was so dangerous that the state had a right to intervene. Indeed, just three years after *Lochner*, in 1908 in *Muller v. Oregon*, the Supreme Court unanimously upheld an Oregon law that limited women who worked in factories and laundries to ten hours of work per day. It did so because it believed that the state had a legitimate interest in protecting women specifically because of their physical differences from men, and also because of the importance of protecting "the performance of maternal functions."[31]

In his dissent in the *Lochner* case, Harlan outlined the dramatic industrial transformations that had overtaken the country during the preceding few decades and the parallel increase in the number of dangerous trades. The state, he explained, had therefore increased the scope of its oversight to keep up with these broader transformations: government "has doubtless been greatly expanded in its application during the past century owing to an enormous increase in the number of occupations which are dangerous, or so far detrimental to the health of the employees as to demand special precautions for their wellbeing and protection." While the state could not legally enact oppressive measures, "it may be lawfully resorted to for the purpose of preserving the public health, safety or morals, or the abatement of public nuisances."[32]

Harlan was even more pointed in recognizing the ways in which the Court's decision in *Lochner* was a tool for maintaining traditional power relationships between master and servant, employer and worker. He pointed out that the original New York State law limiting bakery workers' hours "was enacted in order to protect the physical wellbeing of those who work in bakery and confectionary establishments. It may be that the statute had its origins, in part, in the belief that employers and employees . . . were not on an equal footing, and that the necessities of the latter often compelled them to submit to such exactions as unduly taxed their strength."

Supreme Court justice Oliver Wendell Holmes Jr.'s dissent also provided a telling critique of the Court's majority decision. He pointed out that the Court had essentially endorsed laissez-faire economic doctrine, giving enormous power to the already powerful. The case, he argued, was "decided upon an economic theory, which a large part of the country does not share." Further, the Constitution "is not intended to embody a particular economic theory, whether of paternalism . . . or of *laissez-faire.*" The legislature of New York, perhaps reflecting the growing unrest among the state's workforce in general and its bakers in particular, had seen fit to limit the hours of labor and improve the conditions of work. The Court had no right to countermand New York legislators' judgment that the work was too dangerous. Holmes took issue with the notion that the Fourteenth Amendment was in any way an endorsement of "Mr. Herbert Spencer's *Social Statics*," a reference to the British sociologist and philosopher's 1851 book, which contained the genesis for his later ideas that the government should not act to interfere with the economy or act to help those in need in society because doing so would disrupt what he claimed was the natural evolution of the social order based on "survival of the fittest."[33] The Fourteenth Amendment, a document born of the Civil War and meant to protect Black freedmen from infringements on their civil rights or their reenslavement by the southern states, was now being used by the Court's majority as a tool to extend wage slavery among predominantly white workers in the North and as a means of, in effect, permitting the further occurrence of sometimes horrible injuries and debilitating health for those same workers. For Holmes and Harlan, state governments should have the power to protect the public's health, but it would be several more decades before the Supreme Court agreed that states and the federal government did indeed have that power.

The doctrines of "assumed risk"—that the employee, by taking the job, had assumed the risks inherent in it—and "fellow servant"—that mistakes of others on the job were not the responsibility of the employer but of the fellow workers involved—dominated nineteenth-century legal decisions and largely led to judgments that favored employers and corporations rather than workers when they suffered injury or death. By the end of the nineteenth century, however, the doctrines of assumed risk and fellow servant were beginning to lose their sway with juries, who were learning of and witnessing the injuries resulting from a growing number of industrial accidents and deaths in the factories, railroads, mines, and mills of the nation. Further, as the historian Melvin Urofsky noted, by 1906 twenty-five states had either abolished the fellow-servant rule or had modified it significantly.[34] Only with the passage of workers' compensation legislation in the second decade of the twentieth century were decisions about workers' injuries taken out of the courts and placed in the hands of administrative bodies that were not required to determine responsibility, only that an injury had occurred and was job-related. While the system provided relatively fast compensation to injured workers, the amounts awarded were small, and ultimately the process itself protected companies from potentially huge verdicts.

As noted earlier, the application of the doctrines of assumed risk had never been total, especially when it came to women and children. As a result of *Muller*, in which the Supreme Court upheld Oregon's protective legislation for women, and despite the "free labor" ideology of *Lochner*, by the start of World War I twenty-seven states were regulating some aspect of women's working conditions. "Six states had an eight-hour day and a forty-hour week for most women. Thirteen states limited the work week to fifty-four hours with no more than nine hours per working day," summarizes Alice Kessler-Harris. But even these laws were limited in their scope, she has shown, excluding from protection women agricultural and domestic workers, many of whom were women of color: those who were the most exploited and paid the least. Further, protective legislation generally excluded women from higher-paying jobs, specifically night work (where the wages were generally better and the hours shorter). Women printers, for example, were generally unable to get work because newspapers were printed at night when women were restricted from working.[35] Protective legislation also divided workers by gender, which in itself weakened the power of the labor movement. Creating women as a separate class, however, did promote awareness of the deteriorating conditions of industrial work and the need for legislation to protect men as well, although legislation to that effect would not occur for another two decades.[36]

If the courts in decisions like *Farwell* and *Lochner* tried to enshrine inequality under the guise of nominal market equality in exchanges between employees and employers, other forces were also at work to challenge this formulation. For one thing, as we have seen, courts presumably would allow consideration of the potential effect on the general public's health. Thus protecting the public's health was one wedge of reform. In addition, because industrialization came with mechanization, speed-ups, massive factories, and other changes that increased the dangers that workers faced on the job, one could argue that workers could not secure their own safety and therefore needed protection. Skilled workers, for example, could no longer depend on the knowledge and skills they had acquired in the production of shoes and clothing or cast iron stoves to protect themselves from injury and death. Dangerous machinery and the introduction of toxic new chemicals and high-powered pneumatic chisels, drills, and sandblasters created life-threatening dusts that sapped the health and strength of the workforce.Individual workers could not protect themselves from these dangers.

The toll of accidents at the turn of the twentieth century is one way to gauge the impact that America's industrialization of work was having on its workforce and its health. Frederick Hoffman of the Prudential Life Insurance Company estimated that 25,000 workers died on the job in 1908 alone, but Mark Aldrich, author of *Safety First*, cautions that Hoffman had "advanced [this number] as little better than a guess, for no comprehensive, accurate statistics existed." Aldrich estimates that between 1890 and 1900 over 11,000 workers died mining coal in the country, a rate that was at least twice that of England. Between 1885 and 1907, exploding boilers killed 7,000 workers in the United States but only 700 in Great Britain. Charles P. Neill, the first U.S. commissioner of labor statistics, declared in 1913 that America's industries were the most dangerous in the world. He told the National Safety Council that the country was the leader in the "maiming and mangling and killing of those who attempt to earn their bread."[37] Overall, in the early twentieth century, one estimate is that nationally there were 35,000 job-related deaths every year and 2 million injuries, of which 500,000 were severe enough to cause workers to miss work for at least a week.[38]

In the wake of such injuries and fatalities year after year, combined with low wages and long hours that left workers susceptible to injury, unions began to fight for safer working conditions, better pay, and shorter hours. The movements for shorter workdays began in the early to mid-1800s with agitation for, first, the ten-hour day and then, in the late 1800s, the eight-hour day, perhaps most famously by those who led the demonstration in Chicago that became known as the Haymarket Riots. But reform was uneven and often gendered. As Kessler-Harris relates, "by the 1890s cigar makers, builders and machinists regularly worked only fifty hours a week but there were precious few women among them." Those who worked in textile and garment factories and those who worked in laundries, "all heavily women-employing, still averaged twelve-hour days, and five-and-a-half or six-day weeks," between sixty-six and seventy-two hours a week.[39]

The fight for better wages was tied to better health. As Theda Skocpol relates:

> Minimum wages became a central demand for labor, rationalized as a means of both providing better income but also to improve the health of workers and their families. [In 1912] [s]ocial reformer Florence Kelley pointed to the health benefits that higher wages would provide: "Tuberculosis can be warded off when wage-workers can more universally afford a nutritious dietary, and the tuberculosis crusade may thus become a less hopeless undertaking. Those cases of insanity which arise from worry over insufficient wages combined with physical depletion due to a too low standard of living may reasonably be expected to diminish when wages are rationalized. And the same reasoning applies in great measure to alcoholism among wage earners."[40]

The American Federation of Labor, newly formed in 1886, made health insurance, work conditions, and wages central demands in its negotiations with management. Further, immigrant workers organized fraternal societies that provided "contract doctors," physicians who for a small sum per person would provide medical services to particular groups, and they arranged for burial benefits for breadwinners who died from accidents on the job. Basic reforms such as Social Security, minimum wages, and limits on hours would await the New Deal. It would not be until 1938 that the Fair Labor Standards Act established an eight-hour workday, a forty-four-hour workweek, and a minimum wage. Labor and social reformers had been pushing for these reforms since the late nineteenth century, but their progress had been stymied by the argument that such laws infringed "on rights of free contract."[41]

The growing attention to working-class life and labor in national magazines and among social reformers in late-nineteenth-century America was, in no small measure, a response to the dramatically changing economics of the time. The economic historian Thomas Piketty has detailed the flesh-and-blood meaning of the growing inequality in his massive, definitive economic history, *Capital in the Twenty-First Century*.[42] He sees the changing distribution of wealth as part of a larger story of the social, political, and economic history of nations (specifically, the United States, Britain, and France) during this period. Despite the enormous leap in production and wealth in the late nineteenth century in the industrializing world, Piketty points out, "workers' wages stagnated at very low levels" during those years. Those wages were "close or even inferior to the levels of the eighteenth and previous centuries."[43] While the banker and financier J. P. Morgan lived in a mansion of forty-five rooms, including twelve bathrooms, on Madison Avenue in New York in the 1890s, the housing of Polish, Russian, and Italian immigrants as well as African American residents of the city's Lower East Side was essentially unlivable, as Jacob Riis vividly described in *How the Other Half Lives* (1890): "Crazy old buildings, crowded rear tenements in filthy yards, dark, damp basements, leaking garrets, shops, outhouses and stables converted into dwellings, though scarcely fit to shelter brutes, are habitations for thousands of our fellow beings in this wealthy, Christian city."[44]

How did one explain and justify the obvious inequalities in wealth, income, and power and consequently health that marked the relationship between owners of capital and those they worked often to exhaustion, sometimes to death?[45] Some industrialists like Andrew Carnegie, who had sponsored Herbert Spencer's tour of the country promoting social Darwinism, thought that the "success" of the wealthy was a result of their own hard work and intelligence and argued that the fate of those at the bottom was to be found in their own personal failings. Progressive labor activists, reformers, and radicals of all stripes saw instead injustices that demanded attention. The existence of rampant injustices provided the basis for their broad critique of industrial capitalism's impact on democracy and the lives of working people both inside and outside the factory system. It was obvious to reformers and workers themselves that there was nothing inevitable about most accidents and many other harms; they arose from specific decisions by factory owners and others to construct the world most conducive to their own profits. As we will detail in the next chapter, the harms also resulted from the economic power of corporations to shape the economy and often the police powers of the state.

In the first few decades of the twentieth century, injuries on the job came to embody the imbalances of power and control in the developing economy, and debates about responsibility and liability for those injuries went to the heart of industrial capitalism. In the face of the huge increase in unskilled factory employment and the efforts by factory owners to streamline production at the expense of workers' control and workers' lives, the logic underlying the 1905 *Lochner* decision began to dissipate. Juries, despite the legal doctrines of fellow servant and assumed risk that had shielded industries from painful verdicts in much of the nineteenth century, even began to side with workers in lawsuits against owners who claimed no responsibility for the death or injuries of the worker.[46] Jury members often knew all too well the terrible conditions that existed inside the huge factories where they or someone in their family toiled.[47] If they themselves had not experienced assembly-line speed-ups, or witnessed a railroad accident or mine explosion, they learned of them from journalists, who provided graphic descriptions of the maiming and killing of workers in many industries.

Journalists increasingly reported on labor activism throughout the country. In 1892 the Amalgamated Association of Iron and Steel Workers in Homestead, Pennsylvania, went on strike against the Carnegie Steel Company and were brutally repressed. Lead miners in Colorado also struck in 1903–1904, as did coal miners in West Virginia in 1912–1913. Organizing drives in Chicago were shut done by National Guardsmen in 1886; Pinkertons hunted down the Molly McGuires in Pennsylvania in the period between 1862 and 1876. Workers went on strike against the Pullman Company in 1894, as did mill workers and lumberjacks in Minnesota in 1916–1917. Journalists from the Hearst newspapers, the "yellow press," reported on the jaw-dropping murders of strike leaders, as did reporters in the morning and afternoon editions of newspapers throughout the country. There were newspapers in English, Italian, Yiddish, Czech, Polish, and Hungarian, along with other immigrant languages, that informed readers in New York, Boston, Chicago, San Francisco, and many other cities of various labor activities in the last decades of the nineteenth and first decades of the twentieth centuries. Muckrakers wrote about what one journalist called the "Death Toll of Industry." Socialists published the "Death Calendar in Industry" detailing daily deaths in the Pittsburgh mills, and they wrote books like *Work-Accidents and the Law* (see figure 4.1), in which they described the horrendous cost of the new industrial world that capitalists had created.[48]

Given that the law was not supporting efforts to create a safer industrial world, workers, both men and women, in industries as varied as bakers, needle trades, and steel mills, went out on strike for wages, hours, and working conditions in these same decades. In May 1909, 3,000 Jewish bakers struck, and less than a year later 4,000 German bakers followed suit.[49] The bakers' union identified unsanitary workshops and the spread of infectious disease with nonunion bakeries. They insisted "on proper ventilation and sanitary conditions" and demanded that "the great bread eating public of this country should see to it that the bread they eat bears the bakers' union label."[50] Their ability to link unsanitary working conditions to the health of the public gave their strike tremendous appeal and power.

The prevalence of contagious diseases such as diphtheria, influenza, tuberculosis, and typhoid spurred consumer groups to take up the issue of health conditions on the job as well as in the home. In part, their appeal was prompted by fear that the middle class and wealthy might be infected by goods tainted by sick workers. In the growing garment industry of New York, for example, many dresses, shirts, and trousers were sewn on a piecework basis in tenement slums, raising the specter that the same diseases infecting those in tenements would be transmitted to the men, women, and children of the middle class.

It was this terror that led the National Consumers League, the organization founded in 1899 by Jane Addams and initially led by Florence Kelley, to mobilize consumers to use their purchasing power to pressure employers to improve conditions for workers. The league became

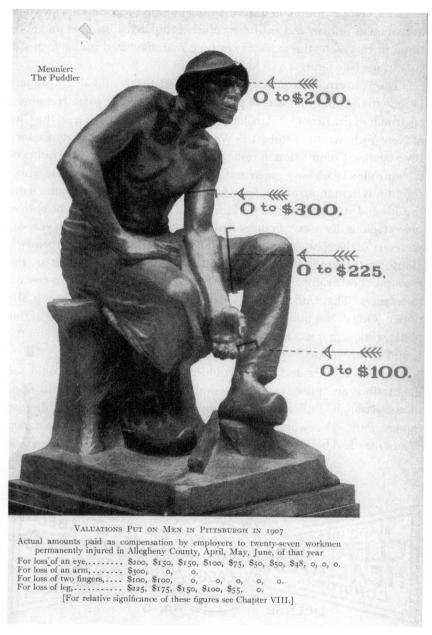

Meunier:
The Puddler

O to $200.

O to $300.

O to $225.

O to $100.

VALUATIONS PUT ON MEN IN PITTSBURGH IN 1907

Actual amounts paid as compensation by employers to twenty-seven workmen
permanently injured in Allegheny County, April, May, June, of that year

For loss of an eye,........ $200, $150, $150, $100, $75, $50, $50, $48, 0, 0, 0.
For loss of an arm,........ $300, 0, 0.
For loss of two fingers,.... $100, $100, 0, 0, 0, 0, 0.
For loss of leg,........... $225, $175, $150, $100, $55, 0.

[For relative significance of these figures see Chapter VIII.]

FIGURE 4.1 "Valuations Put on Men in Pittsburgh in 1907," illustration in Chrystal
Eastman, *Work-Accidents and the Law* (New York: Russell Sage, 1910), 126.

involved in a wide variety of labor-related issues, including fire safety, workers' compensation, and occupational disease legislation, as well as in tenement reform and antituberculosis campaigns. Its label on goods came to represent the mark of clothing manufactured under hygienic conditions (see figure 4.2).[51]

The concern with public health also led the National Consumers League to confront the issue of piecework in tenements. Mary H. Loines, chairman of the Brooklyn Auxiliary of the Consumers League of the City of New York, wrote to Robert F. Wagner of the New York State Factory Investigating Commission in 1912 that work at home led to "long hours of uncontrolled labor for women and little children—often under far worse conditions than those of regulated factories." This in turn undermined the "health and strength" of the workforce and therefore spurred the spread of contagious diseases.[52] Frances Perkins, who had served for two years as secretary of the New York City Consumers League as well as at Greenwich House Settlement, in 1913 condemned the system of home work as "the most practical example which we have of the ability of industry to enslave its workers." That work also had a deleterious effect on public health, she noted: "One of the things which I noticed in regard to the system of this home work is that it is a menace to the health of the community and the health of the worker."[53]

If New Yorkers and others could not read, in 1911 they could see illustrations and photographs of women jumping from the ninth floor of the Triangle Building in downtown Manhattan near Washington Square Park. The women had been locked in a burning sweatshop where they had been sewing blouses, then called shirtwaists. Reporters,

FIGURE 4.2 National Consumers League label (1913).

photographers, and graphic artists documented how women, faced with the prospect of being burned alive, chose to jump to their deaths from a factory whose owner had locked exit doors. Out of these striking images and reports of industrial workplace horrors arose further reform efforts.[54] Alice Hamilton, Eleanor Roosevelt, and Frances Perkins, as well as a number of other women reformers who are remembered more often for their roles in the New Deal and after, emerged from this earlier period dedicated to addressing the terrible conditions of work and life for the industrial workforce, both female and male, child and adult.

Muckrakers, reformers, socialists, and enlightened capitalists wrote of conditions in the stockyards of Chicago, the steel mills of Pittsburgh, and the foundries of Detroit. Politicians and industrialists promoted a workers' accident compensation system, thereby acknowledging the ubiquity of dangers in the new industrial workplace and the threat that breadwinners' injuries posed to the families that were dependent on their wages and ultimately social order. Upton Sinclair's *The Jungle*, published in 1906, is generally remembered for its role in the development of consumer protection of the food supply and the passage of the 1906 Pure Food and Drug Act. In it he describes workers falling into vats and coming out as Durham's Pure Leaf Lard, of rotting meat mixed in with the entrails of dead cows and even rats to create sausage. The novel also depicts the horrifying conditions of life and work in Chicago's meatpacking industry more generally. Sinclair told the story of how Jurgis Rudkis, a vibrant, strong Lithuanian immigrant worker, was destroyed in body and soul by the production process and capitalism itself. As Sinclair later wrote: "I aimed at the public's heart, and by accident I hit it in the stomach."[55]

In some cities, residents, among them bakers and cloakmakers, could walk down the street and hear Socialist orators like "Golden Tongue" Baruch Vladeck, a leader in the Socialist Party, or Joseph Barondess of the Cloakmakers Union in New York admonishing members at times to walk off their jobs and at other times not to.[56] Social workers from Henry Street, Hull House, and other settlement houses in the heart of immigrant and working-class neighborhoods in New York, Chicago, Boston, and elsewhere regularly publicized that they were there to aid the victims of a new industrial state that was forcing people into poverty and wretchedness. Jane Addams, Florence Kelley, and Alice Hamilton agitated for children who needed protection from long hours in factories or from the lead pigment manufacturers whose poisons stunted their mental ability and growth and shortened their lives. In New York State, a Factory Investigating Commission, of which Frances Perkins was a member, did studies that led to fire and building codes to prevent disasters like the Triangle Fire.

In 1891, the Massachusetts Bureau of Statistics of Labor identified the two prevalent approaches to the regulation of work.[57] "In the first case the principle of *laissez faire* has ruled; in the other the principle of State regulation of the employment of labor has prevailed." But, contrary to some who saw these approaches in conflict, the authors of the 1891 report argued that they "were mutually dependent." "Unrestricted competition . . . necessitated governmental interference with individual action." It was no longer simply Christian charity that led to the need for the state to intercede and play a more active role in controlling forces that had been released.[58] Government had to intervene in laissez-faire capitalism because "the preservation of society demanded the establishment of rules under which the new relations between the employer and the employed might continue."[59]

The authors of the report gave a trenchant analysis of the political tensions that the growing power of large corporations had wrought in nineteenth-century America. Business leaders objected that new labor legislation represented "State paternalism, [and] interference on the part of the State with the so-called freedom of contract." But, the report countered,

> such legislation is identical in character with statutes which aim to establish and maintain favorable moral and sanitary conditions in society. It is perfectly true that men cannot be legislated into health or happiness, but it is also true that the social conditions surrounding them have much to do with their mental, moral, and physical development. If it is proper to guard against the maintenance of nuisances which may endanger the health of a community, it would seem equally proper to guard against such industrial conditions as tend either to illiteracy, physical degeneracy, crime, or pauperism; and labor legislation as a rule has had no other object. Indeed, this seems at last to be generally recognized.[60]

Given the long history of government resistance to the enactment of laws protecting workers, it is remarkable that this broad historical analysis came from government officials focused on the experience of workers—not social elites, moralists, or charity workers—in the new industrial state. The report recognized that shorter hours, better pay, and improved working conditions were essential for improving the health, not only of the workers themselves, but also of their families. Perhaps all the efforts at reform had made clear that protecting workers would be good for everyone, or at least would prevent strikes and other forms of rebellion. "The modern industrial world is so closely bound together that the common welfare depends in no slight degree upon the similarity of the conditions under which production is carried on in different communities."[61] It was necessary to establish "rules" that "experience has shown to be necessary,"[62] and such "experience" included not only horrible conditions at work but also an increasing number of violent strikes that spread across the United States in the last third of the nineteenth century and after.

Concerted efforts to reform labor practices, including legal reform, did result in significant changes and improvements in health. States across the industrial North and Midwest enacted various reforms in the closing decades of the nineteenth century and first decades of the twentieth century. Perhaps the most widely adopted were workers' compensation laws. In 1900 no state in the nation had a workers' compensation law on the books, but, as discussed earlier, by 1915 most highly industrialized states had passed an act for some form of workers' compensation aimed at quelling some of the most obvious economic damage that families faced when the breadwinner was laid up because of an industrial injury.[63]

On the federal level, in 1913 Congress established the Department of Labor, which included active women's and children's bureaus devoted to protecting their lives and health. In addition, in 1912 the Public Health Service was empowered to address occupation-related diseases.[64] The advent of World War I made occupational safety and health a national priority as business, political, and labor leaders emphasized the need to protect the workforce, especially in war-related industries. This emphasis led to legislation that gave authority to the Public Health Service to protect the health of laborers in plants with government contracts.

The concern with the unknown effects of new toxic chemicals such as TNT and picric acid made the Public Health Service, with its established laboratory and technical expertise, the locus of authority.

As we have seen, the transformation of American society in the decades following the Civil War was profound. From an overwhelmingly rural, agricultural society in 1860, it became one of the world's leading industrial powers. The infectious diseases that wracked the growing cities and slums in the middle decades of the century were slowly being addressed by the building of aqueducts and laying of pipes to bring pure water, as well as by the introduction of sewer lines, indoor plumbing, and improved sanitation. The infectious diseases of the middle decades declined, giving way to new diseases created by the evolving industrial economy.

The unsafe conditions created by corporate capitalism remained to be addressed. Late in the nineteenth century, demands by labor in the form of strikes and other actions resulted in the passage of laws that greatly improved working conditions. Union negotiations and state legislation resulted in better wages, and shorter hours gave workers more time at home to recuperate. These victories lowered accident rates in some industries. But, as we will see in the next chapter, the world created by the new industrial economy would employ processes, materials, and products that would cause disabling injuries, new diseases, and new risks to health. Americans would learn of disfiguring diseases, some acute and some chronic. Phossy jaw, lead poisoning, silicosis, asbestosis, radium poisoning, and the like would begin to make headlines. As always in our history, there would be a fight to limit the effects of speed-ups, assembly-line production, and other tools of industrialists who were more interested in profit than in health.

CHAPTER FIVE

Gasping for Breath

Creating New Diseases and Inequalities

"The gums become swollen and purple, the teeth loosen and drop out, and the jawbones slowly decompose and pass away in the form of nauseating pus."

CONGRESSMAN JOHN ESCH (R-WI), 1912

In mid-nineteenth-century Britain, a simple invention—a short wooden stick with a blob of highly flammable white phosphorous at its tip—stimulated the marketing of the "cigarette," or shredded tobacco wrapped in paper, which is arguably responsible for the worst epidemic of disease in modern history. (The historian Allan Brandt credits the cigarette's growing popularity to the development of the automatic cigarette rolling machine in the late nineteenth century.) Soon a booming cigarette industry was established along with a matchstick industry that employed thousands of very poor workers, mostly young women, working for ten hours a day to cut the sticks, dip their tips in phosphorous, and pack them in boxes to be sold alongside packs of cigarettes to the growing number of smokers. With little protection and with great danger, these young women and some men breathed in or ingested the deadly phosphorus material. After repeated exposure over several years, this work resulted in "phossy jaw," a disfiguring disease of the face in which the jaws and their bony structures dissolved, leaving its victims disfigured and unable to eat; the disease often ended in death. The growth of the tobacco and match industries would, in coming decades, create twin public health disasters: the "phossy jaw" scandal and, later, a lung cancer epidemic among consumers that has cost millions their lives from the mid-twentieth century to today.

The story of these two diseases of human creation began in 1888 with the dismissal of a young woman by Bryant & May, one of the nineteenth century's match companies, for having taken too long a break. The dismissal sparked the anger of fifteen hundred coworkers, who went on strike to support the dismissed worker and to protest low wages and the working conditions that required them to stand on an assembly line hour after hour while dipping the ends of sticks into the toxic phosphorous. The strike resulted in a journalist bringing phossy jaw and the horrifying conditions of work at the company's factory to the attention of the public and politicians. Soon the disease became a symbol of the terrible price in human lives that was fueling modern capitalism.[1]

In some respects, the strike at Bryant & May began as a traditional job action over wages and control of the workplace (see figure 5.1). But it soon became a strike about the horrifying reality of the disease to which workers were susceptible because they were exposed to the phosphorous in the company's product, "Lucifer Matches."

Other scandals followed about the conditions in the workplace that led to the disfigurement of the young women, and eventually Parliament initiated an investigation, led by the renowned British occupational health physician Sir Thomas Oliver, who, in 1899, produced *Reports . . . on the Use of Phosphorus in the Manufacture of Lucifer Matches*.[2] Oliver concluded that if companies were to continue to use white phosphorus, "men and women should not be allowed to remain more than a few weeks at a time in any one department."[3] But he also recognized that the young girls' social position or class had a major impact on why they were so ravaged by the white phosphorus. "Girls born and bred in the slums of our large cities, reared upon improper and insufficient food, anaemic, undergrown, and ill-clad," were especially vulnerable to its devastating effects; they were sometimes affected in a matter of months and sometimes over the course of several years.[4]

After Bryant & May declared bankruptcy in the 1890s, the American Diamond Match Company acquired the company and its patents and brought the technologies to the United States.[5] As reports of

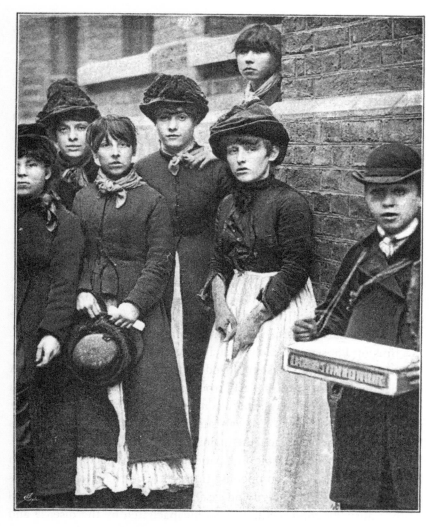

MEMBERS OF THE MATCHMAKERS' UNION

FIGURE 5.1 Young girls in the match girls' strike, London, 1888.

disfigured and dying young women and men flooded the newspapers, newspaper and magazine columnists and editorial writers took note of the huge cost in human suffering that accompanied the expansion of the American match industry. Voices from within labor, reform groups, and even congressmen demanded regulations to limit the use of white phosphorous in match factories.[6] With the development of phossy jaw, "the gums become swollen and purple, the teeth loosen and drop out, and the jawbones slowly decompose and pass away in the form of nauseating pus," Congressman John Esch (R. WI) graphically explained.[7] One 1912 article in an Oklahoma newspaper claimed that a harmless substitute for phosphorus could be used but wasn't because it cost 6 percent more. Greed, then, was the central reason lives were being destroyed, and reform was, as the headline blared, "DEMANDED BY HUMANITY."[8] Meetings were held in which doctors reported that they "had removed the lower jaw bone of six patients and the upper jaw bones of three patients," and "in numerous other cases parts of the jaw bones were removed."[9]

Diamond Company executives drew praise from some local doctors and newspaper editorialists for their efforts to keep their workers safe from phosphorous poisoning by employing a dentist to check employees' teeth and gums. But labor advocates did not believe that such efforts addressed the real problem: the use of phosphorus in the first place.[10] *Labor World* in Duluth, Minnesota, under the headline "Victims of 'Phossy Jaw' Help Match Trust Pile Up Millions," told the story of "Mr. H.," who was employed in a Wisconsin match factory. A married man of forty-six, he "had trouble with his teeth" and went to a dentist, who diagnosed *phosphorous necrosis*, the more formal term for phossy jaw. Referred to a Chicago surgeon, the match worker had his "upper and lower Maxillae" (the major jaw bones in the face) removed. While on the operating table "the patient swallowed his tongue," which led the surgeon to "cut an opening through his throat" to prevent his suffocating. In another horrifying case, "Little Anna M . . . a healthy girl [with] unusually good teeth," was so incapacitated by the disease and ensuing operations that, incapable of swallowing, "she slowly starved to death." As John B. Andrews of the American Association for Labor Legislation and others continually pointed out, the disease was produced by the greed of the match companies, in this case the Diamond Match Company.[11] In the absence of legislative ability to ban or control private industry directly, Congress passed the Esch Act, the White Phosphorus Match Act of 1912, subsequently signed by President William Howard Taft, which imposed a tax on the use of white phosphorous in matches, thereby discouraging its use by increasing its costs to Diamond and other match manufacturers. That legislation resulted in development of the modern-day "safety match," which avoided the use of white phosphorous in the head and used red phosphorus, a less damaging variant, on the striking surface of the box.[12]

THE STRUGGLE OVER THE FACTORY

The struggle over the ravages of phossy jaw revealed the increasing power of giant corporations and their ability to shape the lives and deaths of working people. In the decades following the Civil War, a greater and greater percentage of the wealth of the country was concentrated in the new captains of industry, including steel baron Andrew Carnegie, oil magnate John D. Rockefeller, and railroad tycoon Cornelius Vanderbilt, who ruled over increasingly large corporations. By 1910 the top 10 percent of the population was getting over 40 percent of the total annual income and controlled over 80 percent of the wealth, up from about 58 percent of the wealth one hundred years before.[13] Rich and poor, North and South, urban and rural—social and economic divisions became more and more apparent throughout the country, no more so than between workers and owners in the urbanizing East and Midwest. These divisions also increased disparities in the health of Americans, and as the country's industrial economy developed, new diseases grew in prominence, exacerbated by increases in the speed, intensity, and dangers of the industrial workplace.

As we have seen, by the end of the nineteenth century it was impossible to ignore the abject poverty of so many people living in close quarters in substandard housing in America's rapidly expanding industrial cities.[14] And, while mortality rates were generally improving nationwide as sanitarians, public health workers, and, to a degree, physicians were cleaning up the city, providing families with access to pure milk and fresh food, and developing housing codes that provided fresh air in tenements, certain groups experienced a decline in their health and an increased mortality from accidents and disease associated with the new industrial order.[15] The new industrial workplace exposed millions of Americans to the dust created by high-speed drills and power tools such as sandblasters. Minerals such as lead, used in mass-produced products like lead paint and ultimately in gasoline, produced epidemics rarely seen before or much more prevalent and devastating for much larger portions of the population. Silicosis, asbestosis, childhood lead poisoning, and chronic diseases of long latency joined phossy jaw in a parade of new conditions created by the industrial environment. Long-term disease joined accidents as a plague for the industrial worker.

Accidents, particularly in the mines, were the most immediate symptom of the country's rush to industrial might. On June 17, 1890, 30 miners lost their lives in an explosion at the Dunbar Furnace Company's Hill Farm Mine in Connesville, Pennsylvania; the next year, in Pratt City, Alabama, a mine explosion in the No. 1 Shaft killed 11 miners, including 10 convicts (both white and African American) who were leased to the company under the state's convict lease system; two years later, 100 men died in an explosion in Krebs, Oklahoma. The turn of the century did not lead to lower accident rates. In 1902, 216 miners died in Fraterville, Tennessee, and two years later another 179 men died in Harwick, Pennsylvania. And the beat continued. In 1905, 112 died in a mine explosion in Virginia City, Alabama; and, in 1907, in Monongah, West Virginia, estimates of the dead varied from a low of 362 to over 500, which is widely considered to be the worst mine disaster in U.S. history. The explosions, fires, cave-ins, rock slides, runaway carts, and snapped ropes continued through the first decade of the century as 239 died in Pennsylvania (1907); 57 in Birmingham, Alabama (1907); and 259, including children, in Cherry, Illinois (1909). In 1911 in the Banner Mine in Littleton, Alabama, 128 convict laborers, almost all of them African American, died.[16]

The Monongah mine disaster killed both women and children as well as men: miners, paid by the load, regularly brought their families into the mine to help with loading coal ingots in the carriages that brought the coal to the surface. Because of poor ventilation and the use of explosives and water-driven drills, huge amounts of coal dust and methane gas were poured into the air of the mine, setting off an explosion that instantly killed most of the miners. The timbers that supported the roof of the mineshaft were blown out as well, killing those not immediately killed by the explosion. Others were suffocated by "blackdamp," a gas composed of CO_2 and nitrogen. The victims were largely immigrant workers—Italians, Poles, Czechs, Slovaks, Russians, Hungarians, and Ukrainians.[17] At the time, most of the news stories blamed the workers for the disasters, but mine owners here and elsewhere did not use safety precautions that were already in use in Europe. There miners were given shielded lamps instead of open candles, provided with controllable explosives rather than cheap dynamite, and required to conduct tests that could detect explosive methane gas.

The mechanization of work and the migration of millions of people from rural parts of the country and Europe to the growing industrial cities and rural mining communities presented new challenges as the country began to deal with chronic conditions previously unknown to many. William Attaway, in *Blood on the Forge* (1941)—his proletarian novel about race, ecology, and human-made destruction caused by early-twentieth-century capitalism—recounts his own experience as part of a Black family traveling from rural Kentucky to the steel mills around Pittsburgh. In his novel-cum-biographical-portrait, the hardships of sharecropping and rural poverty are replaced with the harsh realities of the steel mill, where he experienced the physical pain and personal humiliation of foremen who, like the white overseers he escaped back in Kentucky, forced him into hot, body- and soul-destroying work shoveling "slag," waste that fell below the ovens where the metal was melted and poured into casts. In the shadow of the mill's polluting smokestacks, soot of various chemical combinations burned the lungs of every living thing. Both humans and the natural environment were sacrificed. Pollution, dirt and dust, disease and disability—all produced by the industrial plants of the growing industrial cities—defiled everything.[18]

The work of chimney sweeps and lead miners, among others, had long been identified as especially hazardous. Bernardo Ramazzini, the Italian physician and author of *De Morbis Artificum Diatriba* (Diseases of Workers) (1713), and Charles Thackrah, the nineteenth-century British surgeon and author of *The Effects of Arts, Trades and Professions on Health and Longevity* (1832)—both identified as "fathers" of industrial medicine—documented many such workplace dangers.[19] But most of what they identified as problems were acute conditions whose injuries and symptoms appeared relatively soon after a specific event or exposure. Certainly, it was known that miners often developed lung problems and even lead poisoning, chronic conditions that might often appear months or years after exposure. But the high-speed drills and power tools exacerbated the health risks in ways not immediately understood.

Names for the acute symptoms of toxic poisonings worked their way into the lexicon of injury and accident descriptions as journalists and others related the effects of exposure to, for example, phosphorus in the match industry, radium among watch-dial workers, and lead among pigment and paint workers.[20]

Phosphorous and radium poisoning disfigured and killed young women. Lead poisoning caused reproductive disaster for young women and also caused convulsions, paralysis, and death in male and female workers alike. Persistent exposure to mercury, used in the hat-manufacturing companies of Danbury, Connecticut, and elsewhere to transform the fur of small animals into felt, drove hatters insane. It became clear that some processes that once affected a relatively few artisans were now destroying many more lives as manufacturing expanded and moved into large factories.

At particular risk in some of the new factories were women, who were recruited to work at low wages in shoe, rubber, tin can, pottery, and candy factories, where they were exposed to not only a host of traditional chemicals but new ones as well, particularly glues and benzene, methanol, and carbon tetrachloride. Alice Hamilton, considered the founder of occupational medicine in the United States, outlined the different experience of women compared to men in unorganized potteries. The rate of lead poisoning in one pottery was 19.3 per 100 employees for women, for example, and only 4.89 for men.[21] The historian Claudia Clark points out that because women were underrepresented in unions, especially in the "lighter" industries, they were "denied the opportunity to redress poor working conditions through collective pressure." Because women were poorly paid—especially younger, unmarried women—they were more likely to live in substandard housing and have inadequate diets and thus were "more susceptible to any disease, including industrial diseases." Citing much of Alice Hamilton's work in support of protective legislation for women, Clark notes the contemporary arguments that women, being of smaller physical stature than men, and, if younger either pregnant or lactating, were at increased chance "of injury from chemicals because of the stress on their bodies and because of risks like miscarriage."[22] Other factors, such as different levels of exposure and differing jobs within the factory, were also involved.

One of the most dramatic instances of the particular risks women faced on the job occurred in the 1920s when young women who were exposed to considerable radium became the first victims of radiation poisoning. The "radium dial" workers, women in their late teens and twenties, were employed to paint the dials of wristwatches so that they would glow. To get a fine point on their brushes, the women typically licked the tip of the radium-infused hairs, thereby ingesting small amounts of radioactive material. Over time, they developed anemia, weakened bones, cancers, and a horrifyingly disfiguring condition in which their jaws, like those of the matchmakers, slowly dissolved, making them the object of shocking newspaper images and public spectacle.[23]

These new industries were creating environments and building worlds that bred new diseases on a scale never before encountered. Soon phossy jaw, radiation poisoning, silicosis, and asbestosis, to name a few, were added to the medical lexicon. Later in the century, mesothelioma, acroosteolysis, angiosarcoma of the liver, and other diseases of the new industrial world would join them.

LABOR CONFRONTS THE HEALTH CRISIS IN THE WORKPLACE

Phosphorous, radium, lead, and mercury poisoning quickly became as important as accidents and injuries in the class politics of the early twentieth century, leading to growing attention to the industrial environment as a source of suffering among laborers. Headlines and reports in publications sympathetic to workers (see figure 5.2) began to view these poisonings as the product of the developing system of corporate capitalism.

At the turn of the twentieth century, there was an explosion of job actions, labor unrest, and strikes that cannot be understood without looking into the degradation of the work environment. With the rise of Taylorism (the management techniques that broke down work in the factory to discrete tasks that could be performed by unskilled or semiskilled labor and that could be used to lessen the dependence of management on the skilled workforce) and, soon, with the multiplication of assembly lines, the work environment was becoming more socially integrated, though not in a way that was always appreciated.

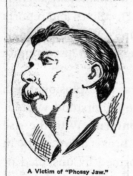

A Victim of "Phossy Jaw."

FIGURE 5.2 "War on Phossy Jaw," *San Juan Prospector*, June 17, 1911.

The growth of industry drew not only on "natural" population increase but also on continuing migration from the countryside and from overseas, especially from southern and eastern Europe. These new immigrants for the most part were non-English-speaking, of darker hue, and from different religious backgrounds, which made them the object of scorn. When there was an increase in accidents and acute diseases that paralleled the intensification of work, long hours, and low pay, employers and some elites blamed the workers themselves for their ignorance, inattention, or a poor work ethic. Labor advocates, on the other hand, blamed the dangerous conditions of the workplace and called repeatedly for factory inspection, decent wages, "fresh air into our shops," and other factory legislation to address the problem of workers' health.[24]

Campaigns for greater safety measures in factories and mines were typically led by labor unions, government investigative commissions, muckrakers, social welfare reformers, and settlement workers rather than by public health and medical professionals. In a 1911 article published in the popular weekly *The Outlook*, one muckraking author described the constant inhalation of dust among other "work that kills."[25] In Illinois, for example, the state factory inspector in 1913 pointed to the deleterious effects of dust on workers in metal polishing, buffing, and grinding, and in New York State, the Factory Investigating Commission that was organized following the Triangle Shirtwaist Fire held hearings in the same year on the dust conditions in a number of upstate industrial concerns.[26] While individuals in the public health movement such as C.-E. A. Winslow and Alice Hamilton participated in these larger movements, participation was not viewed as an intrinsic part of the mandate of public health departments until the second decade of the twentieth century.[27] Before that, the public health community had focused on causes of infectious disease, and it was only beginning to pay attention to the factory as part of its mandate. Even then, it rarely considered dangerous factory conditions other than those related to control of tuberculosis and other infectious diseases among the industrial workforce.[28] (Of course, the influenza epidemic of 1918–1919 was of major concern to public health authorities at the time because it killed an estimated 50 million people worldwide and an estimated 675,000 in the United States, although even here public health was not focused on the factory workforce.)[29]

By the first decades of the twentieth century, however, people began to take note of new as well as previously little-recognized chronic diseases, many related to workplace conditions. The ill-health effects of dust from the use of high-powered tools in the mining of coal, the carving and quarrying of granite and other silica-bearing rock, and the use of sand in the sandblasting of industrial molds in foundries began to generate considerable attention. The use of steam-powered drills in the Vermont granite quarries and in the Appalachian coal mines, as well as of sandblasters in the foundries of Ohio and other midwestern industrial states, all highlighted new ways that unchecked industrialism and the failure of employers to install basic health and safety measures killed and disabled members of the workforce. Power tools and employer schemes such as pay by the piece rather than by the hour, as well as twelve- and fourteen-hour shifts, made work time more productive and efficient from management's point of view, but from labor's perspective, these practices undermined the ability of workers to control the work process, thereby imperiling their health.

Writing in 1906, the social worker Graham Taylor saw four "characteristics of employment" that put workers at risk: "insanitary conditions," "low rate of wages," "fatigue," and "long and irregular hours." Under the heading of "insanitary conditions," Taylor identified two major subcategories, "[un]hygienic surroundings which are not inherent in the trade itself and those conditions which are to a certain extent necessitated by the character of the trade." Among the latter, he wrote that the dusty trades, particularly "those in which the dust-particles [were] very irritating," made their workers susceptible to tuberculosis by weakening the lungs and providing an opportunity for the tubercle bacillus to wreak its havoc. Taylor identified stonecutters, grinders, cigar workers, and lead and copper miners, among others, as at risk. These workers were usually "strong well-developed men," he noted, but they suffered from enormous death rates from tuberculosis, although many of these cases were likely lung diseases of industrial origin associated with the breathing of silica and coal dust, among other industrial dusts.[30]

As John Andrews, the secretary of the American Association for Labor Legislation, put it in March 1914, "we begin to realize how much of the modern labor problem is a health problem," and of course, how much of a health problem was a modern labor problem. While certain industrial diseases, such as phossy jaw, had received considerable attention, there was a much broader array of health problems resulting from the "disastrous effects of unhealthful conditions of employment." These conditions included large amounts of dust, general uncleanliness, long hours, and inadequate pay that limited the foods that workers could afford. Curtailing the scourge of occupational diseases could not be left to the worker, the employer, or even to the medical professional alone, Andrews argued. "The prevention of occupational diseases is properly the function of government," as governments were the only force that could counter the power of large corporations.[31] Individual states, especially those in the Northeast and Midwest, had begun to address these issues in the first decade of the twentieth century, but it would take several more decades for the federal government to step in.

PINPOINTING THE SOURCE: PHTHISIS, CONSUMPTION, AND TUBERCULOSIS

A flashpoint for conflict over chronic disease and work was disagreement over the causes of consumption, "phthisis," and tuberculosis, previously noted in chapter 3 as a collection of discrete conditions whose symptoms included violent hacking, coughing, wasting away, spitting of blood, loss of weight, and ultimately suffocation. For many reformers, consumption was caused by poverty, poor housing, inadequate diet, and overcrowding—all aspects of the world created by industrial capitalism—as much as it was due to the presence of the tuberculosis bacillus, for example. Others saw the array of symptoms not as infectious but as directly linked to the workplace, especially the dusts produced by modern tools and machinery.[32] The social welfare reformer Graham Taylor declared that "disease[s] of the working classes" were a product of "everything which makes the life of the workingman harder." "Everything which is attendant upon poverty, makes for the increase of this disease."[33] Such ideas made the industrial workplace one place to consider when thinking of remedies.

It is ironic that even though dust in the workplace had been identified as a source of disease for much of the nineteenth century, developments in medicine late in the century obscured that relationship, and it had to be "rediscovered" in the early twentieth century.[34] Since antiquity, observers had recognized that workers developed serious breathing problems when they inhaled the dust of certain rocks and minerals. Throughout most of the nineteenth century, doctors and laymen alike had accepted dust as a source of phthisis or *consumption*, the descriptive term used to identify those losing weight and being "consumed" by the disease. In descriptions of various dusty trades, it was commonly pointed out that phthisis and consumption were caused by the specific conditions in the industry. *Miners rot* and *glassblowers phthisis* were terms used to describe workers' lung diseases in the popular as well as the professional press. One study from 1881 described the sources of "grinders' consumption" in the axe industry as "the constant inhalation of the grit and bits of steel thrown off in the process," which caused disease and even death.[35]

It was Robert Koch's discovery in 1882 of the tuberculosis bacillus, perhaps the most dramatic confirmation of the significance of the concept of the germ, that more than anything else resulted in a neglect of the industrial causes of lung diseases. According to Ludwig Teleky, a noted industrial physician and author of the first history of industrial hygiene, after Koch's discovery "the study of the effects of dust stopped. All cases [of phthisis] were diagnosed as tuberculosis." Researchers "mocked at all those 'curiosities' of quartz lungs, coal lungs, and iron lungs, 'all of which belong [more] in a cabinet of curiosities than in industrial hygiene.'"[36]

Just as the medical field was developing unanimity regarding how to define and explain "true" phthisis, however, Thomas Oliver, the turn-of-the-century British physician whose work was important in documenting the phosphorous poisonings in Britain and who was a preeminent expert on industrial hygiene, published along with other governmental investigators a series of studies that would have a major effect on some American reformers, public health workers, and statisticians. Oliver and his colleagues argued that noninfectious cases of lung disorders were more important than medical professionals were positing. In 1902, Oliver, in a famous treatise on the "dangerous trades," noted that "the tendency of modern pathology is to look upon all pulmonary phthisis or consumption as tuberculosis, but the fact remains that phthisis can be caused by dust." Though these pneumoconioses had been neglected, he said, they were significant illnesses in their own right among large cross-sections of the working population. "The affected workman is regarded as the victim of consumption, but the disease is not necessarily tuberculosis," he warned.[37] Workers in the dusty trades, themselves generally isolated from the new ideology of medicine and public health, continued to see their suffering as rooted in the terrible conditions of work, particularly the inhalation of dust. They were correct, it would turn out, as would be evident in the struggles of workers in Vermont's granite quarries, among other places.

Early in the twentieth century, officials of the Granite Cutters' Union in Barre, Vermont, complained that consumption was "claiming almost every granite cutter in this vicinity, before he reaches the age of fifty." In the quarries of rural Vermont, jackhammers, commonly called "widow makers,"[38] replaced sledgehammers and picks, and among the sculptors in the sheds, steam-powered chisels and drills replaced hand chisels.[39] It was obvious to the skilled workers who made up the union that the cause of the epidemic was the granite dust inhaled while carving, chipping, and finishing monuments, gravestones, and building facades. Local physicians agreed that the workers were suffering from consumption, but they differed from their patients in the understanding of its cause. The physicians assumed that the workers' consumptive symptoms were caused by germs that spread among the workforce as a result of poor personal hygiene and unsanitary living conditions. Although the physicians had begun to refer to consumption as tuberculosis, the Granite Cutters' Union and the workforce insisted on using the older nineteenth-century terms *consumption* and *phthisis* to describe the condition. Physicians "have given the old-time consumption a new name," the union observed, "and talk learnedly about it, but what does that amount to when men are dying in our midst almost daily of this fell disease?" Writing that the rate of disease should "strike terror to the heart of every granite cutter," the union declared that the focus of attention should be on preventing the dusty conditions and controlling the speed of work because "the men work at a faster clip than the constitution of any human machine is able to stand up to," thus weakening the ability of the workers to fight off infection.[40]

Throughout most of the nineteenth century, the death rate from consumption fluctuated between 30 and 40 per 10,000 population, and after the 1880s it began to decline because of the various housing and sanitary reforms described in the last chapter. In the nation overall, the death rate from consumption continued to decline in the first decades of the twentieth century, from 19.5 per 10,000 in 1900 to 9.7 in 1922.[41] Between 1896 and 1918, Vermont granite cutters, concentrated in Barre, saw the rate of tuberculosis, to which workers exposed to silica dust were especially susceptible, rise from 25.7 per 10,000 to an astounding 95.3 per 10,000 despite a decline among the general population, for the same period, from 20.7 to 9.6 per 10,000. In Barre itself, the death rate from pulmonary tuberculosis was, as late as 1919, over 23.3 per 10,000 persons, compared with 9 per 10,000 for the rest of the state, and the rate was still going up, despite the relatively healthful home conditions of the granite workers.[42] Thus, in spite of nearly identical rates in 1896, the granite cutters' rate rose 400 percent, while the general population's rate declined more than 50 percent.[43]

What accounts for these vastly different experiences? Again, in the first two decades of the twentieth century, steam-driven equipment replaced hand drills and sledgehammers in granite quarries throughout the nation. These quarries produced the large blocks of granite that would be chipped, carved, and crafted into the ornamental stone used for building facades, monuments and gravestones, columns, mantelpieces, doorsteps, and hearthstones. From cavernous pits in the earth's surface, men would cut the giant blocks of stone that would be hoisted, loaded, and transported to the carving sheds where the craftsmen and operatives would cut, shape, and engrave the stone.

In the first decade of the twentieth century, the *Granite Cutters' Journal*, the publication of the granite workers' union, contained numerous articles about "stone cutters' consumption," closely linking its increase to the recent introduction of power tools and the continuing problem of poor ventilation in the sheds. In July 1905, an article entitled "About the Dust Question" pointed out that, during the summer, when the sheds were open, the use of the pneumatic tools that had been introduced over the course of the past decade was tolerable. But during the winter months, when the windows were closed to conserve heat, dust in the sheds was everywhere. The workers in Northfield, a granite center about 10 miles from Barre, voted in November 1909 that they would not use the pneumatic tools until May 1, 1910, when warmer weather would see the sheds opened up and ventilated. In response, the owners fired or locked out the workers, leading to a much wider job action in the granite sheds throughout the Barre area.[44] An agreement reached in February 1910 between workers and the area's employers provided for an immediate pay increase and for the pneumatic tools not to be used until April 1.

In addition, employers had until June 1 to install dust removal equipment or the tool was to be permanently retired. Just before the June 1 deadline, the Barre granite cutters wrote to the national union that "it will be good-bye to the notorious trouble-making disease-breeding, hand surfacer tomorrow, unless properly equipped with suction fan or other device to remove the dust. . . . The hand surfacer is only a man killer at best, and the scrap heap where many of them will be consigned to is a fitting end for all such inventions."[45] In the first decades of the twentieth century, after insurance company officials like Frederick Hoffman of Prudential Life Insurance Company visited the granite quarries, companies began to implement reforms in the granite shed such as better ventilation, suction devices to remove dust at the point of production, masks, and wetting devices to keep dust down. It was only in the 1920s that researchers in Barre were able to show that the granite dust was producing silicosis, which at the time was seen as a form of consumption, not produced by a bacillus but by silica dust itself, and that it was this disease that was the cause of the suffering and health problems that had been afflicting the granite cutters (see figure 5.3).[46]

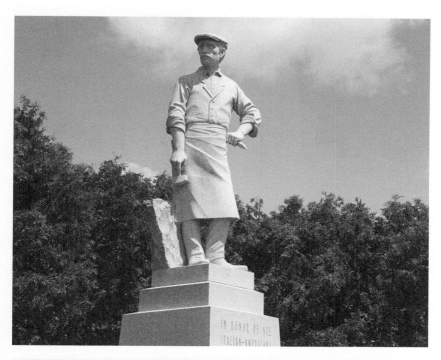

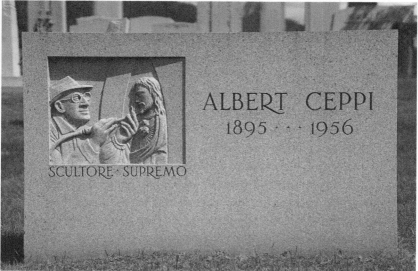

FIGURE 5.3 Headstones in the Hope Cemetery in Barre, Vermont. Headstones in the cemetery sometimes depicted deaths in the arms of loved ones, chiseled by Italian granite cutters who saw their fate slowly unfold. Images from LocalCemeteries.net; photos courtesy of the author.

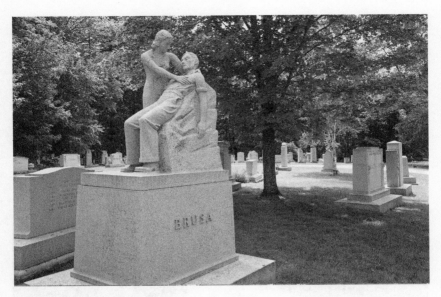

FIGURE 5.3 (*Continued*)

Emery Hayhurst was one of the leading investigators of industrial disease. Working out of the Ohio State Board of Health, he asserted in 1915 that "consumption is the principal terminal occupational disease. . . . Conservatively put, over 50 per cent of all deaths among occupied persons are preventable. This amounts to about a quarter of a million lives a year in the United States."[47] The studies in Barre showed that because the long-term inhalation of silica dust damaged workers' lungs, they were much more susceptible to contracting tuberculosis as well. The work done by statisticians and reformers in Vermont, Ohio, Illinois, and elsewhere on documenting the impact of the new industrial work conditions on the health of the workforce had a broad effect in the early twentieth century. In 1915, the United States Public Health Service was for the first time granted authority by Congress to investigate "occupational diseases and the relation of occupations to disease," and the group organized a Section of Industrial Hygiene and Sanitation to address the issue. Shortly thereafter, the American Public Health Association formed its own section of Industrial Hygiene.

The crises of Barre were but some of the headline-grabbing events that linked industrial production to the incidence of disease in the twentieth century's early decades. Rising concern over the extent of industrial illness merged with growing awareness of new forms of environmental and community dangers created by old industrial poisons. In the years following World War I, lead, the known cause of serious neurological disease among workers in a host of old and new industries, emerged as a bellwether for future environmental dangers as the expanding auto and petrochemical industries became the backbone of the American industrial system. Along with the growth of the auto industry and the creation and expansion of industries for war production, life both in cities and in the countryside was changing. As Henry Ford was expanding his Michigan-based automobile plants, even small cities and rural communities saw the markets expand for mechanical means of transportation and factories to produce them. In Elmira, New York, for example, a local bicycle manufacturer who became an auto parts manufacturer before World War I became the area's largest employer during the war. In the immediate postwar years, he employed 6,300 workers in a plant that spread over 74 acres.[48]

By the 1920s, the automobile industry was already highly competitive. In addition to national manufacturers such as Ford, General Motors, and Studebaker, local companies such as Elmira's former bicycle manufacturer competed for special markets. Ford had dominated the pre-1920 market, producing nearly half of all cars bought by Americans. Its Model T, small and cheaply produced, was the standard for the industry. In the 1920s, though, General Motors developed a number of marketing and stylistic innovations that enabled it to replace Ford as the country's number one producer by the end of that decade. Alfred Sloan, president of General Motors, explained that its profit strategy called for creating demand "not for basic transportation, but for progress in new cars for comfort, convenience, power and style."[49]

Central to the creation of the large, powerful automobiles envisioned by corporate heads like Sloan was the development of a more efficient fuel that was capable of driving cars at greater speed. Fortuitously for them, in 1922 Thomas Midgley and coworkers at the General Motors

Research Laboratory in Dayton, Ohio, discovered that adding tetraethyl lead to gasoline raised the compression, that is, the power, and hence speed, by eliminating the engine "knock." This discovery allowed for the development of the "modern" automobile that would be produced over the next fifty years. General Motors quickly contracted with DuPont and Standard Oil of New Jersey to produce tetraethyl lead, and leaded gasoline was placed on sale in selected markets on February 1, 1923. The following year, DuPont and General Motors created the Ethyl Corporation to market and produce its final product. While producing tetraethyl lead may have made sense to General Motors, Standard Oil, and DuPont given their interlocking directorates and their stake in the use of fossil fuels, they were fully aware that there were safer non-fossil-fuel alternatives already available at the time, such as ethanol-based fuels based on corn.[50] They proceeded to market lead despite the fact that industrial hygienists such as Alice Hamilton had long since identified lead as a dangerous toxin.[51]

In the same year that Midgley and his coworkers at General Motors Research Corporation heralded the discovery of this powerful anti-knock compound, scientists in and outside of government warned that tetraethyl lead in gasoline might be a potent threat to the public's health. In October 1922, William Mansfield Clark, a professor of chemistry, wrote to A. M. Stimson, assistant surgeon general at the Public Health Service, warning of "a serious menace to the public health." He feared that tetraethyl lead's use in gasoline would result in environmental pollution, which could cause chronic lead poisoning, theorizing that "on busy thoroughfares it is highly probable that the lead oxide dust will remain in the lower stratum" of the atmosphere.[52] Two months later, H. S. Cumming, the U.S. surgeon general, wrote to P. S. DuPont, chairman of the board of the DuPont Company, asking whether the public health effects of tetraethyl lead manufacturing and use had been taken into account. He was answered by Thomas Midgley himself, who allowed that although the question "had been given very serious consideration . . . no actual experimental data has been taken." While acknowledging that lead in high quantities could cause damage to workers, Midgley argued that the amount of lead coming out of the tailpipes of cars was harmless. Despite the lack of experimental data, GM and DuPont were confident that "the average street will probably be so free from lead that it will be impossible to detect it or its absorption."[53]

Industry assurances of leaded gasoline's safety were undermined by a horrifying disaster that occurred in the Standard Oil Company's laboratories at its processing plant in Elizabeth, New Jersey. Between October 26 and October 30, 1924, of the forty-nine workers in the tetraethyl lead processing plant, five workers in the labs there died and thirty-five others experienced palsies, tremors, hallucinations, and other serious neurological symptoms of organic lead poisoning. Thus, by the end of October 1924, over 80 percent either died or were severely poisoned. On the first day after the poisonings, the *New York Times* quoted the company doctor as suggesting that "nothing ought to be said about this matter in the public interest," while one of the supervisors at Standard Oil's Elizabeth facility was reported to have said that "these men probably went insane because they worked too hard."[54]

After the initial revelations about the disaster, every major newspaper in New York began to report on conditions at the plant. Day after day, the *New York Times*, the *New York World*, and other newspapers revealed deaths and occupationally related "insanity" due to what the newspapers called "looney gas."[55] The company continually sought to deny management's responsibility for the tragedy, with Thomas Midgley blaming the workers for their own ill-health. At another plant, he said, "the men, regardless of warnings and provision for their protection, had failed to appreciate the dangers of constant absorption of the fluid by their hands and arms."[56] Despite Standard Oil's attempt to shift blame to workers, others were reaching different conclusions. The Union County, New Jersey, prosecutor asserted that he was "satisfied many of the workers did not know the danger they were running. I also believe some of the workers were not masked nor told to wear rubber gloves and rubber boots."[57]

Continuing controversy over the deaths and the acute lead poisoning that the workers experienced led to new concerns about the potential public health dangers from the lead that would be spewed from vehicular exhaust pipes. New York City, New York State, Philadelphia, and many other municipalities and states went further: they banned the sale of leaded gasoline, called "ethyl."[58]

As a result of these continuing revelations and public disquiet, the surgeon general of the Public Health Service announced at the end of

April 1925 that he was calling together experts from business, labor, and public health to assess the tetraethyl lead situation.[59] The conference convened the following month in Washington, DC, with every major party—industry, labor, public health and government officials, scientists and engineers—represented. At the conference, the ideologies of the different participants were clearly and repeatedly laid out, thus providing an important forum in which to evaluate the scientific, political, economic, and intellectual issues surrounding this controversy. In the words of one participant, the conference gathered together in one room "two diametrically opposed conceptions. The men engaged in industry, chemists, and engineers, take it as a matter of course that a little thing like industrial poisoning should not be allowed to stand in the way of a great industrial advance. On the other hand, the sanitary experts take it as a matter of course that the first consideration is the health of the people."[60]

The conference opened with statements from General Motors, DuPont, Standard Oil, and the entity that those companies had created to manufacture tetraethyl lead, the Ethyl Corporation, outlining the history of leaded gasoline's development and the reasons why they believed its continued production was essential. Three themes emerged as the companies' central arguments. First, the manufacturers maintained that leaded gasoline was essential to the industrial progress of America. Second, they maintained that any innovation entails certain risks. Third, they stated that the major reason that deaths and illnesses occurred at their plants was that the men who worked with the materials were careless and did not follow instructions. C. F. Kettering, of GM and Ethyl, and Robert Kehoe, scientific consultant to the industry, both stressed the importance of tetraethyl lead as a means of conserving motor fuel. But it was Frank Howard, representing the Ethyl Gasoline Corporation, who provided the most complete rationale for the continued use of tetraethyl lead in gasoline. Automobiles and oil were central to the industrial progress of the nation, if not the world, he argued. "Our continued development of motor fuels is essential in our civilization." Noting that at least a decade of research had gone into the effort to identify tetraethyl lead, he called its discovery an "apparent gift of God." This was a theme that would recur time after time with the introduction of new, untested chemicals—progress was essential even if it meant introducing untested, potentially harmful chemicals into the bodies and environment of millions of people. "What is our duty under the circumstances?," he asked. "Should we say, 'No, we will not use'" a material that is "a certain means of saving petroleum? Because some animals die and some do not die in some experiments, shall we give this thing up entirely?"[61]

Industry continued to maintain that tetraethyl lead was key to America's economic prosperity and that any great advance required some sacrifice. H. C. Parmelee, editor of *Chemical and Metallurgical Engineering*, for example, asserted that the companies did their best to safeguard the workers, but in the end, the "casualties were negligible compared to human sacrifice in the development of many other industrial enterprises."[62]

The final part of the industries' position was that workers, rather than the companies, were at fault for other poisonings identified among workers at Standard Oil's tetraethyl lead facility in Elizabeth, New Jersey; DuPont's Deepwater plant in southern New Jersey; and General Motors's Dayton laboratories. Acknowledging that there were "certain dangers" inherent in tetraethyl lead's production, the companies asserted that those dangers were being blown all out of proportion. At one press conference, Midgley dramatically "washed his hands thoroughly" in what he said was pure tetraethyl lead and proclaimed, "I'm not taking any chance whatever, nor would I take any chance doing that every day." He performed this act even though only a year before he had taken a prolonged vacation in Florida to cure himself of lead poisoning.[63]

Those who opposed the introduction of leaded gasoline disagreed with every fundamental position of industry representatives. First, opponents pointed out that what are now called inorganic lead compounds were already known to be slow, cumulative poisons that caused tremors, convulsions, comas, and ultimately death and that they should not be introduced into the general environment. Second, they believed that, because of what they saw as industry's reckless disregard for workers' and the public's health, the federal government should step in and assume responsibility for protecting the health of the nation. Third, they rejected the notion that the workers were the ones responsible for their own poisoning because they had been simply following standard protocols. Fourth, and most importantly, because they believed that the public's health should take precedence over the drive for corporate profits, they argued that the burden of proof should be on the companies to prove that tetraethyl lead was safe rather than on opponents to prove that tetraethyl lead was dangerous.

The strongest and most authoritative critic of industry was the Yale physiologist Yandell Henderson. He told the conference that lead was as serious a public health menace as were the infectious diseases then affecting the nation's health. He expressed horror at the thought that hundreds of thousands of pounds of lead would, over time, be deposited in the streets of every major city in America. Henderson's warning to the conference of the long-term dangers to consumers and citizens exposed to polluted air would prove to be an accurate prediction: "conditions would grow worse so gradually and the development of lead poisoning will come on so insidiously . . . that leaded gasoline will be in nearly universal use and large numbers of cars will have been sold . . . before the public and the government awaken to the situation."[64]

Opponents of leaded gasoline were most concerned about industry propaganda that equated the use of lead with industrial progress and the survival of American civilization itself. Reacting to the Ethyl Corporation representative's statement that tetraethyl lead was a "gift of God," Grace Burnham of the Workers' Health Bureau pointed out that by 1925 many more workers had been poisoned or died at DuPont, Standard Oil, and General Motors facilities. She said that it "was not a gift of God when those 11 men were killed or those 149 were poisoned." She angrily questioned the priorities of "this age of speed and rush and efficiency and mechanics"; "the thing we are interested in the long run is not mechanics or machinery, but men," she insisted. But it was Yandell Henderson who most succinctly summarized the opponents' position and delineated an appropriate course for future public health policymakers. In a private letter to R. R. Sayers of the Bureau of Mines before the conference, he said, "In the past, the position taken by the authorities has been that nothing could be prohibited until it was proved to have killed a number of people. I trust that in the future, especially in a matter of this sort, the position will be that a substance like tetraethyl lead cannot be introduced for general use until it is proved harmless."[65]

For the vast majority of public health experts at the conference, the problem was how to reconcile the opposing views of advocates of industrial progress and those concerned about the potential for disastrous health consequences. How could you make the use of leaded gasoline safe in a way that would ensure that the public would not become poisoned? Although everyone hoped that science would provide an answer to this imponderable dilemma, the reality was that all evidence on this point was ambiguous. One major problem was that, in the 1920s, no one had a model for explaining the apparently idiosyncratic occurrence of lead poisoning.[66] Specifically, public health authorities were just beginning to understand the slow evolution of chronic diseases, that it could take years for symptoms to develop when someone was exposed to small quantities of a toxin. Further, they were slow to understand how much more vulnerable certain populations, in this case children, were to the effects of these toxins.

As one of the country's foremost authorities on lead, Alice Hamilton expressed her belief that the environmental health issues of leaded gasoline were much more far-reaching than the occupational health and safety issues involved, adding that she doubted that any effective measures could be implemented to protect the general public from the hazards of its widespread use. "You may control conditions within a factory," she said, "but how are you going to control the whole country?" In an extended commentary after the conference on the issues that it raised, Hamilton stated, "I am not one of those who believe that the use of this leaded gasoline can ever be made safe. No lead industry has ever, even under the strictest control, lost all its dangers. Where there is lead some case of lead poisoning sooner or later develops, even under the strictest supervision."[67]

Most public health professionals did not agree with Henderson and Hamilton, however. In the face of industry arguments that oil supplies were limited and that there was an extraordinary need to conserve fuel by making combustion more efficient, most public health workers acceded to industry's argument that there should be overwhelming evidence that leaded gasoline actually harmed people before it was banned.

Despite widespread ambivalence on the part of public health professionals and the opposition to any curbs on production on the part of industry spokespeople, the public suspicions aroused by the disasters at Standard Oil's refineries in Elizabeth, DuPont's Deepwater plant, and General Motors's Dayton labs, as well as what was revealed at the conference itself, led to a significant victory for those who opposed the sale of leaded gasoline. At the end of the conference, the Ethyl Corporation announced that it was suspending the production and distribution of leaded gasoline until the scientific and public health issues involved in its manufacture could be resolved. The conference also called upon the surgeon general to organize a blue ribbon committee of the nation's foremost public health scientists to conduct an investigation of leaded gasoline. For Alice Hamilton and other opponents of leaded gasoline, the conference appeared to be a major victory because it forced industry to bow to the pressure and agree to wait until further research had been conducted before deciding on the future of such a consequential poison.[68]

Initial euphoria over the apparent victory of science over political and economic self-interest was short-lived, however. The blue ribbon committee, mandated to deliver an early decision, designed a short-term, very limited study of garage and filling-station attendants and chauffeurs in Dayton and Cincinnati. As a result of the study, the committee concluded seven months after the conference that "in its opinion there are at present no good grounds for prohibiting the use of ethyl gasoline, provided that its distribution and use are controlled by proper regulations." It suggested that the surgeon general formulate specific regulations with enforcement by the states.[69] Although it appears that the committee rushed to judgment in only seven months, it must be pointed out that this group saw its study as only an interim report, to be followed by long-term studies in ensuing years. In its final report to the surgeon general, the committee warned: "It remains possible that if the use of leaded gasoline becomes widespread conditions may arise very different from those studied by us which would render its use more of a hazard than would appear to be the case from this investigation. Longer experience may show that even such slight storage of lead [in the human body] as was observed in these studies may lead eventually in susceptible individuals to recognizable or to chronic degenerative diseases of a less obvious character."[70] No follow-up government studies were conducted, however, and from 1926 until the 1980s leaded gas spewed from the tailpipes of millions of cars all across the United States. It is estimated that in the sixty years following its introduction, at least 7 million tons of lead were burned and spread over the environment by the millions of cars that were sold.[71] The subsequent studies of the use of tetraethyl lead were conducted instead by the Ethyl Corporation and scientists employed by them, and it was not until the 1960s and 1970s that independent researchers did studies that demonstrated widespread lead pollution in America's cities and the devastating effect that pollution had on children, especially children of color living in poor communities.[72] From the 1920s through the 1970s, children suffered severe neurological damage, seizures, and even death; beginning in the 1980s, in conjunction with the auto industry's adoption of the catalytic converter, which could be ruined by a car's use of leaded gasoline, unleaded gasoline was introduced into the marketplace, lowering lead emissions and perhaps leading to less incidence of dramatic, but still life-altering, lead-induced effects of fuels, including attention deficit/hyperactivity disorder, neurological damage, and loss of IQ. The development of cars and the lead-based fuels that powered them was justified on the basis of their service to society. But, as public health advocates revealed the flaws in that argument, warning of dangerous health and environmental threats that these innovations posed, the economic self-interest of an emerging, giant industry ultimately triumphed over the health of future generations.

INDUSTRIAL HEALTH DISASTER AT GAULEY BRIDGE

In the early years of the Great Depression of the 1930s, hundreds of thousands, if not millions, of workers left their homes and their families in search of work so that they could send some money back home. Among them, one group of over four thousand left the South for West Virginia, having heard that there was work there building a water tunnel near Gauley Bridge. A subsidiary of the Union Carbide and Carbon Company hired the workers and told them that their job was to drill through a mountain. What it didn't tell them was that the mountain was made up of almost pure silica, which was known at the time to cause a debilitating lung condition called silicosis that destroyed the essential tissues of the lung, making it impossible for sufferers to breathe. Over the course of the project, about three thousand workers toiled in the tunnel, where the danger of silicosis was most severe, about 75 percent of them African Americans.

Usually, silicosis takes years or even decades to manifest itself, but exposures in the Gauley Bridge tunnel were so extreme that within a few months workers started complaining about breathing difficulties. Company doctors told the workers there was nothing to worry about; they just had "tunnelitis." The company apparently hoped that because silicosis usually took so long to manifest itself, the workers would be long gone by the time they became ill. A subsequent congressional investigation uncovered damning evidence that despite their reassurances to the workers, company officials and engineers would wear masks when they entered the tunnel, a precaution that was denied to the workers. Hundreds of workers actually died on the job, and many, especially the African Americans among them, were buried in unmarked graves. That the vast majority of workers who died were migrants and far from their loved ones apparently led the company officials to believe that they could cover up their deaths. In fact, families who inquired about deceased workers were lied to, being told that the workers had "moved on." According to estimates from the physician and author Martin Cherniack, as many as fifteen hundred were killed as a result of their exposure to the silica in the tunnel project.[73]

The company had built three camps to house the tunnelers and others. These were segregated by race, with the facilities for African American workers—no surprise—much more crowded and lacking electricity and other amenities. Whereas shanties that housed white workers had one bunk bed for two workers, for Black workers there were usually two or three bunk beds housing four to as many as ten workers. Workers were roused from their accommodations at the start of each shift by armed overseers and were not allowed to remain in the bunk even if they felt ill. As Cherniack quotes one surviving African American worker of the Gauley Bridge tunnel project, "If a colored man was sick and really couldn't go to work in the morning, he had to hide out before the shack rouster came around. That fellow had two pistols and a blackjack to force men to go to work."[74] Intimidation was also used to force Black workers back into the dusty confines of the tunnel but was not used against white workers. As one white engineer later told the congressional committee investigating the disaster, "I have heard quite a few times that they used pick handles or a drillstead and knocked them in the head with it."[75]

It is conceivable that this tragedy, perhaps the worst industrial health disaster in U.S. history, would have landed in the dustbin of history but for Vito Marcantonio, a radical U.S. congressman from New York's

Italian barrio on the Upper East Side who held hearings that elicited testimony from workers, journalists, company officials, and government personnel. Thanks to these hearings, newspapers and magazines made the deaths and disease from silicosis of these workers a national story, with one magazine titling its account "Village of the Living Dead."[76] Although this industrial catastrophe overwhelmingly affected Black workers, the racial dimension of the tragedy was nonetheless muted by the news media. Following the hearings, the U.S. Department of Labor, headed by Frances Perkins, organized the National Silicosis Conference, which made silicosis a national public policy issue, leading to its inclusion as the first chronic lung disease in workers' compensation legislation and stimulating many lawsuits on behalf of injured workers.

Although the tragedy of Gauley Bridge was really a manifestation of acute silicosis because of how rapidly it killed and disabled its victims, the publicity about it served to awaken the nation to the effects of breathing toxic dusts in a variety of industries, including coal and hard-rock mining, construction of subway tunnels, and iron and steel foundries.

LEAD, ZINC, AND SILICA IN THE MIDWEST

If the issue of silicosis and other chronic diseases resulting from work with little or no regard for elementary safety equipment was first raised in the Barre quarry sheds and places like Gauley Bridge, and if concern about the impact of low-level environmental exposures was highlighted by the tetraethyl lead controversies in the 1920s, the two issues—silicosis and environmental lead poisoning—were joined in the Tri-State region of Missouri, Kansas, and Oklahoma in the 1930s.

Lead and zinc—critical minerals used in products ranging from steel and brass alloys to batteries, munitions, and gasoline—were central to the emergence of the United States as the world's leading industrial power. Lead and zinc are often found in the same location and extracted from the same mine. In the mid-nineteenth century, lead and zinc ores were discovered in the sparsely populated agricultural countryside of southwestern Missouri. Mining communities soon flourished in the area around Joplin, Missouri, and by the 1910s the area had become the world's leading producer of lead and zinc ores.[77] At first, the industry was highly competitive, with hundreds of mines owned by scores of different producers. In the early twentieth century, larger and better-capitalized companies, using dynamite, more sophisticated machinery, and power tools, were able to drive out smaller competitors as the center of the industry shifted from Joplin to richer deposits around Picher, Oklahoma, and Treece, Kansas. The new techniques created immense amounts of very fine dust composed largely of silica, which was embedded in the rock that contained the sought-after mineral ores.

By 1915, soon after the introduction of power tools and dynamite blasting, miners and their families in the Tri-State region of southwestern Missouri, northeastern Oklahoma, and southeastern Kansas were, like the workers at Gauley Bridge, developing debilitating and life-threatening lung conditions. Provided with little other than the occasional use of "wet drills" to dampen the dust and a kerchief and sometimes a mask to filter out some of the larger particles, miners in the Joplin area were at greater risk of dying from disease than from accidents. Further, because silicosis left miners unusually susceptible to tuberculosis infection, some among them carried tuberculosis back into their homes and spread it to their families. The families were especially vulnerable to contracting the disease because they were undernourished and living in shacks surrounded by chat piles of silica and lead wastes. One mine owner told the U.S. Bureau of Mines that he had employed 750 men between 1907 and 1914. By 1915, he reported, "only about 50 of these were still living, and all the others except not more than a dozen were said to have died" from tuberculosis.[78]

Worsening work conditions and the increasing prevalence of lung diseases spurred union organizing drives in the Tri-State area. As ownership of the mines passed from entrepreneurs working in small teams to giant corporations such as the Eagle-Picher Lead Company, labor-management relations deteriorated. The Western Federation of Miners (WFM), then affiliated with the syndicalist Industrial Workers of the World, organized a local in Joplin as early as 1906.

During the Great Depression, conflict over deteriorating health conditions reached a climax as employment in the Tri-State mines plummeted from over 7,000 in 1929 to 1,331 in 1932. The International Union of Mine, Mill, and Smelter Workers (an outgrowth of the WFM) began a concerted organizing effort that stressed the hazards of silicosis and tuberculosis as well as inadequate wages, speed-ups, and other harsh working conditions. Inspired by Section 7(a) of the National Industrial Recovery Act, which provided legal protections for workers who organized unions, Mine-Mill representatives organized broadly, seeking to unionize "nearly everyone in the [Tri-State] district." In a 1935 letter to Secretary of Labor Frances Perkins, James Robinson, the secretary-treasurer of the Mine-Mill international, noted that a census study that examined miners, both working and unemployed, found 205 cases of silicosis in 544 homes in the city of Picher. He charged that "the mining companies in this district make no effort to alleviate this condition."[79] The international was well suited to organize the Tri-State area because of its commitment to industrial unionism and mass organizing, and it sought to organize the larger community to counteract mine owners' control of the economic and political life of the region.

The problems of working conditions transcended the workplace, reaching into the home and community. The mine owners, in neglecting to protect their workers adequately from silicosis, in effect destroyed the miners' health and their ability to support their families, and in some cases they brought tuberculosis into the home. Writing to Eleanor Roosevelt, the secretary of one union local offered to send "plenty of factual and documentary evidence that men are dieing like flies and that 8 out of every 10 women in this district are widows, 75 percent of the children orphans." The union claimed that mine owners preferred to spend money "to buy tear gas, munitions, and to hire thugs and gunmen to terrorize union men and women" rather than install "air cleaning devices" to combat silicosis.[80] With silicosis rampant, the union argued that it was impossible to separate the issues of work and community; the Tri-State Zinc and Lead Ore Producers Association maintained instead that those issues were unrelated, and they refused to bargain with a union that represented "a host of unemployed and relief workers."

By the late 1930s, the issue of silicosis had in a way transcended the domains of professionals, management, insurance, and labor. The groundwork had been laid for liberal and left-wing political groups to transform silicosis into a symbol of exploitation. Just as the Scottsboro case represented lynch justice in the South, so silicosis in the Tri-State area represented corporate greed that was causing the slow death of working-class communities. The major propaganda effort on behalf of the workers was spearheaded by the National Committee for People's

Rights, a left-wing organization based in New York whose leadership included such well-known Popular Front figures as the artist Rockwell Kent. In the fall of 1939, the committee issued a report publicizing living, working, and health conditions of the Tri-State region. It described the substandard housing, reminding readers that poor housing contributed to the high tuberculosis rate found in the area and that poor sanitation exacerbated health problems there.[81] The report also illustrated how the organization of work in the Tri-State mines affected workers' health. Because miners were paid on a piece rate, for example, time taken for health or safety practices cost the miners rather than the owners. In many mines, the shovelers were responsible for wetting down the slag heaps to cut down on silica dust, but they rarely took the time to do so, as a shoveler's pay was based on "how many ore cans he has been able to load on each of his shifts." Wetting the dust was thus "tantamount to asking them to finance the [company's] mine dust control program."[82]

The national media picked up on the report. *Time* magazine, in a December 1939 article titled "Zinc Stink," noted that silicosis was not only an occupational disease but also "a public health menace," because the miners lived in overcrowded houses and the father, who was a miner and was suffering from tuberculosis, often shared "the same room or even the same bed with his children, even though he is continually showering the air with germs when he coughs." The *New Republic*, in an article titled "American Plague Spot," suggested that the report should be "compulsory reading for all those who, under the pressure of news of wholesale misery abroad, have forgotten that we have our share of it at home." Even *Business Week* devoted a major article to what it called "a sizzling report detailing desperate living conditions among the miners."[83]

In early 1940, as war production was being ratcheted up, the U.S. Department of Labor[84] hoped that federal power and publicity could be used to counter the enormous influence of mine owners at the state and local level.[85] In April 1940, a two-day conference was convened in Joplin, Missouri, presided over by U.S. Secretary of Labor Frances Perkins, the first woman appointed to a president's cabinet. It was the culmination of forty years of debate over silicosis, tuberculosis, and responsibility for disease in the Tri-State area. Labor strife had forced government, management, union officials, and others to attend, and the relationship of health and disease to the broader labor struggle dominated discussion at the conference.

The position papers and conference proceedings revealed the intense politics that shaped the debates over disease and public health. In the course of the conference, a new and much more fundamental debate over the very notion of chronic disease emerged as well. The mine owners promoted the view that industrialization had made the traditional dichotomy between the healthy and the diseased meaningless: the common understanding of medicine and public health had not kept pace with the revolutionary industrial changes people experienced with their exposure to man-made dusts and chemicals. In modern societies, dust in the environment was no longer exceptional. The presence of dust in workers' lungs was not as such pathological, so the argument went; only the existence of "excessive" amounts that limited their activity—work—could be considered pathological. Management argued that the boundaries between normal and abnormal, healthy and diseased, had to be redrawn to accommodate these new industrial realities. Labor representatives and their advocates in the Department of Labor argued that the presence of toxic dust and chemicals in the environment, however prevalent, could not be considered normal because in humans, dust produced physiological changes that were part of a disease process. Such changes in working and living conditions indicated a fundamental imbalance between humans and their environment. Such imbalances were not natural but the product of conscious social decisions, and it was the role of social workers, public health and labor officials, and particularly company management to control and regulate the environment to protect the public.

Management and labor were thus debating how chronic industrial disease posed a host of new problems for the medical and public health community. The causes and effects of such disease (unlike the causes and effects of accidents) were rarely clear-cut. Except in cases of acute poisoning or death, chronic disease might not show symptoms for years, even decades, after exposure to toxins. Some workers were affected by relatively limited exposures to toxic materials, while others were far more tolerant. Some workers showed physiological changes without exhibiting behavioral symptoms; others showed no apparent physiological change yet found themselves losing strength. In the case of silicosis, diagnosis of the disease did not preclude conflicting opinions about its importance in the life of a worker. Some medical and public health experts believed that mild silicosis rarely interfered with the workers' ability to earn a living and thus the condition was of little significance from their point of view. Others believed that physical limitation, whether affecting work or not, was unacceptable and should be redressed.

Management's position was laid out by Evan Just, secretary of the Tri-State Zinc and Lead Ore Producers Association, who sought to downplay the effects that industrial substances had on the workforce. He held that inhalation of silica per se was not dangerous. The body could defend itself from minute silica particles by surrounding them with tissue, creating a benign "condition known as fibrosis." He asserted that "almost every adult person has some." Silicosis was, according to Just, merely an advanced case of a normal fibrotic condition that substituted "non-functional tissue for functional tissue." He minimized the problems of silicosis by claiming that since a person had "considerably more lung capacity than [he/she] needs," the loss of some of that capacity because of silicosis "does not result in noticeable disability." Disability only occurred "in very advanced cases."[86] Further, he claimed, the health status of area residents compared "favorably with the average."

Just maintained that the focus of the conference was wrong. The real problem of the Tri-State area was tuberculosis, an infectious disease caused by poor living conditions, not silicosis, an industrial scourge. Further, the widespread prevalence of tuberculosis was the product of the free choices workers and their families made about how to spend their wages. The companies paid "adequate wages," but "many people who can afford better homes, prefer to live in small, unpainted two or three room shacks and spend their surplus funds on automobiles and radios." Workers' lifestyle was thus the root cause of the health crisis, he maintained, and only the workers could change it. One company-affiliated physician, Jesse Douglas, reiterated the owners' position that tuberculosis was the real problem and that its prevalence had little to do with the mines. He held that "the American stock has carried along with it tuberculosis," and that the Tri-State area "had been well seeded with the tuberculin bacilli."[87] In other forums, Just went on to claim that the real problem was that most of the area's workers were independent-minded old-stock Americans. Turning common nativist arguments on their head, Just claimed that the "principal difficulty is that this type of worker—unlike 'a foreign-element' will not take orders. . . . Because of their ignorance it is almost impossible to educate them in a sanitary way of living."[88]

In opposition to the mine owners' positions, officials in the Department of Labor and union representatives presented medical, political, and social arguments. They saw the incidence of silicosis and tuberculosis as inextricably related to management's control over the work process and community life. The Department of Labor's critique of Just's analysis was sharp and trenchant.[89] To the Department of Labor, there was nothing "normal" about extensive dust in the workplace or silicosis among workers: "In plain English, silicosis is a disease of the lungs [and] . . . is strictly an occupational disease." There was little need to argue about the appropriate response. Silicosis could be prevented with little new research or theoretical study, as industrial hygienists had developed a variety of techniques to protect workers—wetting down the dust, exhausting the dust at the point where it was produced, isolating dusty practices, and, as a last resort, requiring workers to wear positive air respirators so that they were not breathing the dust.[90]

The Department of Labor's view of silicosis was in part a product of its own history, established as it had been during the tumultuous period of labor unrest in the first decades of the twentieth century and in part a product of the experiences of those who headed it. Secretary of Labor Perkins had led New York's Department of Labor, perhaps the most important and progressive labor department in the country, and she had been reared in the tumultuous decades of the new century in which attention was focused on the impact the expanding industrial system was having on the well-being of workers and their families. During that period, some of the most important pieces of federal legislation concerning workers had become law, including federal workers' compensation legislation, laws protecting women and prohibiting child labor, laws regulating hours and wages, and laws requiring safety and health measures. Furthermore, it was during her early years, in the 1910s and 1920s, that the Triangle Fire and various mine explosions occurred. In addition, formal studies of the impact of industrialization showed increases in accidents, deaths, and illnesses among Pittsburgh's steelworkers, Chicago's meatpackers, New York's garment workers, West Virginia's miners, and New Jersey's dial workers. All made headlines around the country.

Perkins had been one of the inspectors who toured New York's industrial towns as a member of the New York Factory Investigating Commission, documenting the dangerous conditions of the factory and its human costs in terms of accidents and poor health. In its survey, the commission visited 3,385 workplaces, interviewed 472 witnesses, and held 59 public hearings in communities around the state, all in a period of two years, 1911–1912. As an inspector of factories in the groundbreaking 7,000-page *Report of the New York Factory Investigating Commission*, of which only the *Pittsburgh Survey*, a six-volume pioneering sociological study documenting the effects of industrialization in that city, could compare, Perkins came to the job with a focus on the effects of industrial accidents and disease on workers and the communities that depended on them.[91]

As a labor advocate, Perkins saw occupational accidents and disease as a reflection of the exploitative relationship between factory owners and their employees that necessitated political and regulatory actions. This viewpoint led her to establish within the U.S. Department of Labor the Division of Labor Standards, a division whose positions came into conflict with the emerging consensus of many professionals in state departments of health as well as in the federal Public Health Service. The new Division of Labor Standards combined traditional labor concerns over hours and wages with a new focus on health and safety conditions. This was a serious effort to integrate occupational safety and health into a broader, more traditional conception of working conditions that emphasized hours and speed of work and to place the authority of the department behind this potentially radical effort.

The new division challenged older conceptions of the role of the state in the relationship between owners and workers, a role that had largely precluded government involvement on behalf of labor in strikes, walkouts, lockouts, and slowdowns during periods of conflict. Perkins recognized the radical nature of her new focus on injuries and disease as symptoms of the inequalities in power in the industrial plants, mines, and mills that were now employing larger and larger numbers of workers. "As the head of the Department of Labor in New York," Perkins recalls in her oral history, "I knew that we had never heard from the U.S. Department of Labor, that we never saw any of them, never heard anything from them. We didn't even get their publications unless we asked for them. In other words, there had never been the slightest effort on the part of the federal government to bring any knowledge to bear upon the problems of labor legislation in the State of New York, or . . . Massachusetts, or . . . New Jersey." Perkins felt that the federal department she headed needed to be more responsive to the needs of labor and of the states where activist departments of labor were eager to intervene to protect the workforce and their families.[92]

Secretary Perkins arrived in Missouri for the April 1940 conference well prepared and received tremendous local publicity as she first made a whirlwind tour of the mines in the Tri-State area. In a photo display and article in the *St. Louis Post-Dispatch*, she was shown descending into a mine in miner's garb, speaking with local residents and addressing an evening meeting of the International Union of Mine, Mill, and Smelter Workers. In her opening address to the conference, Perkins adopted a conciliatory tone. She left to others in her department the task of analyzing the deficiencies in management's presentation on silicosis. But when it came to larger public health issues and specifically the impact of tuberculosis in the region, she took a personal interest, revealing her frustration with management protestations of helplessness to combat disease. She objected to management's attempt to focus attention on the lifestyle of employees as the cause for the high incidence of tuberculosis and to the assertion that the area was "seeded" with the tuberculosis bacillus. Perkins found such explanations simplistic, noting that they undermined effective public health measures, such as better housing and improved pay for the workers, and diverted attention from the occupational and environmental implications of the community's health problems.[93]

The secretary of labor especially objected to the idea, promulgated since the nineteenth century, that certain human "stock" carried a predisposition to tuberculosis. She recounted her own experience as a young public health worker on a street in New York's Lower East Side where tuberculosis rates were so high that it was called the "lung block." She and others at the time believed that because the community was "almost entirely of Irish extraction, [therefore] the Irish, we thought, were the 'seedbed' of tuberculosis. So we could safely ignore the fact that there was so much tuberculosis in that particular area."[94]

Yet when Jacob Riis, Theodore Roosevelt, and other reformers initiated a public health campaign that entailed rebuilding the block, sending in visiting nurses, setting up tuberculosis centers, and increasing medical and social work attention, the tuberculosis rate declined substantially. As a result, Perkins realized that it had been wrong to see the Irish as "the seedbed for tuberculosis"; instead, she and her colleagues began to look for what specific conditions would make the neighborhood "a favorable environment for the growth of whatever seeds might be planted anywhere in the human body."[95] Optimistic about the efficacy of human action to control the disease environment, she laid out a model of disease causation and cure that had evolved from her experiences in public health work during the Progressive Era. Perkins believed that disease could not simply be prevented or cured by identifying particular germs and treating specific diseases. Instead, attention to conditions in the overall environment—in the workplace, in the home, and in the community—would ultimately resolve the area's problems.[96]

She realized that "all of us—the American stock and Irish and German and Scotch, and recently the Italian and recent Czech and Slovakian, the whole human race—are all pretty good seedbeds for tuberculosis if we get exposed to it." She argued with the owners' and professionals' view that the prevalence of silicosis and tuberculosis in the area was a problem of bacteriology or the personal behavior of the workers themselves. Rather, it was "very largely the environment in which [people] live that determines whether [they] are disabled and crushed by [disease] or whether [they] manage to lift [their] heads above it and go on."[97]

Perkins maintained that miners' susceptibility to tuberculosis was due to the weakening of their lungs by long-term inhalation of silica dust. The widespread presence of tuberculosis confirmed, rather than excused, the hazardous working conditions and terrible living conditions of the miners and their families. The first problem was preventing the dust from reaching the miners' lungs to begin with, and this meant ensuring the use of long-standing methods of dust control, including better ventilation, drills with the ability to capture the dust these tools generated, and wet drilling. In addition, Perkins and her staff privately advocated for diversifying the economy of the Tri-State region so that the mine owners did not exert such a dominant influence over the area. She hoped that broadening the economic base would give men and women greater opportunity for better-paying jobs and lessen the power of the mine owners over the life of the community.[98]

The labor position closely paralleled Perkins's analysis. Tony McTeer of Mine-Mill told the conference that the problems of the area were intertwined. To prevent disease and premature death in the community—that is, to prevent silicosis and tuberculosis—it was necessary to institute "better dust control and better working conditions in the mines." But addressing the silicosis problem was part of a broader attack needed to address a range of community problems. McTeer called for improvements in the medical care system, specifically hospitals to treat the diseased workers, and adequate housing for miners and their families, in the process rejecting the claim of management that workers "chose" to live in the hovels and shacks surrounding the mines.[99]

The mine owners were not without allies in government and industry who also saw disease as resulting from the personal behavior of the miners themselves rather than as a product of the environment in which they worked and lived. But, by the 1930s, New Deal reforms and the growing labor movement had changed the balance of power in the political and social arenas, and the courts acquiesced to many prolabor initiatives, including actions by the Department of Labor.

While the Department of Labor officials saw industrial disease as a symptom of a broader industrial system that often sacrificed workers in the quest for profits and as a condition that demanded reform of the workplace, the U.S. Public Health Service often took a more hands-off approach, identifying the biological or toxicological sources of illnesses among the workforce and providing information that might—or might not—be utilized by policymakers, factory owners, and others with specific interest in the issue. When it came to labor-management disputes over working conditions, or legislative efforts to address specific issues that threatened the social order in particular communities, public health officials felt that it was not their role as doctors and public health professionals to intervene in the political process—only to provide objective information that could be utilized in remedying the problem.

The Public Health Service approach—seeking solutions to public health problems by addressing the biological sources of infection—represented a transition from a public health past that had been more focused on structural and systemic reform. In essence, the Department of Labor assumed the ideologies that had inspired Frances Perkins and the public health and social welfare activists of earlier in the century.

The story of silicosis in the first decades of the twentieth century, then, is the story of the discovery of chronic industrial disease and its relationship to industrial society. Even though silicosis was not the leading cause of death in the middle third of the twentieth century, it reflected, as the discussions at the Tri-State Conference indicated, the social and scientific assumptions of that era, and it framed the professional, industry, labor, and public understanding of disease. The crisis of silicosis forced the federal government for the first time to play an important role in addressing a disease that was neither an infection nor an immediate threat to the general public.

"THE EVIL EFFECTS" OF ASBESTOS DUST

The Tri-State Conference resulted in some changes in the mines that undoubtedly improved the conditions of work, but silicosis was not the only dust disease that emerged during the Depression. In England, where authorities kept track of such things, government factory inspectors early in the twentieth century had identified another insidious dust, this one causing widespread disability and death in mills that produced blankets made of asbestos, an insulating material used in coating steam engines, boilers, household stoves, and other objects subject to high heat. Like silicosis, asbestosis was a chronic condition, appearing years, if not decades, after workers entered an industry. It raised a host of concerns about how to legislate in a society dominated by corporations and private property holders, as well as how to reduce the corporation's social impact when it conflicted with the health needs and well-being of the community and workplace. In the midst of the Depression, the association of this disease with industrial work in Britain, the United States, and several other countries was bad enough. But policymakers now had to confront whether the "costs" of the disease were to be measured in lost lives or lost jobs. After all, introducing the ventilation equipment and personal protective equipment needed to limit exposure during an economic depression could conceivably put marginal companies out of business.

Concern about the industrial effects of working with asbestos in England go back to 1898, when "Lady" factory inspectors—women assigned by the government in London to inspect the hygiene of the country's textile mills, coal mines, and other industrial plants— journeyed to the northern textile mills where, for a century, cotton was woven and made into clothing and fabrics of all kinds. For at least a century, these mills were the center of the country's industrial revo- lution. But this time the inspectors visited the mills where a variety of asbestos blankets and other insulating materials were manufactured. Here they found workers suffering from what others called phthisis and consumption. "Of all the dusty occupations which specially came under observation in 1898 three . . . stand out on account of their eas- ily demonstrated danger to the health of the workers, and because of the ascertained cases of injury to bronchial tubes and lungs medically attributed to the employment of the suffer[er]s," began one of the Lady Factory Inspectors, Lucy Deane, or, as she was invariably referred to in the report, Miss Deane. She reported specifically on "the evil effects of asbestos dust." She noted that "a microscopic examination of this mineral dust . . . clearly revealed the sharp, glass-like jagged nature of the particles." These particles, when "allowed to rise and remain sus- pended in the air of a room, in any quantity, . . . have been found to be injurious, as might have been expected."[100]

Miss Deane and a colleague visited one asbestos works where "the work (sifting, mixing and carding) appeared to be carried on with the least possible attempt to subdue the dust . . . no sort of ventilation being applied."[101] As with the uncovering of silicosis, the British, with a cen- tralized governmental inspection system, were the first to formally iden- tify the dangers of asbestos dust and its debilitating effects, and in the coming decades they continued to document its dangers.[102] By the sec- ond decade of the twentieth century, Americans began to acknowledge its dangers as well. By 1917 representatives of American and Canadian insurance companies generally refused to offer life insurance policies for asbestos workers because of their increased risk of early death, and by the 1920s *Asbestos*, an American trade journal "Devoted to the

Interests of the Asbestos and Magnesia Industries," reported on workers in England who were dying of "asbestos poisoning."[103]

By the late 1920s, there was little doubt that asbestos was a cause of a newly identified fibrotic lung disease. Pathologists during an autopsy had identified asbestos "bodies" in the lungs of a thirty-three-year-old woman in the United Kingdom who had worked in the textile mills since she was thirteen. Around the same time, newly developed x-ray machines had begun to be used to document fibrotic lungs in living workers in the United States.[104] By 1928, a new disease entity was named, "asbestosis," which the leading medical journal in the United States, the *Journal of the American Medical Association*, warned "deserves more attention than it has had."[105] In 1930, E. R. A. Merewether, Britain's Medical Inspector of Factories, and C. W. Price, Britain's Engineering Inspector of Factories, detailed the results of their study of 363 asbestos textile workers, "21 of [whom] showed signs suggestive of commencing fibrosis. . . . Of these 12 had been employed for less than 7 years, and 6, for between 4 and 5 years."[106] They described asbestosis as causing a scarring of the lung that "gradually and literally strangles the essential tissues of the lung," eventually killing the worker. Asbestos was responsible not only for fibrosis in the long term but also for "pulmonary and bronchial catarrh, asthma, bronchitis, . . . and secondary changes, such as emphysema" and was "a notable factor in the production of the excess mortality rate from pulmonary tuberculosis" as well.[107] This information quickly circulated around the world in professional journals, and, by the early 1930s, reports of asbestosis were flooding in from clinicians and pathologists around the world. It was a growing problem because asbestos was now used in multiple products, sometimes as insulating materials for ducts and pipes and sometimes as cheap filler for grouting and wall sealants as well as "popcorn" ceiling decoration, wallboard, clothing, and mittens. Hollywood used it as "snow" when filming *The Wizard of Oz*, and Christmas trees were decorated with it to mimic snow and icicles. Further, immediately before and during World War II, the U.S. government used it to insulate battleships against fire, and thousands of workers were exposed in private and public shipbuilding yards, leading to studies of the safety measures taken or ignored there and the extent of disease.[108]

As early as 1932, Merewether had identified the origins of the new threat. He noted that asbestosis could result, not only from working with raw asbestos in asbestos textile factories, but also from "the sawing, grinding and turning in the dry state of articles composed wholly or partly of asbestos," such as in the replacement and grinding of "motor car brake[s] and clutch linings, jointings [the British term for what Americans referred to as gaskets], electric insulating materials and some types of electrodes." If a product contained asbestos and that product was manipulated in a way that released the asbestos dust, then those who breathed that dust were in danger, whether they worked in a factory or not.[109] By the mid- to late 1930s, a slew of lawsuits by sickened workers led to judgments that threatened the solvency of companies and led Pennsylvania, New Jersey, Massachusetts, Illinois, and many other industrialized states to include silicosis- and asbestos-related disease in their lists of conditions compensable under newly revised workers' compensation acts.[110]

BIOLOGIC BOMBS WITH A DELAYED TIME FUSE

While the recognition of asbestosis as a chronic condition of long latency was taken seriously, the public health community recognized that it affected fewer workers than silicosis did. But asbestosis soon presented another, even more troubling, problem: the fear that it could lead to lung cancer.[111] In the mid-1930s and early 1940s, a slew of pathology reports showed that asbestosis victims also had lung cancer. This fact raised the specter of cancer epidemics among the workforce and, potentially, the general population because asbestos had been adapted for use in so many products.

Wilhelm Hueper, in his massive tome *Occupational Tumors* (1942), had reported that "since 1935 an appreciable number of cases associated with asbestosis with carcinoma of the lung have been reported from England, Germany and the United States"; they were "suggestive" of a relationship between the two conditions because the number of such reports was "definitely excessive." Soon thereafter, in 1946, Hueper published an even more assertive article in the journal *Occupational Medicine*. He argued that occupational cancers "represent[ed] a challenge . . . to the social conscience of human society." Industrial cancers were like "a biologic bomb having a delayed time fuse . . . placed in the body of the victim without his knowledge and realization and which display[ed] its deadly effect many years later when the conditions connected with its introduction are often forgotten."[112] This was a sharp and quite troubling moral formulation of the growing worries about the impact of industrial work on the health of society, as America began to come to grips with the possible long-term effects of other "bombs," specifically those dropped on civilians in Hiroshima and Nagasaki. During the postwar era, the fear of nuclear power forced an anxious population to confront the health impact of what Dwight D. Eisenhower in his farewell address in January 1961 deemed the emerging "industrial-military complex."[113]

For much of the two decades preceding publication of Hueper's book, from the 1920s on, the public health field had begun a trek away from focusing on reform of the physical environment as the primary means of controlling disease. While the nineteenth century had seen the extraordinary success of infrastructural developments—sewer systems, swamp drainage, housing codes, aqueducts and reservoirs, sanitation departments, and the like—in stemming the onslaught of epidemics, the era after World War I had embraced laboratories, medical breakthroughs, and personal hygiene as keys to forestalling or fighting disease. Drawing inspiration from the remarkable discoveries of bacteriology and its promise of targeted and more precise interventions, as well as the promise of antitoxins, pharmaceuticals, and other medical treatments, public health departments, schools, and the profession more generally had begun an exodus that moved away from nineteenth-century origins and into the lab. For the most part, the issues that arose around the new industrial workplaces were not addressed by the biomedical approach that was increasingly being adopted by the public health community. Rather, it was the United States Department of Labor that filled the void because it saw the issue of occupational health not in biomedical terms but as embedded in the struggles of labor and capital.

Hibbert Hill, a Canadian epidemiologist trained at Johns Hopkins and the author of *The New Public Health* (1916), summarized an important strand of thought in early-twentieth-century public health when he proclaimed, "The old public health was concerned with the environment; the new public health is concerned with the individual. The old sought the sources of infectious disease in the surroundings of man; the new finds them in man himself. The old public health . . . failed because it sought them . . . in every place and in every thing *where they were not.*"

Unlike the "old" public health, which found solutions in tearing down slums, building the water supply system, and addressing the inequalities that plagued the poor in the ever-expanding large cities, the "new" public health, he claimed, was more efficient, even cheaper, focusing on the individual and identifying the diseased and the disease carrier, not expending scarce, expensive resources rebuilding entire communities.[114] Because the new public health advocates were focused more or less exclusively on the biological aspect of disease causation, they increasingly ignored the close interactions among social, environmental, and biological causes of disease. As we have seen in the case of tuberculosis, Frances Perkins saw clearly that relationship and brought her perspective into the Department of Labor when she became secretary.

The most vivid example of this move away from a social and humane understanding of disease within the public health community was the Tuskegee studies that the U.S. Public Health Service sponsored over several decades. In a desperately poor, underserved, and disenfranchised community of Black sharecroppers in Alabama, professionals in the name of science conducted a study of how syphilis affected African American men over time. In the early 1930s, the Public Health Service began an observational study of late latent stages of untreated syphilis in African Americans, even after the development in the 1940s of an effective antibiotic treatment for the disease. This left these men to suffer neurological effects such as stroke and paralysis, along with a host of other deadly consequences such as heart disease. The withholding of treatment for these men became a scandal in the 1970s. The Tuskegee experiment revealed not only the racism embedded in the public health assumptions of the time but also some of the more troubling results of the new ideology of the laboratory and science emerging in the early twentieth century. The emphasis on research and the laboratory, cloaked in an ideology that purported to be "objective," provided legitimacy for racist studies and undermined earlier traditions of public health rooted in activism and social reform.[115]

By the end of the Depression, the same two commingled but distinct approaches to public health in general were being applied to the health of workers. The Department of Labor and the Public Health Service took different positions. The first, as represented by Labor Secretary Frances Perkins and her division of Labor Standards, saw the incidence of disease as a sign of the social inequalities that created the "seedbed" for suffering. Government responsibilities included addressing these inequalities either by improving the conditions in which people worked and lived or regulating the powers that perpetuated the inequalities. The other path, as embodied in the U.S. Public Health Service, focused on identifying particular germs, gathering data, delineating disease pathways, and surveying disease outbreaks. In this view, government took no sides in the social, political, and moral issues that determined who lived and who died.[116]

The predominance of either the social or biological view of disease had deep political implications because it would determine which agencies of government would be primarily responsible for addressing occupational diseases. If occupational diseases were seen as rooted in individuals and their specific susceptibilities to toxins or bacteria, then the primary agency that would be responsible for addressing this issue would be the Public Health Service, most aligned with biomedicine. If those diseases were seen as rooted in the social and economic relationships of the workplace, then the Department of Labor, focused on labor and management relations, would take prominence. This was why Frances Perkins saw disease as within the purview of the Department of Labor. She was not calling for radical redistribution of wealth as the answer to the struggles of workers. She still had faith that, through social reform, the state could at least narrow, if not eliminate, the conditions constructed of great inequalities of resources and power that created so many early deaths and so much suffering. She had participated fully in the New York State factory investigations following the Triangle Fire in the hope that, along with factory safety and health legislation, corporations would voluntarily improve safety conditions; as secretary of labor, she organized conferences that brought labor and management together to discuss how to stop the silicosis epidemic, as we've seen. Yet, despite these efforts, corporate management saw her efforts as prolabor and feared that such efforts could disrupt the status quo in which corporations dominated and profited. They viewed the government's seeming support of labor during the Depression as dangerous. In the coming decades, a new effort to reassert the primacy of management and diminish the role of government would take shape. Postwar prosperity and a more conservative political climate would allow for the suppression of radicals and reformers inside and outside the labor movement. They would also make it difficult for government to support unions and have a say about conditions that affected workers' health and well-being.

The second half of the twentieth century would be marked by growing awareness of the centrality and effect of chronic disease on the health of Americans outside the factory setting. This period was marked by the growing perception that many chronic conditions, such as various types of cancers and heart disease, were shaped by environmental factors that were, in turn, the results of societal decisions about the way we live. It was with regard to silicosis that many of our most basic ideas regarding the relationship between the human environment and chronic disease were formulated. The silicosis crisis of the 1930s brought into question one of the central beliefs of the twentieth century—that technological innovation and the growth of industry would, as a matter of course, provide general improvements in the quality of people's lives. In the post–World War II era, the complexity of chronic illness and its relationship to the environment would call into question the decisions that we as a nation have made about the kind of world we want to live in. They would also undermine a general faith that technology can solve all problems. Following the crisis over silicosis, the federal government began to accept a role in the identification and control of toxins that caused chronic disease, particularly diseases linked to heavy industry. In this sense the government was accepting that it had a responsibility to ensure a better world to live in, one with less disease and death. In the immediate aftermath of World War II, the recognition that work had a direct impact on health was mostly focused on mines, factories, and chemical facilities. Beginning in the 1960s and 1970s, more and more white-collar and agricultural workers began to absorb the lessons of the past.

CHAPTER SIX

Better Living Through Chemistry?

> "Silently and insidiously they creep, like old age, upon their victims distributed over many industries. . . . They are difficult to diagnose and often masquerade as other diseases."
>
> E. R. A. MEREWETHER, 1950

> "Today chemicals pervade so many phases of man's environment we might say the environment has been 'chemicalized.'"
>
> HARVEY F. LUDWIG, "CHEMICALS AND ENVIRONMENTAL HEALTH," 1955

Since at least the early part of the twentieth century and in some cases before, deaths from the main nineteenth-century infections have been declining significantly. The rate of tuberculosis, probably the nation's leading cause of death throughout the nineteenth century, was halved every two decades from the 1880s onward.[1] Typhoid, cholera, and other water-borne diseases were largely controlled through the successful reengineering of the water supply and sewerage systems, the passage of food regulations and housing laws, and other improvements that resulted in better ventilation, rodent control, and flush toilets. Other changes further altered people's health experience as public transportation moved away from reliance on the horse to reliance on electric trolleys and then gas-powered engines and as the construction of subways lowered the density of highly congested cities. In medicine, a diphtheria antitoxin was developed in the late nineteenth century, and a vaccine for the disease became available in the 1920s and 1930s. In the mid- to late nineteenth century, vaccines for smallpox replaced variolation, and in subsequent decades of the twentieth century vaccines were introduced to prevent measles, mumps, and diphtheria. The development and wide use of penicillin in the 1940s and other antibiotics in subsequent years vastly improved the treatment of a host of bacterial infections. Even polio, the terrifying summertime threat, began to lose its ferocity in the public mind with the successful development of the Salk (1955) and then the Sabin (1960) vaccines. Public health and then medical science had seemed to "conquer" infections.

It was in this changing epidemiological context that the nation became more conscious of the prevalence of chronic conditions like heart disease, stroke, and cancer on which the old public health preventative technologies and the newer curative medical miracles seemed to have little or no impact. Cancer went from being the eighth leading cause of death in 1900 to the second leading cause of death (after heart disease) by 1940. In fact, the rate of cancer diagnosis doubled between 1900 and 1950 and continued to rise throughout the rest of the twentieth century. These increased rates could have been a function of better detection methods and more comprehensive screening, but they were also due to the fact that people were living longer. In 1930, the average length of life for men was 58 years and for women, 61.6 years; by 1950, the length of life for men and women had increased substantially. Men on average now lived to 65 and women lived to 70.[2] Nonetheless, many believed that improvements in early detection, surgery, radiation, and chemical interventions (chemotherapies) could treat these conditions. Other chronic conditions like diabetes and asthma also increased in the second half of the century. Two things are notable about this change in the patterns of disease. First, these diseases seemed to be linked to the greatly expanded use of both old and new chemicals and products, affecting both workers and the general public. And second, many of these materials were being introduced into a consumer society with very little attention to their safety. After World War I and increasingly in the post–World War II period, a host of newly identified carcinogenic materials, such as asbestos and tobacco, as we saw in chapter 5, were being linked to lung cancer and mesothelioma. About the same time, these materials were incorporated into thousands of consumer products. Asbestos, for example, was being used in floor tiles, spackle, and the filters of cigarettes. Synthetic organic chemicals such as vinyl chloride were used in hair sprays, piping, and liquor bottles, and polychlorinated biphenyls (PCBs) were used in pesticides, inks, paints, adhesives, the ballasts of fluorescent lighting, and even chewing gum. Tobacco was marketed to millions of people and, especially during World War II, to young men in the armed forces.

Rightly or wrongly, by the mid-twentieth century the great infectious epidemics of the nineteenth century were perceived to be largely over. Americans were able, on average, to add decades to their longevity between 1900 and 1950, with the years of the 1918–1919 flu pandemic as the great exception. In 1900 the average life span of Americans was 46 years. By 2010, the average age at death was over 80 for women and 77 for men. With the exception of the past few years, when Covid-19 and opioids took their toll, the popular and professional story of the past twelve decades has been of increasing longevity. Yet the disparities in death and disease rates between Black and white, Native American, Hispanic, and Anglo, rich and poor—the historic manifestations of the inequalities inherent in the societies we built—remained, although they narrowed some. For example, in 1950 life expectance for whites at birth was 69.1 years, and for African Americans it was 60.8. By 2017, there was still a gap, but it had narrowed. A white child was predicted to live to 78.8 years old, while an African American child was predicted to live to 75.3 years.[3]

In 1800, tuberculosis had risen to 1 death in every 100 people. By 1960 it was fewer than 5 in every 100,000. In 1900 the leading causes of death were predominantly infectious diseases, among them tuberculosis, pneumonia, and diarrhea (with heart disease, kidney disease, and stroke emerging as important). By 1968, given the radically reduced rate of deaths from infectious disease, some experts were declaring that continued focus on infectious disease was misplaced, and even the Public Health Service's surgeon general was said to declare that chronic diseases such as heart disease, cancer, and stroke were the real problems of the future. That same year, a report from the Public Health Service's National Committee on Vital and Health Statistics argued that "the ascendancy of chronic noninfectious diseases as major causes of morbidity and mortality requires new types of data and changes of emphasis in existing types of data."[4] In public and professional minds, lung cancer, diabetes, heart disease, and other chronic conditions had replaced the nineteenth-century scourges of smallpox, tuberculosis, cholera, and typhoid.[5]

In the post–World War II era, Americans began to realize that the environmental hazards of an earlier era had even more ominous repercussions than originally thought. While asbestos and its associated disease, asbestosis, had made physicians and industrial leaders aware of the dangers of chronic disease caused by the industrial environment in the 1930s and 1940s, as we saw in chapter 5, by the 1940s and 1950s asbestos, along with other building materials, was being linked to newer, more menacing threats. In 1950, E. R. A. Merewether, the same person who had written the influential 1930 factory inspectors' report on asbestosis, presented his latest findings to the Canadian Medical Association Section on Industrial Medicine. In a series of pathology reports of over 232 deaths from asbestosis, more than 13 percent "were found on autopsy to have cancer of the lungs." Merewether, by now the dean of the field of dust diseases, began by saying, "It can be said with certainty that a few months' exposure to silica or asbestos dust in gross or, to use Leroy Gardner's happy word, 'insulting' concentrations will inevitably cause death." The problem was not an individual, local, or even national one, he continued; it was global: asbestosis—and therefore asbestos—were linked to lung cancer in countries around the world. "When we go further and think, not of one small country, but of the world and consider the toll of life throughout the ages from [asbestosis and lung cancer] . . ., we may well regard them as one of the major scourges of humanity."[6]

Merewether worried that the modern infatuation with bacteriology and personal health had diverted attention from the terrible costs in human life of insidious diseases of long latency and wondered what could account for it. "When we think of the achievements of medicine in preventing and curing diseases like diphtheria, we cannot help but ask, with something of shame, why mortality from these dust diseases remains so high." After all, he pointed out, "in theory at any rate, they are wholly preventable." He believed the public health community and the broader society needed to appreciate the "urgency" of dealing with chronic diseases of long latency, but he was skeptical that they would. Why? His theory was that "the pneumokonioses"— the generic term for all dust diseases of the lung such as asbestosis, silicosis, brown lung (caused by cotton dust), and black lung (caused by coal dust)—"have no spectacular impact on the community, like accidents or dramatic epidemic diseases which make news headlines: silently and insidiously they creep, like old age, upon their victims distributed over many industries, who fade away with little but local disturbances. They are difficult to diagnose and often masquerade as other diseases."[7]

At the same time that Merewether was making his observations about lung cancer and asbestosis, the British researchers Richard Doll and Bradford Hill were documenting that tobacco smokers also suffered disproportionately from lung disease. In 1948, statisticians in England had noted a dramatic rise in the number of people dying of lung cancer, and the Medical Research Council, Britain's premier medical research unit, sponsored a conference devoted to identifying the causes of this rise. Doll and Hill began a survey and then a controlled study of 650 men in London hospitals and discovered that those who reported being smokers had a disproportionately high incidence of lung cancer. The two epidemiologists next expanded their study to include 750 patients in four other communities with starkly different social characteristics and in different areas of the country—Bristol, a maritime community; Leeds, one of the early centers of the Industrial Revolution; Cambridge, home of scholars and elites; and Newcastle, a city built around coal mining. They identified the same relationship between smoking and lung cancer. The paper, finally published in 1954 in the *British Medical Journal*, was strongly contested by the tobacco industry, leading to years of corporate-sponsored public relations efforts and spurious science meant to create doubt in the mounting evidence of a link between smoking and lung cancer.[8]

By the 1950s, researchers were documenting links not only between smoking and lung cancer, and asbestos and lung cancer, but also the changes in lifestyle that were producing increased rates of heart disease, diabetes, and stroke. The postwar fast-paced economy built around white-collar office work was increasingly seen as a source of stress that led to the changes in diet and behavior that promoted heart disease and stroke. Women, for example, saw a dramatic change in workplace participation. By the 1950s the leading workplace had shifted from domestic work to clerical work.

Two parallel explanations of the rise of heart disease, stroke, and cancer competed in both professional and lay circles: either corporate campaigns stimulated, often even created, demand for products they understood could create disease and so were themselves responsible, or individual lifestyle and personal choices about what we ate, drank, or smoked and how we lived largely determined these diseases. Was lung cancer, for example, the result of a ravenous tobacco industry convincing millions of teenagers to buy its brand and thereby hooking them on tobacco, or was it a personal free choice made by soldiers, young adults, and others who exercised their freedom to choose? Was the industry targeting specific groups, like women, who were told that smoking Virginia Slims was a feminist act? Or was it targeting African Americans, as the historian Keith Wailoo documents, telling them that the manufacturers of Kool cigarettes were supporters of African American culture?[9] See figures 6.1 and 6.2.

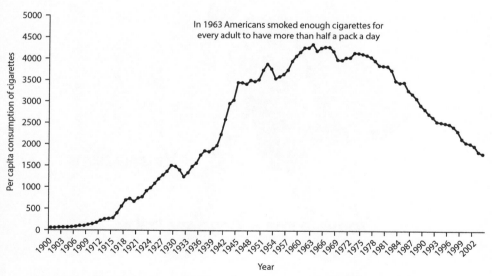

FIGURE 6.1 Per capita consumption of cigarettes among adults ages eighteen years and older from 1990 to 2004. Source: Institute of Medicine, "Epidemiology of Tobacco Use: History and Current Trends," in National Academies of Sciences, Engineering, and Medicine, *Ending the Tobacco Problem: A Blueprint for the Nation* (Washington, DC: National Academies Press, 2007), 42.

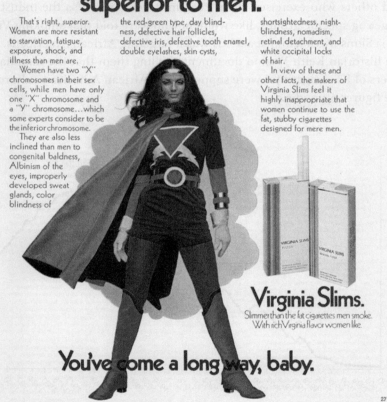

We make Virginia Slims especially for women because they are biologically superior to men.

That's right, *superior.* Women are more resistant to starvation, fatigue, exposure, shock, and illness than men are.

Women have two "X" chromosomes in their sex cells, while men have only one "X" chromosome and a "Y" chromosome...which some experts consider to be the inferior chromosome.

They are also less inclined than men to congenital baldness, Albinism of the eyes, improperly developed sweat glands, color blindness of

the red-green type, day blindness, defective hair follicles, defective iris, defective tooth enamel, double eyelashes, skin cysts,

shortsightedness, nightblindness, nomadism, retinal detachment, and white occipital locks of hair.

In view of these and other facts, the makers of Virginia Slims feel it highly inappropriate that women continue to use the fat, stubby cigarettes designed for mere men.

Virginia Slims.
Slimmer than the fat cigarettes men smoke.
With rich Virginia flavor women like.

You've come a long way, baby.

27

FIGURE 6.2 Two cigarette ads from the 1970s and 1980s targeting women and African Americans: (*A*) Virginia Slims; (*B*) Kool.

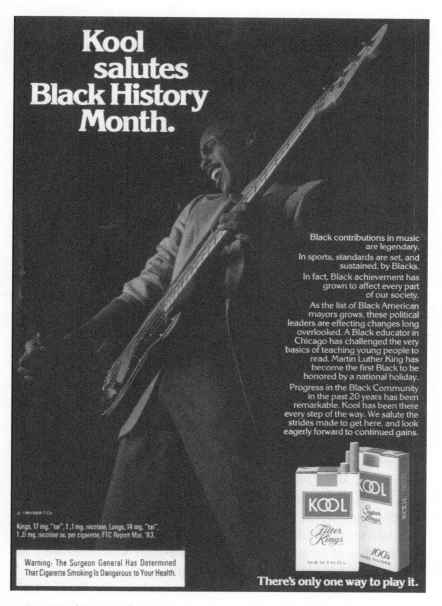

FIGURE 6.2 (*Continued*)

Was alcohol advertising and availability to the young something to regulate more strictly, or would such government action intrude in the "free market" and place an unjustified limitation on individual liberty? Were the rising rates of Type II diabetes due to what consumers "wanted," or were they due to a restructured agricultural and marketing economy that promoted junk and fast food?

The way these questions were answered had enormous implications for industries that were dependent on mass-produced chickens, fast food, tobacco, chemical additives, synthetic fibers, and plastics—and for Americans' health. Many in U.S. industry argued that industrial progress was fulfilling the promise of the American dream by offering consumers a wide variety of products to stock their refrigerators, fill their garages, and spray on their lawns. But others cautioned that this bounty was coming at a cost: not only did all not share in it equally, but the use of new, often untested materials and the expanded use of old toxins were already having deleterious effects on both the environment and on human health.

Despite the growing awareness of the dangers to health from older toxins, some companies moved headlong to develop new, often untested synthetic products. The defeat of Germany and the destruction of the European chemical industry in World War I allowed American companies to expand largely unimpeded in the 1920s. Companies took over German patents and developed in the lab new synthetic resins from hydrocarbons and carbon disulphide to make a host of new synthetic fibers, including rayon, nylon, cellulose, and synthetic threads. These were used to make clothes, "fake silk" stockings (figure 6.3), cellophane, and even kitchen sponges.[10] Others saw the development of pesticides and herbicides as useful in the expanding agricultural market—DDT (figure 6.4), Aldrin, and other chlorinated hydrocarbons became ubiquitous in the American environment.

Questions about the introduction of new technologies and chemicals into the environment arose in the 1940s and 1950s in the context of a number of social and political realities that Americans were just beginning to understand. The United States came out of World War II as the dominant industrial and military nation, but with that came new threats. The Cold War and the Soviet Union's explosion of its own atomic bomb fed an underlying fear that new technologies—particularly atomic

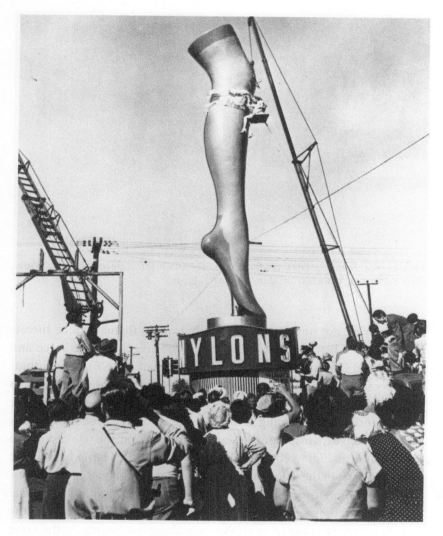

FIGURE 6.3 Marketing nylon, Los Angeles, California, 1946. Movie star Marie Wilson is shown suspended from a crane next to a 30-foot-high reproduction of her calf. Courtesy of the Hagley Museum.

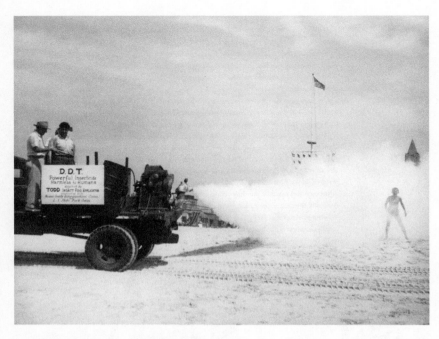

FIGURE 6.4 Spraying DDT for mosquito control on Jones Beach on Long Island, New York, 1945. Courtesy of Alamy/Pictorial Press.

energy—were not unmitigated goods, but might themselves be threats in ways never before experienced. The Women's Strike for Peace and the National Committee for a Sane Nuclear Policy (SANE), both antinuclear organizations active in the 1950s, addressed not only the threats to world peace but also the health effects of nuclear testing, including the radiation that was spreading across the globe.[11] In the 1960s Americans witnessed the expansion of the war in Vietnam and the use of napalm on civilians, including children, and they eventually learned about the toxic fallout from the use of Agent Orange to defoliate Vietnam's forests. Protesters pointed to the increasing power of the "military-industrial complex," and they specifically targeted those industries that made the materials that went into America's war-making machinery. At the same time, there was anxiety that the investment in technology and "progress" drew away resources needed to address social problems. A reinvigorated civil rights movement brought the nation's attention to poverty, segregation, and racism, further sensitizing people to the inequities in power that plagued the country. In the 1970s, the nuclear accident at Three Mile Island near Harrisburg, Pennsylvania (along with the popular movie *The China Syndrome*), further raised public awareness of the possible impact of technological change on the nation's well-being.

The late 1950s through the 1960s was a period when Americans were both becoming more aware of dangers to the environment and growing increasingly suspicious of the motives and trustworthiness of America's industrial corporations. It was not long before armies of environmentalists, consumer activists, and labor unions joined to challenge corporate arguments concerning industrial production, particularly pollution, and pointed to corporate actions and policies that threatened Americans' health. The chemical industry, as one of the fastest-growing sectors of the economy and the purveyor of many of the newest toxic substances, was soon confronted by these environmental, consumer, and labor groups that pressed for the creation of federal agencies to act to control industry and protect the health and welfare of workers and the public.

POISONS, POLLUTION, AND PUBLIC HEALTH

The total amount of capital in the chemical sector of the U.S. economy grew about 1,000 percent between 1899 and 1948, far more than any other sector of the economy except for the transportation sector, which had ballooned because of the phenomenal growth of the automobile industry.[12] In the decades following World War II, the chemical industry argued that emissions from its plants and the chemical substances they produced at worst constituted a nuisance, not a health hazard. Further, just as the automobile and oil industries had argued when lead in gasoline was introduced in the 1920s, they argued that the substances were a small price for the country to pay for economic progress and the good things that industry made possible.

As the growing environmental, consumer, and labor movements in the 1960s expressed distrust of the chemical industry's claims of limited (if any) harm, some within the industry itself privately viewed environmental pollution as a very serious hazard that companies ignored at their own peril.[13] But publicly the chemical corporations remained united in assuring Americans that they could be trusted to protect community residents and the natural environment as well.

Following World War II, the chemical and electrical industries produced massive advertising campaigns in which they proclaimed for themselves a special role in America's newfound affluence. The E. I. du Pont de Nemours and Company (DuPont) announced that the "American century" was made possible by "Better Things for Better Living . . . Through Chemistry," while the General Electric Company advertised over and over that "Progress is our Most Important Product." For the first half of the twentieth century, despite particular environmental crises and increased scientific concern about pollution, many Americans, fairly hypnotized by a parade of technological advances, had remained largely unaware of the ecological and health costs of such progress. Most were eagerly incorporating the plastic chairs, radio casings, toys, and wall coverings, products of the chemical industry, into their lives. Meanwhile, General Electric and Westinghouse were providing the seemingly unlimited energy and equipment to run appliances like electric ranges and refrigerators, as well as motors for new gizmos of every type. Few among the public initially thought that polyethylene, vinyl chloride, and chlorinated biphenyl, among other increasingly ubiquitous substances, could possibly pose a danger. Fascination with this seemingly good life depended on a shared set of values that equated the progress of a society with the technological progress from the production of electric motors to the production of atomic bombs—as well as ignorance of the health consequences of the products and how they were manufactured.[14]

Americans were also largely indifferent to the dangers posed by smokestacks and oil rigs.[15] A tragedy that occurred in Donora, Pennsylvania, in 1948 began to wake them up. According to a report put out by the Pennsylvania Department of Environmental Protection, this small factory town near Pittsburgh, home to a number of smelters and steel mills, including the American Steel and Wire Company's zinc works, was enveloped in "a poisonous mix of sulfur dioxide, carbon monoxide and metal dust . . . from the smokestacks from the local zinc smelter where most of the town worked." An air inversion turned the street dark at noon. "Twenty residents died and half the town's population—7,000 people—were hospitalized over the next five days with difficulty breathing."[16] For those five days, a cloud of toxins sat over the town.[17]

Meanwhile, Americans were beginning to notice the effect of pollution on the environment. The rapid growth of Los Angeles and its dependence on the automobile raised worries among the public about smog and its long-term effects on American health, and therefore new worries for industry.[18] Smog, in the words of one industry trade journal, "cease[d] to be a joke to industrialists."[19] Overseas, as early as 1930, industrial pollution was identified as responsible for the Meuse Valley Fog in Belgium that sickened several thousand people and caused the death of an estimated sixty people. The Great London Fog of 1952 raised even greater concerns when a heavy smog, caused primarily by the burning of coal, blanketed London and caused the death of apparently twelve thousand people.[20]

Understanding that air pollution's effect on health was potentially a significant political issue, the Manufacturing Chemists' Association, the trade association of the chemical industry, sought to depict air pollution as "a nuisance problem and not a health problem."[21] The American Petroleum Institute (API), the trade association of the portion of the chemical industry that was primarily concerned with petroleum refining, also addressed the growing fear that air pollution from industry was linked to serious diseases. Seeking a way to reconceptualize the health issue as one of annoyance and nuisance, John C. Ruddock, a former lead researcher and the chair of the API's Subcommittee on Atmospheric Pollutants, argued repeatedly that with the exception of incidents at Donora, London, and Meuse, so far no one had been able to prove "aggravation of such diseases as asthma, tuberculosis, bronchitis, etc., nor does air pollution particularly affect the aged or very young." He agreed that air pollution should be reduced, and he was, he said, "sympathetic with all those who do not like 'smog.' As true Americans, we do not like our rights infringed upon, whether it is the inability to see as far as we desire, or whether it is the discomfort and eye-smarting that occurs with air pollution." Certainly, there were many "poisonous and noxious fumes" in polluted air. But, he argued, they were only dangerous when they exceeded "a certain density and are either inspired or ingested."[22]

"We have found no single case, nor have we found any pathological effect attributable to atmospheric pollutant per se," the API claimed.[23] Yet, at this very time (the decade of the 1950s), studies had begun to appear documenting the impact of smog from industrial pollution and automobiles on human health. Studies following the London smog of December 1952 documented that people died from the chemicals in the air they breathed. In London, 370 tons of sulfur dioxide were converted into 800 tons of sulfuric acid, while 140 tons of hydrochloric acid, 2,000 tons of carbon dioxide, and 14 tons of fluorine compounds were held responsible for the over four thousand deaths that are believed to have occurred in a four-day period.[24] Studies of Los Angeles in the 1950s similarly heightened awareness of the dangers of industrial and automobile smog by documenting where most of the pollution came from and showing that it was produced not just by cars but by the burning of fossil fuels anywhere.[25]

"EVERY VENTURE INVOLVES SOME RISK"

The chemical industry was clearly worried about what would be made of the growing body of research on the health effects of pollution. In early 1962 the Manufacturing Chemists' Association (MCA)'s Public Relations Advisory Committee expressed a sense of "urgency of the situation confronting us."[26] The MCA began to introduce into its argument about the benefits of the chemical industry the idea of "acceptable" risk. "Whether public health officials will admit it or not," Dr. E. O. Colwell of the Aluminum Company of America told the Air Pollution Abatement Committee, "there is a place for the term 'calculated risk' in this human health business." Echoing the argument made nearly thirty-five years earlier by the General Motors representative who declared that leaded gasoline was a "gift of God," Colwell asked, "What price are we willing to pay for absolutely clean air?" It was both impractical and unnecessary "to make the air so clean that the most sensitive individuals will be comfortable if such is not economically sound," he said. "The public we must satisfy would better risk a few cases of bronchitis or even emphysema than to risk mental and physical ills that would accompany the economic failure of an industry, a community, or a country"—as if a few pollution control devices and improved practices would bring down everything from a company to a country. From the industry perspective, the economic interests of the chemical industry were synonymous with the interests of the country,[27] or, as Charles Wilson, president of General Motors and later secretary of defense, was quoted to have said, "what was good for our country was good for General Motors, and vice versa."[28]

The publication of Rachel Carson's *Silent Spring* in September 1962 decisively undermined the chemical industry's reassuring overall message. Carson biographer Linda Lear has written that industry and others recognized *Silent Spring* as "a fundamental social critique of a gospel of technological progress." Some quarters were so threatened by Carson's book that they attacked her personally. Ezra Taft Benson, the secretary of agriculture in the Eisenhower administration and later a leading elder of the Mormon Church, asked "why a spinster with no children was so concerned about genetics," suggesting that it was because she was "probably a communist."[29]

Silent Spring was certainly not a "communist" tract. But it did provide a telling critique of the chemical and agricultural industries' drive to reshape the world through chemistry and corporate greed. The book argues that the twentieth century, with its creation of the industrial machine, was "the moment of time" when "one species—man—acquired significant power to alter the nature of his world," and that chemicals were "the sinister and little-recognized partners of radiation in changing the very nature of the world."[30] Explicit in the book was a critique of modern farming practices and specifically the concentration of American agriculture in a few large companies following World War II. Carson argued that the creation of single-crop farming—huge, corporately owned tracts devoted to one grain or plant that could be efficiently planted, fertilized, sprayed with pesticides, and harvested—had destroyed the natural, diverse, balanced environment that had evolved over eons of time. Small farmers, by intermingling diverse crop species among one another, as nature had done, minimized the threat posed by insects that thrived on one particular grain: they could not destroy an entire ecosystem of plants to which they were ill-suited. Now one species of bug could.[31]

Rachel Carson's publication, *Silent Spring* (1962), was the culmination of more than twenty years of research that had documented the ways that chlorinated hydrocarbons had endangered the environment and the general ecology. Her book, written as a popular text, explained to the general public the enormous body of scientific literature that showed that DDT and other chlorinated hydrocarbons were persistent in the environment, causing death and disease among vertebrates and invertebrates alike. Most significantly, she also documented the damage and long-term threats to mammals, among them human beings. She explained that it was impossible to know the long-term effects of the accumulation of small amounts of these chemicals, both alone and in combination. She also hypothesized that cancer was associated with exposure to chlorinated hydrocarbons. The book set off a firestorm of controversy because she put together in one place an extensive scientific literature. But more importantly, she wrote in a prose that was accessible to scientists and the general public alike, and she helped spur the development of a popular environmental movement that would make the accumulated science, previously of little popular impact, relevant and central to broad policy debates.[32]

The early reaction of industry to the concern about pesticides was simple: put the responsibility for danger on the back of the customers: by "educating" them. All that was needed was "a strong program of education for customers and the general public in the appropriate use of products."[33]

Despite the willingness of some chemical industry representatives to keep their heads in the sand, the chair of the MCA's Environmental Health Advisory Committee, James Sterner, acknowledged in 1967 that the available data indicated that problems attributable to chemical pollution would soon be approaching apocalyptic proportions. Given that sulfur dioxide contamination in some urban areas was already a serious problem, in the future it was likely to become extremely dangerous, he suggested. Water pollution from industrial plants and the runoff from the pesticides used on farms, as well as the waste from hogs and other animals raised there, had already caused the near death of major rivers, such as the Cuyahoga River in Ohio; some rivers would "in another decade . . . have zero dissolved oxygen." While some on his committee might think his predictions too extreme, he noted, "there is a growing procession of thoughtful and critical scientists and citizens whose initial skepticism has changed to concern and even alarm."[34]

In 1969 the MCA did finally acknowledge that air pollution was a health problem and not merely a nuisance, but still the industry downplayed the dangers. It agreed that some people, already suffering from respiratory disease, could be "adversely affected" by air pollution, but people in good health, "even though temporarily discomforted," would quickly recover from acute exposure to chemical pollution "without residual damage." It was "unlikely" that air pollution was "a sole or principal cause of any disease entity," and at worst it could accelerate the death of those previously ill, particularly among the elderly. But the industry conceded no clear health risk from long-term exposure, no relationship between allergic asthma and air pollution, and no clear relationship in the United States between bronchitis and air pollution, despite the gathering evidence from studies of Los Angeles and other major cities.

By 1969, the federal bureaucracy included over eighty agencies that dealt with air or water pollution and other problems of the environment. That year, Congress passed the National Environmental Policy Act (NEPA) and created a Council on Environmental Quality to provide an "exhaustive study" of the environmental impact of any proposed federal project.[35] The President's Advisory Council on Executive Organization, appointed by President Richard Nixon and chaired by Roy Ash, the former CEO of Litton Industries, recommended in the spring of 1970 that an Environmental Protection Agency (EPA) also be established as "an independent body concerned with pollution abatement and with jurisdiction over all monitoring, research, standard setting and enforcement."[36] In early July of that year, Nixon formally proposed the EPA as part of a reorganization plan, thereby outflanking the Democrats, who had staked out the environment as one of their major issues.

In January 1970, the need for the EPA was confirmed as the nation learned of a massive oil spill off the coast of Santa Barbara, California. Millions of viewers of the evening news saw huge numbers of birds covered with oil struggling in the water, dead seals washing up on shore, and dead fish covering the beach.[37] Three months later the first Earth Day demonstrations took place around the nation.[38] The EPA was established that same month as a cabinet-level agency.[39] In the short span of a decade, then, the chemical industry, which had become the leading symbol of the country's industrial and technological progress, was the subject of considerable suspicion. In 1965, Americans had ranked environmental pollution near the bottom of the ten most important problems facing the nation, but by 1970 pollution had become the second most pressing issue in public opinion polls, ranking just below crime reduction.[40]

By the late 1960s, the chemical industry was also tied in the public's eye to the "military-industrial complex" and the divisive controversies of the Vietnam War. When Dow Chemical Company produced napalm as a weapon to use against civilian populations and created herbicides to defoliate the forests that were said to hide North Vietnamese and National Liberation Front troops, students protested on college campuses across America. They accused the chemical industry of complicity in "ecocide" in Southeast Asia, and protests on campus carried signs declaring "Dow = Death."[41] More generally, the prosperity of the 1960s, the technologies that appeared to be at its core, and their use against peoples in a far-off land had ironically led Americans to become far less naïve about the deleterious effects of modern technological and industrial progress.[42] The growing skepticism about corporate America's involvement in the military-industrial complex fed suspicion of the impact of consumerism and chemicals on the environment and on health.

During the 1960s, new conservation and environmental groups were attracting younger, more politically activist members.[43] As the historian Samuel Hays explains, this period marked a transition in the history of environmentalism in the United States. Older groups, like the Sierra Club, the National Wildlife Federation, and the Audubon Society, which had focused primarily on outdoor recreation, forest preservation, and the maintenance of open spaces, now turned to a consideration of air and water pollution. Later, in the 1970s, they turned to safe and sustainable forms of energy and the deleterious effects of toxic chemicals, radiation, and other threats on the environment and human health.[44] The traditional environmental movement, which focused on conservation and environmental preservation, was primarily middle class in constituency and orientation, with participants often seeing the city, the factory, and even those who worked in it as natural enemies of a pristine, natural environment. It would take the challenge of working people, both white and Black, to transform environmentalism in the 1980s into a more radical and anti-establishment movement.

LABOR JOINS THE FRAY

As the 1960s saw the beginnings of a trend toward greater federal involvement in environmental protection, labor and consumer activists joined together to push for the passage of two significant pieces of federal legislation. The Coal Mine Safety and Health Act of 1969, the first wide-ranging and strict federal legislation covering the mine industry in the United States, included provisions for annual inspections of coal mines, mandatory fines for safety and health infractions, and compensation for miners afflicted with black lung disease. The second significant piece of legislation was the Occupational Safety and Health Act (OSHAct) of 1970, establishing the Occupational Safety and Health Administration (OSHA) in the Labor Department and the National Institute for Occupational Safety and Health (NIOSH) in the Department of Health, Education, and Welfare. Never before had the federal government established an agency such as OSHA, with a mandate to protect the health of the nation's workers. In fact, before this time, especially in the early years following World War II, an implicit labor-management "accord" virtually eliminated issues of workers' safety and health from the formal agenda in contract negotiations. While wages and hours were negotiable, safety and health issues were seen as a challenge to management's prerogative to maintain control over the work process. Although the labor movement of the 1960s was viewed as conservative because of its identification with the military and its blue-collar disdain for the youth movements of the day, there were indications of a more activist strain within it. It was the Vietnam War, in fact, that placed new pressures for production on American industry, resulting in speed-ups, long hours of required overtime, and a resulting increase in the number of industrial accidents, all of which laid the groundwork for greater rank-and-file attention to issues of health and safety.[45] In 1966 and 1967, the number of strikes reached a decade-long high, and declining productivity coupled with an increasingly militant labor force spelled potential trouble for business.[46]

When Anthony Mazzocchi, the head of the Oil, Chemical and Atomic Workers International Union (OCAW) local on Long Island, became the legislative director of the union in 1965, he "started getting tons of calls" about a range of health and safety issues. At the union's convention in 1967, concern was so great that the delegates passed a resolution that identified the dangers that members of the union faced from working with benzene and other chemicals.[47] OCAW was an unusual union, however, and didn't restrict concern to its own workers. Instead, it recognized that the same hazards that affected workers also posed a threat to the community. Mazzocchi pointed out that the "very pollutants that are contaminating our environment emanate from the workplace."[48]

Unlike the steel mills, mines, and foundries where the dangers from accidents, extraordinary heat, dust-laden air, and odious fumes were fairly obvious, the new chemical plants looked clean and modern. "But," Mazzocchi warned, "the industry we work in has a danger that most people are unaware of, and it's insidious."[49] The chemical industry exposed workers to not only traditional and known toxins, but also to thousands of new untested and unregulated chemicals.[50] "Exposing a person to a toxic chemical that shortens his life is tantamount to murder, in my opinion," Mazzocchi said.[51]

Mazzocchi recognized that the workers who labored with such dangerous materials were the true repositories of information about unhealthful workplace practices, and they had knowledge of the ways their companies were trying to hide the danger to the community. Workers reported "being instructed to permit certain emissions, into the air and into sewers, after dark but not during daylight hours." They were instructed by management to curtail dumping activities when the media were around or when inspectors were present. "Workers in some plants tell of being ordered to inject perfumes into exhaust gases going up the stacks so that people in the vicinity cannot smell the gases."[52]

One of the most important labor organizing efforts of the mid-twentieth century combined the health concerns of both workers and consumers. In the late 1960s and the early 1970s, Cesar Chavez and Dolores Huerta, two Chicano agricultural workers in California's Central Valley, organized the largely migrant farmworkers into one of the most prominent unions in the country, the United Farm Workers (UFW). The farmworkers organized a national boycott of grapes and lettuce over working conditions for the largely Mexican and Filipino field workers and over the potential health hazards that pesticides sprayed on the crops posed to both the workforce and consumers.[53] In 1969, the United Farm Workers won a contract that included "language banning DDT, DDE, and dieldrin . . . covering union farms in and around Delano, and the use of other dangerous pesticides altogether."[54]

By the mid-1960s, the threat of chemicals to the general public had been firmly established in the public mind. Childhood poisoning from lead paint had become a symbol of the damage done to low-income African American and Hispanic children in their poorly maintained tenement housing. Automobile exhaust, with its toxic stew of sulfur, lead, and carbon monoxide, was now understood as an important component of urban smog, affecting children in crowded neighborhoods where cars stalled in traffic released these chemicals into the air. Smokestacks from the chemical, oil, and heavy industries, once symbols of economic progress, were now more likely seen as symbols of the excesses of the new industrial order. Pesticides were widely viewed, not as a great advance but as a potential cause of cancers and environmental destruction affecting rich and poor alike, if to different degrees. It was in this context that consumers and workers joined in parallel struggles to address industrial threats to human health.

Over the course of the twentieth century, agriculture had undergone a fundamental reorganization, with giant industrialized farms replacing many of the family farms that had been the basis of American rural life in the nineteenth and early twentieth centuries. In 1949 Herbert Abrams, the chief of California's Bureau of Adult Health, explained the health consequences of this transformation. A new class of pesticides had been used with increasing frequency—organophosphates, which were highly toxic and already shown to cause illness and even death among farmworkers.[55] In 1960, Edward R. Murrow aired his classic documentary, *Harvest of Shame*, which depicted the horrendous conditions under which migrant workers on the East Coast labored virtually all their lives. Through moving interviews with Black and white fruit and vegetable harvesters, he documented how a completely isolated, migrant workforce lived without the protections and labor laws that other regulated industries offered. They had neither workers' compensation protections nor unemployment insurance. Their housing lacked running water and indoor toilets, and they were reduced to sleeping on beds infested by lice, mice, and even rats. As Murrow notes, the migrant workers, many of whom had worked in the fields with their parents from the time they turned eight years old, were among the most exploited people in the country, with no political power and no means of escaping their poverty. Working from dawn to dusk and traveling in overloaded trucks from one field to another, they labored for a dollar a day, which allowed them to buy milk for their children only once a week. One line in the documentary captures the exploitative relationship between the owners of the farms and their workers: "We no longer own slaves," he remarks; "now we rent them."[56]

Despite the documentary's powerful impact, it is telling that little was mentioned of the hazards these families faced from the agricultural chemicals they came in contact with every day, month after month, year after year. Even though Rachel Carson's book alerted the nation to the perils of pesticides two years after the Murrow documentary was aired, it would not be until the late 1960s that the sixteen thousand pesticides registered in California for use by or near farmworkers would become a national concern, thanks largely to the efforts of the California farmworkers themselves.[57]

During the early to mid-1960s, the United Farm Workers was organizing mostly Mexican and Filipino agricultural workers, whose demands included addressing the unsanitary housing and working conditions that existed in the fields and communities in which they lived.[58] Then, in 1968 nineteen orange-grove harvesters became very sick as a result of heavy spraying of the pesticide parathion in the field where they were working. Other illnesses came to light shortly thereafter, and by the following year the UFW had made worker health and safety the primary demand for their organizing drive, even more important than the recognition of the union. Through their organizing efforts, the historian Linda Nash writes, pesticide poisoning came to "symbolize the ways in which the modern environment could permeate the body."[59] A UFW pamphlet declared that "motivated by profit [growers] continued to subject our people to systematic poisoning."[60] Like Mazzocchi and the chemical workers, however, the UFW made clear that "the polluted agricultural landscape posed risks not only to farmworkers but also to everyone who passed through it or consumed its products." As part of the union's organizing strategy, it launched a boycott of lettuce and grapes to alert consumers to the risks posed by pesticides and to engage consumers in its labor struggle. As a result, Nash notes, "farmworkers and environmentalists now wielded disease to demand the reorganization of the local environment and the larger society."[61] In 1969 the union signed a contract with one grower banning the use of DDT and dieldrin, among other pesticides, years before California or the U.S. government provided protections for these workers.[62] The following year, the union signed contracts with 150 grape growers covering thirty thousand grape harvesters that, according to environmental historian Chad Montrie, gave "workers the power to approve use of organophosphates, refuse dangerous work, and determine reentry periods for workers laboring in sprayed vineyards."[63] Industrialized agriculture had replaced family farms as the locus of food production, and just as consumers had come to reevaluate the place of the chemical industry as a positive force in American life, they now came to see that the fruit orchard, once a symbol of a healthy life, was replaced by an industrialized agriculture "that could produce disease and sometimes even death."[64]

OSHA, EPA, AND INDUSTRY RESISTANCE

Out of efforts of the UFW, Mazzocchi and the chemical workers, and other labor activists in the 1960s came the movement to enact the groundbreaking OSHAct of 1970. It established the principle that workers, including agricultural workers, had a right to a safe and healthful workplace. The large proportion of agricultural workers were Black and Latino and had been excluded from coverage in the Social Security Act. The OSHAct also established that the federal government had a responsibility to ensure the health and safety of workers through inspection, regulation, and the establishment of safety standards. The act guaranteed workers access to information previously held to be proprietary trade secrets about the substances they worked with and the possible harmful results from exposure to them. The act held that OSHA should "set the standard which most adequately assures, to the extent feasible, on the basis of the best available evidence, that no employee will suffer material impairment of health or functional capacity even if such employee has regular exposure to the hazard dealt with by such standard for the period of his working life."[65]

Passage of OSHAct and EPAct and, perhaps surprisingly, Richard Nixon's signing of them into law can be seen as key moments in the country's industrial history, establishing the authority of the federal government to directly intervene in private industries' traditional control over the production process. Previous to these acts, standards for toxic exposures in the workplace and disposal of waste products through chimneys, hazardous waste dumps, or release into streams and rivers were largely established either by voluntary or industry-friendly groups such as the American National Standards Institute, the American Conference of Governmental Industrial Hygienists, the Lead Industries Association (representing the lead industry), and the National Paint, Varnish and Lacquer Association (NPVLA) (representing the broader paint industry); by local and state authorities; or by the informal, and often irresponsible, practices of the factory managers or corporations themselves. Through new standard-setting rules established by OSHA, the government highlighted industry's failures to establish safe workplace standards (many of which were decades old) and began to revise downward levels of exposure considered safe for a variety of toxins, including asbestos, lead, silica, cotton dusts, a variety of carcinogens, vinyl chloride, and PCBs.

Asbestos, because it had gained enormous attention in the previous decade in both the medical press, from Paul Brodeur's article in the *New Yorker*, and in other reports in the popular press, was among the first substances that federal agencies sought to regulate.[66] By the 1960s it had been shown to be the cause of three terrifying diseases—asbestosis, first named in the 1920s; lung cancer, clearly linked to asbestos exposure by the 1950s; and mesothelioma, an extremely rare cancer of the lining of the lungs that was linked to asbestos by 1960.[67] Asbestos-related diseases were no longer solely occupational. Household members, including children, were documented as developing mesothelioma from the asbestos that was brought home on workers' clothing.

OSHA set out to address a number of long-standing workplace hazards as well. Silica, perhaps the historical mother of the dust-caused diseases, was, as we saw in chapter 5, long identified as a cause of silicosis, the severe fibrosis of the lungs. It had killed and disabled thousands of workers in granite cutting, foundries, construction, potteries, glassblowing, hard-rock mining, and scores of other processes where granite, sand, and other silica-bearing rock products were used in far-flung corners of the nation.[68] Lead, long identified as a cause of neurological and other diseases among factory workers, and lead paint in particular, long marketed as a child-friendly means of brightening up homes and children's rooms (figure 6.5), were by the 1970s having a devastating effect on children, particularly poor Puerto Rican and Black children living in rental housing unmaintained by their absentee landlords, where they

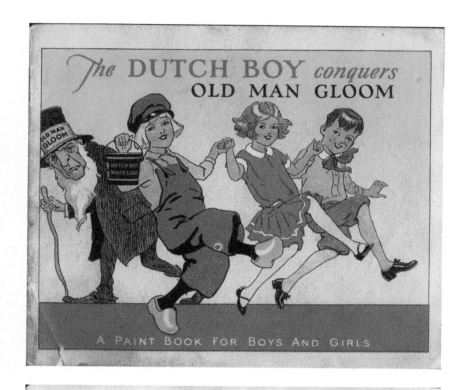

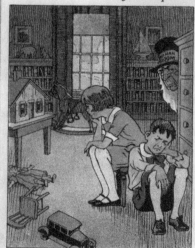

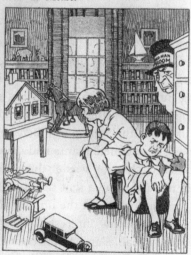

Give Coupon to Father or Mother

The girl and boy felt very blue
Their toys were old and shabby too,
They couldn't play in such a place,
The room was really a disgrace.

All gray and old with nothing bright,
It surely was a sorry sight,
And yet that poor neglected room
Was the delight of Old Man Gloom.

FIGURE 6.5 *The Dutch Boy Conquers Old Man Gloom: A Paint Book for Boys and Girls* (National Lead Company, 1929). Courtesy of the author.

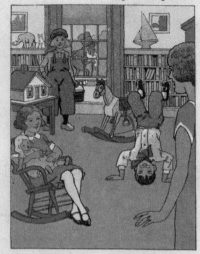
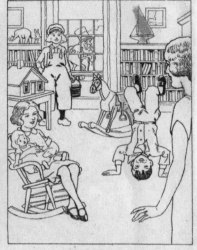

Give Coupon to Father or Mother

And when the Dutch Boy closed his stay
That happy home was bright and gay,
For he had beautified each room
And fairly routed Old Man Gloom.

He said, "I'd really like to tell,
That I paint outside just as well
And houses shine where'er I spread
Their outside walls with Dutch Boy Lead."

FIGURE 6.5 (*Continued*)

were exposed to lead from crumbling paint on the walls. They were also exposed to the exhaust of cars that burned leaded gasoline.[69] Vinyl chloride, the building block of polyvinyl chloride (PVC), a major plastic being introduced into every living space in the nation in the form of piping, wall coverings, house shingles, toys, bottles, countertops, and the like, was the source of much concern when it was discovered that workers in chemical plants had developed angiosarcoma of the liver in 1970. Vinyl chloride was at the center of a scandal the following year when it was revealed that the chemical industry had previously lied to the government about the finding of cancers in rats exposed to it.[70]

For physicians interested in working with workers, OSHA represented a viable and important employment alternative to being a company doctor doing annual checkups in factories. For young physicians and people concerned with workers' health and that of their families, OSHA presented a fresh, previously unavailable opportunity for meaningful, socially responsible work. Some physicians went into the field of occupational health inspired by the vision of Mazzocchi, while others were inspired by doctors like Quentin Young in Chicago or Jack Geiger in Boston, both of whose histories were shaped by the civil rights and occupational health movements.[71] Dave Kotelchuck, professor emeritus at the City University of New York, completed his doctorate in physics at Cornell and then received a master's in public health from Harvard. Following this elite education, he went to work with the United Electrical, Radio and Machine Workers of America, as director of health and safety in the research department.[72] Similarly, Jeanne Stellman received her doctorate in physical chemistry but joined the OCAW as presidential assistant for job safety and health and went on to an illustrious career bringing attention, through her landmark books and advocacy, to women's health in the workplace.[73]

OSHA also attracted some strong and often very progressive administrators and scientists. Eula Bingham, the daughter of a railroad worker injured on the job, became the head of OSHA in 1977. Anthony Robbins, previously head of Vermont's and Colorado's health departments, was appointed by Jimmy Carter to head NIOSH in 1978. The Chamber of Commerce attacked Robbins as a "social activist" with a "radical antibusiness posture" for his advocacy for workers' rights and suggested that he had "turned his research agency into a zealous enforcement arm" of OSHA.[74]

At the same time, the EPA actively encouraged legislation to protect the nation's air, water, and general environment. It established standards and regulations that had the force of law to control emissions into the atmosphere of toxic vehicular and factory exhaust and to curb indiscriminate dumping of toxic waste on the ground and into streams. In its first years, the EPA moved to enforce the newly passed Clean Air Act by "establishing limits on air pollutants and enforcing them," and soon thereafter, in June 1972, the EPA banned the application of DDT in the entire country.[75]

In most states, individual companies that were found to have polluted water supplies or dumped waste on public lands could get away with modest fines or no fines at all. Now, however, federal officials were looking over their shoulders; and companies started to realize that they could face real penalties, both financial and political, for misdeeds. The passage of the two acts establishing OSHA and the EPA was a direct challenge to a host of companies that had previously escaped much accountability for their actions even when those actions were causing disease and, in some cases, death.

THE POWELL MEMORANDUM: INDUSTRY'S RESPONSE

With their corps of relatively young activists, OSHA and the EPA went about their work with an enthusiasm and energy that sent shivers up the spines of many corporate leaders. What may have at first seemed like abstract and distant threats to the autonomy of industry suddenly became quite real and palpable. Despite the fact that William Ruckelshaus, the first administrator at the EPA, and George Guenther, OSHA's first head, were Republicans, the new agencies' focus on both the internal workings of the factory and the external impact of its products on the health of the nation appeared to some conservatives to be part of a larger attack on the American "free enterprise" system. In this view, the environmental and occupational health movements seemed of a piece with social protests over the military draft and the war in Vietnam, the unrest that accompanied the late civil rights movement, the growing women's movement, and student protests over the military-industrial complex. Some saw these movements as real threats to capitalism itself, threats that demanded concerted action to suppress.

Yale professor Charles Reich attacked "our system of justice" in *The Greening of America*, first published in 1970 in the *New Yorker* and then in expanded form as a book. The 50-page *New Yorker* article opened with these words: "There is a revolution under way. It is not like revolutions of the past. It has originated with the individual and with culture, and if it succeeds, it will change the political structure only as its final act. . . . [I]t is spreading with amazing rapidity, and already our laws, institutions, and social structure are changing in consequence."[76] In the piece, published just as OSHA, EPA, and NIOSH were being organized, Reich described the environmental movements, much as conservatives feared, as part of the efforts to stop the war in Vietnam, end poverty and racism, oppose the war machine, regulate technology, and execute control over corporate power.[77]

The modern corporate state, in Reich's view, was destroying democracy itself, and the driving forces in this process were business organizations.[78] Corporations "need stability, freedom from outside interference, constantly increasing profits. . . . The medium through which these imperatives operate is the law. The legal system acts as an instrument of corporate-state domination, and it acts to prevent the intervention of human values or individual choice."[79]

The "imperative" for profit put the environment, workers, and consumers at special risk. Corporate practices often harmed workers and the environment, but there was no requirement that they pay the costs associated with those harms, what economists call the "externalities." As Reich explained, "A manufacturer would dump wastes into a stream but pay nothing to take care of the pollution, leaving the public to share in the costs but not the profits. The manufacturer fought against having to pay for accidental injuries to workers, although they were statistically predicable, leaving the costs to be borne for, sometimes, an entire lifetime, by the unfortunate individual and his family."[80] Reich argued that the contemporary generation saw "a society that is unjust to its poor and its minorities, is run for the benefits of a privileged few, lacks its proclaimed democracy and liberty, is ugly and artificial, destroys the environment and the self, and is, like the war it spawns, 'unhealthy for children and other living things.'"[81]

Industry was not going to stand for this characterization of itself. Lewis Powell, a partner in Williams, Gay, Powell, and Gibson, a Virginia law firm that represented the Tobacco Institute, saw this as a direct threat to the future of the American state and social order. The blueprint of mainstream industry's response to what was seen as a broad attack on the capitalist system was issued in a detailed memo written by Powell in August 1971, shortly before he was nominated to become a Supreme Court justice. Written under the heading "CONFIDENTIAL MEMO: ATTACK ON AMERICAN FREE ENTERPRISE SYSTEM," the memo was addressed to the Education Committee of the U.S. Chamber of Commerce. It began with the direct statement that "no thoughtful person can question that the American economic system is under broad attack. This varies in scope, intensity, in the techniques employed, and in the level of visibility."[82]

Powell continued:

There always have been some who opposed the American system, and preferred socialism or some form of statism (communism or fascism). Also, there always have been critics of the system, whose criticism has been wholesome and constructive so long as the objective was to improve rather than to subvert or destroy.

But what now concerns us is quite new in the history of America. We are not dealing with sporadic or isolated attacks from a relatively few extremists or even from the minority socialist cadre. Rather, the assault on the enterprise system is broadly based and consistently pursued. It is gaining momentum and converts.[83]

It was not "the Communists, New Leftists and other revolutionaries who would destroy the entire system, both political and economic," Powell argued. "The most disquieting voices joining the chorus of criticism come from perfectly respectable elements of society: from the college campus, the pulpit, the media, the intellectual and literary journals, the arts and sciences, and from politicians. . . . [T]hese often are the most articulate, the most vocal, the most prolific in their writing and speaking." Powell was bewildered by the "paradoxes of our time," including "the extent to which the enterprise system tolerates, if not participates in, its own destruction." The media, college students, even members of the business community were willing participants in this giant effort to overthrow the existing order. He argued that attacks on banks by the Weather Underground were an outgrowth of the wide acceptance of revolutionary ideas in the broader society, including "respectable liberals and social reformers." "It is the sum total of their views and influence which could indeed fatally weaken or destroy the system," Powell added. Ralph Nader, author of *Unsafe at Any Speed*, an exposé of the Chevy Corvair's design flaws, and considered one of the modern founders of the consumer rights movement, came under singular attack as "perhaps the single most effective antagonist of American business." He had "become a legend in his own time and an idol of millions of Americans." Nader was of special concern because his popularity suggested an acceptance of his belief that not only "fly-by-night hucksters" but "a great many corporate executives belong in prison—for defrauding the consumer with shoddy merchandise, poisoning the food supply with chemical additives, and willfully manufacturing unsafe products that will maim or kill the buyer."[84]

Powell described the problem as he saw it and ways to address it: "The painfully sad truth is that business, including the boards of directors and the top executives of corporations great and small and business organizations at all levels, often have responded—if at all—by appeasement, ineptitude and ignoring the problem." They have "not been trained or equipped to conduct guerrilla warfare with those who propagandize against the system, seeking insidiously and constantly to sabotage it."[85]

In an argument that appears all too prescriptive, Powell laid out a detailed plan for counteracting this "threat." Corporations and businesses must wage continual lobbying campaigns in the halls of Congress and the political arena. But more important, it was essential to launch efforts to win the intellectual war, counter leftist ideologies, and reorient the intellectual life of the nation to ideas consistent with business beliefs. He proposed that the Chamber of Commerce support conservative scholars in the social sciences "who believe in the system" as well as like-minded speakers, a speakers bureau, and a system of evaluating, and censoring, textbooks based on their adherence to traditional American business beliefs: "If the authors, publishers and users of textbooks know that they will be subjected—honestly, fairly and thoroughly—to review and critique by eminent scholars who believe in the American system a return to a more rational balance can be expected." He was particularly piqued that more than one hundred speeches by "avowed Communists" (at least according to the FBI) had been given on campuses but there had been "no corresponding representation of American business, or indeed by individuals or organizations who appeared in support of the American system of government and business."[86] With little acknowledgment of any truth to the critique of industry as a threat to the environment or the health of the nation's population, Powell decried "the stampedes by politicians to support almost any legislation related to 'consumerism' or to the 'environment.' "[87]

While changing the direction of the university and reshaping what could be learned through lectures, books, and television were long-term solutions to the problems facing American businesses, Powell declared that "business must learn the lesson, long ago learned by labor and other self-interest groups. This is the lesson that political power is necessary; that such power must be assiduously cultivated; and that when necessary, it must be used aggressively and with determination—without embarrassment and without the reluctance which has been so characteristic of American business."[88]

In short order, a series of think tanks were founded in the 1970s to roll back progressive reform efforts and to create an intellectual and political cadre to "protect" free enterprise and promote libertarian ideas and antigovernment ideologies.[89] Among those think tanks still influential today are the Cato Institute (1974), the Heritage Foundation (1973), the Manhattan Institute (1977), the Free Congress Foundation (1977), and the Ethics and Public Policy Center (1976). As Sheldon Whitehouse has explained in his book, *The Scheme: How the Right Wing Used Dark Money to Capture the Supreme Court,* many of these institutes were established in light of Powell's "blueprint" and were, and still are, funded by industrial and right-wing "dark money" donors, including the Koch Brothers, to create doubt about the human sources and consequences of environmental damage that were despoiling the world's natural habitats.[90]

Powell's call to arms did not go unheeded by the business community. Over the course of the next decade, increasingly sophisticated efforts were made to reshape American attitudes and political power, culminating in the election of Ronald Reagan as President and a concerted effort by an empowered Republican right wing to undercut the legislative and regulatory advances of the 1960s and 1970s. Many in the business community saw OSHA and EPA as institutional manifestations of the broader attack on the "free enterprise" system that Powell described. The trade associations for the asbestos, chemical, and plastics industries, as well as the automobile and petroleum industries, began to lobby Congress, to attack critics, and to publicly pillory and ultimately undermine the EPA, OSHA, and other agencies that, by establishing protections for American workers and the environment, could threaten their corporate profits and interests. OSHA in particular came in for massive attacks as a prime example of government intrusion into the "free market" system and as a purported cause of the economic downturns that marked much of the 1970s and early 1980s.

A brief review of a few of the substances that OSHA identified for early regulation will demonstrate the increasingly sophisticated efforts of American industry to stymie these early efforts at structural reform. As we have seen, in the middle decades of the twentieth century, asbestos was widely distributed throughout the American landscape. By the time OSHA and NIOSH were organized in 1970, thousands of articles and news reports had made asbestos a focus of their attention.[91] Because this literature was so extensive and because asbestos was so dangerous, the first action that OSHA took in 1971 was to enact an "Emergency Standard" for asbestos.[92]

Groups like the Friction Materials Standards Institute (FMSI), a trade association that included numerous brake and clutch manufacturers, and the Cosmetics, Toiletries and Fragrance Association (CTFA), which represented the manufacturers of numerous talcum powder products found in facial powders, baby powders, and body deodorants, perceived themselves as under attack by government itself. The reaction of industries with an interest in profiting from asbestos in their products was swift. A new trade association, the Asbestos Information Association (AIA), was formed in response to the establishment of OSHA in late 1970 as a promotional and informational service, but it quickly became an advocacy group to lobby against government efforts to regulate asbestos use. Matthew Swetonic was a graduate of Columbia University's journalism school who first worked in the publicity department of the giant Johns Manville asbestos company and then became executive secretary of the new AIA. He explained to members of the Asbestos Textile Institute in 1973: "In our original concept the Association would limit its activities to providing accurate, unbiased information on asbestos and health to the press, the public and to interested politicians and other government officials. . . . [But] *fortunately—and properly—the Association has had the wisdom to alter its original limited concept of its proper functions, and now endeavors to assume whatever activities and responsibilities it deems necessary to protect the interests of the asbestos manufacturing industry in the United States vis-à-vis asbestos-health* [emphasis added]."[93]

At first, the trade organizations' response to the threat of regulatory action was defensive and fairly disorganized—sometimes trying to cooperate with OSHA while lobbying for industry-friendly standards; sometimes organizing to attack the scientists who delivered bad news about the safety of their product; sometimes ignoring the agencies, summarily dismissing and flouting their authority; and sometimes challenging the science and scientists that identified asbestos fibers in their products. The AIA then launched efforts to stifle the new agencies and their older siblings from limiting AIA's behavior.

In a speech to the Asbestos Textile Institute, Swetonic depicted the asbestos industry as the "victim" of federal regulation. He began, "I am sure that many of you have asked yourselves . . . why has the asbestos industry seemingly been singled out as the prime target for so many assaults by government, labor, the press, certain segments of the medical profession, and by various environmental and consumer activist groups?" "Why us? Can asbestos really be all that bad? Are the products we produce truly going to kill millions of Americans. . . . Or is there some sort of nefarious conspiracy afoot to destroy the asbestos industry?"[94] His answer was clear: from the industry's point of view, the industry was a victim and had to fight back. While it is undoubtedly true that industry was generally successful in scaling back regulations, new pollution controls and worker safety protection added substantially to industry's costs. Some companies like Altria, formerly Philip Morris, have now coopted critics' arguments to their own ends and claim to have moved "beyond smoking," marketing themselves as a "harm reduction company."[95] Other industries like asbestos, while not completely dead, have had their markets substantially restricted by regulations and lawsuits and have most recently been banned.

THE GROWING FOCUS ON CHRONIC DISEASES AND THE THREAT FROM NEW CHEMICALS

In the changing environmental, epidemiological, and political context of the 1970s, a rising chorus of health professionals had begun to point to a range of industrial chemicals and toxins—"old" threats to workers—as new or ignored threats to the general public. Among the most significant classes of these new chemicals were the chlorinated hydrocarbons—chemicals that contain hydrogen along with chlorine atoms attached to a ring of six linked carbon atoms. Chemicals of this class that had become major concerns in the postwar era included DDT and other pesticides, persistent pollutants such as polychlorinated biphenyls (PCBs), and a wide range of plastics, such as polyvinyl chloride (PVC). As one Monsanto scientist noted, when he came into the business in the 1940s, all chlorinated hydrocarbons were considered toxic in their production and/or in their use.[96] Although some of these substances had been developed earlier, in the years following World War II many, including DDT, Lindane, and other pesticides, as well as PCBs, entered the environment in huge quantities.

In the midst of America's Great Depression, the Monsanto Chemical Company, one of the nation's largest, identified polychlorinated biphenyls—PCBs—chemicals first synthesized in Germany in the nineteenth century, as immensely useful. Previously of seemingly little practical import to industry, PCBs, it came to be realized, had qualities that made them excellent candidates for insulating material for coating wires, protecting generators, and ensuring the proper operation of transformers and capacitors. Transformers are large pieces of equipment that regulate the voltage transmitted through electrical cables coming from everything from dams and power stations to the electricity coursing through the wires on a residential block. Their widespread deployment was essential for the emergence of the electrified consumer world following the end of the Depression and World War II. Capacitors are smaller units that stored and turned electrical energy into a usable power source for everything from electrical equipment and industrial machinery to light bulbs, vacuum cleaners, washing machines, and other appliances in the postwar years.

Two companies, General Electric and Monsanto, seized on the enormous possibilities of PCBs, identifying Swann Chemical, a small company in Anniston, Alabama, as the sole producer of PCBs in the nation. Less than six years after Swann began producing PCBs in 1929, Monsanto purchased the company and began mass production. The chemical stability of PCBs and their fire-resistant qualities made them useful in buildings where space limitations sometimes gave them an advantage over mineral oil, which had been the fluid of choice for insulating transformers and capacitors in the 1930s.

The early years of the Depression were an ideal time for Monsanto to invest in the Swann Chemical Company, as Franklin Roosevelt's New Deal was working to bring electricity into every town and hollow in the nation.[97] In the course of a few years, tens of thousands of workers laid tens of thousands of miles of electrical cable, creating a huge market for companies that provided the wire, the cable, the transformers, and the capacitors that lay at the heart of the electrical revolution that we still benefit from, and struggle with, today.

Even in the 1930s and 1940s, it was recognized that, as chlorinated biphenyls, PCBs were considered potent toxins for those who came in contact with them, particularly the workers in electrical equipment manufacturing, wire making, and chemical plants. Industries had every reason to worry about the effects on workers of PCBs because they were based on a combination of benzene rings chemically wedded to chlorine, and from early in the century, benzene alone—a colorless, odorless, flammable liquid that is sweet to the taste—had been identified as an acute poison. When inhaled at particularly high concentrations, benzene caused "death within a few minutes." Textbooks related the terrible consequences of concentrated benzene exposure: "Acute exposure to benzene produces rapidly increasing symptoms of tightening of leg muscles, dizziness, excitation, and pallor, followed by flushing, weakness, headache, breathlessness, apprehension of death, and constipation in the chest. The pulse becomes rapid, and the color blue. Visual disturbances, tremors, and muscle weakness are encountered. Convulsions are fairly frequent. Death may occur almost at once or several hours to several days following exposure."[98]

While the acute effects of benzene were terrifying, recognition of the varied and poorly defined effects of chronic exposures further alarmed the industrial hygiene community. One report, written under the direction of Harvard's Cecil Drinker in 1948, told of the problem: the relationship between the exposure and the symptoms was much less exact than was the case with the more widely recognized bacterial diseases, whose symptoms were often more precisely identified. "The different humans reacted differently to benzene. Some excreted much of it, other retained it and metabolized it into dangerous phenols." With long-term exposure "a variety of reactions may be encountered," Drinker observed, "and there is little correlation between the degree and duration of exposure and the severity or nature of the findings in the blood on microscopic exam." Chemists and industrial hygienists were identifying questions for clinicians in an era when bacteriology, the science of identifying a viral or bacterial cause for specific symptoms and diseases, still held sway but was of limited relevance to the effects of these new toxins. Benzene, for example, did not produce one specific or universal change in the blood of a worker. Indeed, some workers developed leukemias, while other were not affected at all.[99]

The varied symptoms and pathology of benzene were troubling enough. But it was widely recognized that chlorinated hydrocarbons—benzene molecules joined to chlorine—were an even more potent danger.[100] Drinker, only a few years before he wrote his textbook, had investigated the deaths of three workers who had died in a Halowax plant where workers produced a mixture of PCBs and naphthalene, another waxy material.[101] With the support of the Monsanto and Halowax companies, Drinker identified PCBs as a systemic poison that caused at least two well-documented conditions: yellow atrophy of the liver, whose symptom, jaundice, announced the destruction of the liver; and chloracne, a debilitating skin rash among workers who either inhaled PCB fumes or came in physical contact with its fumes.[102] Chloracne was a long-known problem for those exposed to chlorinated hydrocarbons: Karl Herxheimer, a German-Jewish dermatologist, had identified it by 1899.[103] By the late 1930s, reports of workers in Monsanto's Anniston, Alabama, PCB plant and in the Halowax plant were leading to papers and conferences about PCBs' deleterious health effects.[104]

These observations of Drinker and others came at a time when industrial hygienists and physicians, as well as lab workers, were becoming aware of the dangers of fast-emerging chemical products that were increasingly present in the general environment. In the United States in the 1920s, public health officials first identified the potential for widespread damage from the introduction of leaded gasoline as a fuel for the auto industry, as we saw in chapter 5. Once perceived as a threat to the health of workers, in the 1920s public health officials and labor activists began pointing to the possible damage that such a known industrial toxin as lead might pose when introduced into motor fuel whose exhaust would pollute the wider environment and its populace.[105] Also by the 1920s, aniline dyes, used commercially to dye wool, silk, and other fibers, had been identified as a cause of bladder cancer, raising the specter of epidemics of other noninfectious, deadly diseases linked to industrial production, while investigations of new synthetic materials like rayon (whose use of carbon disulfide in the production process posed severe dangers to workers) led to suspicions of potential health dangers in the new world of synthetic compounds.[106]

At DuPont, the possibility of danger to health from new chemicals in use had led to the creation in 1934 of the Haskell Laboratories. The toxicologist Wilhelm Hueper, who had emigrated from Germany in the mid-1930s, became its head and discovered that DuPont itself had an unusual number of workers who had died of bladder cancer. Despite efforts by DuPont to censor his work, in 1942, after being fired from DuPont, Hueper went on to publish *Occupational Tumors and Allied Diseases*, an 896-page textbook identifying thousands of published studies that linked occupation and cancer, as noted in chapter 5. Beginning with a discussion of the impact of "the new artificial environment" on humans, the book contained extensive sections on organic chemicals, including chlorinated hydrocarbons, which he described as suspected carcinogens.[107]

Notwithstanding chlorinated hydrocarbons' possible link to cancer, Monsanto saw a huge market for its new product. Not only were PCBs effective insulating materials, but they also were useful plasticizers—additives to plastics that gave them flexibility, pliability, and strength—that could be used by the booming petrochemical industry of the postwar world. Almost from the start of their mass production, PCBs were touted for use in everything from the millions of miles of wire and cable, transformers, and capacitors to tape and shower curtains, paint, and even chewing gum. There were unlimited uses for PCBs in plastics, paints, and other consumer products, a *Saturday Evening Post* advertisement bragged (figure 6.6).[108]

Soon PCBs had become some of Monsanto's major products. They were sold as well to General Electric and Westinghouse for use in their transformers and to GE and Sylvania for use in capacitors in fluorescent bulbs. Hundreds of millions of small amounts of PCBs were distributed in homes, offices, schools, and factories throughout the country as General Electric promoted its messages that "progress . . . is our most important product" and that GE "brought good things to light."[109]

In the waning years of the Depression and during World War II, Monsanto had shown some interest in finding ways to protect its workforce from possible danger in the manufacture of PCBs. But, as its market began to expand and profits from the product increased, the company came to see public health concerns as hindrances to its marketing goals. By the early 1950s, virtually all warnings that PCBs were systemic toxins

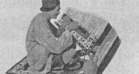

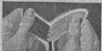
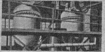

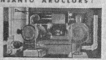
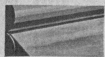
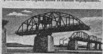

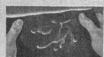
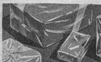
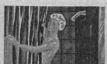

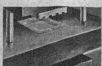
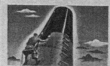
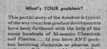

FIGURE 6.6 "Found! Three Industries that Can't Use Aroclors," [Monsanto's trade name for PCBs] advertisement, *Saturday Evening Post*, August 3, 1946.

ceased, and Monsanto conducted no studies on the effects of long-term exposures to even the small quantities of PCBs found in a host of products ranging from paints, caulking, and carbonless copy paper to adhesives, cosmetics, and fluorescent light fixtures.

Although Monsanto was the sole producer of PCBs, it did not investigate, much less warn about, the possible long-term effects of exposure to its almost indestructible product. In general, Americans did not know the various uses that PCBs had, including as insecticides and insecticide extenders, medicinals, and manicure resins, as well as the possibility that they could get into food. Americans remained ignorant of the danger even though throughout the 1940s and 1950s other chlorinated hydrocarbons, specifically DDT, Lindane, Aldrin, and Endrin, came under increasing scrutiny in the press and in congressional hearings for their potential to cause long-term harm to people and the environment.

During World War II, eminent industrial hygienists and physicians such as Alice Hamilton and Wilhelm Hueper noted growing concerns about the chlorinated hydrocarbons. In 1943, the year after Wilhelm Hueper noted that chlorinated hydrocarbons were potentially a human carcinogen, Hamilton wrote "The Toxicity of the Chlorinated Hydrocarbons" in the *Yale Journal of Biology and Medicine*, noting their increasing use as a degreaser for metals, a cleaning agent in dry cleaning, a solvent for rubber, and a thinner in lacquers and warning of their possible health dangers.[110]

Concern about the broad dangers these new chemicals posed came with growing worry that some pesticides, most importantly, the chlorinated hydrocarbon DDT (dichlorodiphenyltrichloroethane), were being sprayed extensively on the fruits people were consuming as well as in neighborhoods to control a host of insects from mosquitoes to beetles. DDT, first synthesized in 1874 and developed as an insecticide in 1939 by Paul Hermann Müller, a Swiss chemist who was awarded the Nobel Prize in Physiology or Medicine in 1948, began to be used extensively to protect troops in the tropics from disease-carrying insects during World War II.[111]

As DDT and other chlorinated hydrocarbons came into general use in the 1940s and 1950s, a body of scientific evidence accumulated that pointed to their chronic toxicity in animals and humans. These studies all noted that this class of chemicals was stored in fatty tissue and was present in the milk of lactating animals; in addition, many of the studies noted the "possibility of chronic poisoning."[112] By 1950 the implications of the studies conducted primarily on DDT and related insecticides led the public health community to worry about the broader category of chlorinated hydrocarbons. That year the *American Journal of Public Health* issued a report by its Committee on Chemicals Introduced in Foods that warned, "The chlorinated hydrocarbons, such as DDT and chlordane, are soluble in fats and are stored in the fatty tissues of the body. These compounds possess a high order of toxicity, and their uncontrolled . . . use is not desirable."[113]

The following year the House Select Committee to Investigate the Use of Chemicals in Food Products, a committee led by James Joseph Delaney, a Democratic congressman from Queens, New York, held hearings at which sixty-two chemicals were identified as being used or proposed for use in food. DDT was included, "as are representatives of a number of organic chlorides used as insecticides."[114] Thus, it was clear in the early 1950s that the health problems with DDT were not unique to DDT. The committee presented manufacturers of other chlorinated hydrocarbons with the information they needed to proceed cautiously in exposing masses of people to their products.[115] Morton Biskind of Westport, Connecticut, author of a number of scientific articles on the chlorinated hydrocarbons, gave one of the most comprehensive statements at the hearings. It was "surprising," he told the committee, that DDT and these pesticides had been "spread indiscriminately over so large a portion of the earth," given that "a large amount of data was already available in the medical literature showing that this agent was extremely toxic for many different species of animals."[116] Biskind declared, "Exposure to this whole group of compounds is now universal in the United States, and it appears that few persons escape storage of these toxic agents in the bodyfat."[117] In addition, he said, the long-term effects of this group of insecticides were particularly troubling because of the potential ecological and agricultural devastation that they could cause.[118]

Concern about chlorinated hydrocarbons grew throughout the 1950s, and more studies were conducted that indicated their toxic effects on human beings.[119] Among the chlorinated hydrocarbons, DDT and other pesticides garnered the most public attention in that period because of their widespread distribution through the food chain.[120] PCBs were sometimes promoted for use along with DDT as a "pesticide extender" because their adhesive qualities could be used to prolong the period of time pesticides would adhere to plants and hard surfaces in the home. Monsanto knew that PCBs were being used with other pesticides on crops that were aimed for the dining room table, use that worried some people in the company.[121] In an internal memo in 1957, the Monsanto scientist L. V. Sherwood sent a letter to P. G. Benignus of Monsanto's Development Department about a Monsanto publication promoting PCBs, marketed as Aroclors, to "increase the insecticidal life of lindane," warning that such use would be reckless. He said, "It is most surprising to see that you are recommending without restriction a use for Aroclor which has not been approved" by the United States Department of Agriculture and the Food and Drug Administration. He noted that "since Aroclors are toxic," the federal government "would require . . . data to show whether or not residual Aroclor is present," and, if so, whether "tolerances for the pesticide in question must be developed." He pointed out that "a tolerance cannot be established until after two-year chronic toxicity feeding tests have been completed for Aroclor."[122] Yet such tests were not even begun for another twelve years.

Evidence of PCB contamination of the environment mounted during the 1960s, especially after 1966, when two Swedish researchers, Soren Jensen and Gunner Widmark, while looking for DDT in the environment, found PCBs in salmon, pine needles, the hair of one of the research scientist's babies, and virtually everything else they looked at. Reports flowed in of leaking storage tanks and spills and leaks in the vessels in which PCBs were shipped, including trucks, railway cars, and drums. Waste PCBs, it was revealed, were regularly dumped in landfills and sewered into streams and other waterways.[123]

The discovery of widespread PCB contamination came at a critical time in environmental history. Rachel Carson's book, *Silent Spring* (1962), had appeared only a few years before the Jensen and Widmark publication, and Monsanto had reacted quickly and aggressively to the positive attention Carson's account received. The October 1962 issue of *Monsanto Magazine* featured a counternarrative entitled "The Desolate Year." "Does the world really need chemical pesticides? . . . Is the world being sold a monstrous bill of goods?" It imagined an apocalyptic future without modern pesticides and other chemical products, in language reminiscent of *The Blob, Invasion of the Body Snatchers,* and other science fiction horror films of the late 1950s and early 1960s. It included a vivid description of the Mediterranean fruit fly, which "turned her stiletto-like appendage into a grapefruit [and] sent an egg inside," launching a vermin-infested nightmare: "Quietly, then, the desolate year began. . . . The bugs were everywhere. Unseen. Unheard. Unbelievably universal. On or under every square foot of land, every square yard, every acre, and county, and state and region in the entire sweep of the United States. In every home and barn and apartment house and chicken coop, and in their timbers and foundations and furnishings. Beneath the ground, beneath the waters, on and in limbs and twigs and stalks, under rocks, inside trees and animals and other insects—and, yes, inside man."[124]

Monsanto's frontal assault on Carson and environmental awareness, however, did little to stem the flow of information Americans received about the potential toxicity of the new chemicals that were pouring out of plants in Louisiana, New Jersey, Illinois, and thousands of other locales across the nation. Nor had its assault assuaged concern about DDT, Lindane, and other chlorinated hydrocarbons on which Carson had focused.

The actions of Monsanto to preserve its markets in agribusiness through its campaign against concerns that Rachel Carson and other scientists raised were focused on pesticides, but Monsanto saw the growing questioning of new chemical products as a broader threat.[125] Monsanto's first response to Jensen and Widmark's discovery in 1966 of widespread PCB contamination was to hope that it would have little impact on America's shores. But information and concern about PCBs only grew in the ensuing months and years as press reports filtered out of Europe. D. H. Hardy from Monsanto's British Division wrote to his counterparts in St. Louis about new findings and new suspicions voiced by representatives from Shell and other major consumers of Aroclors.[126] But, unlike DDT, which Monsanto had also produced from 1947 to 1957 before it withdrew from that highly competitive market, PCBs were manufactured *only* by Monsanto in the United States, and Monsanto alone would be held accountable in this country if it were discovered to be a contaminant. Here was one of Monsanto's signature chemicals at risk, and PCBs were sold not only in the agricultural sector, but now in a variety of products like paints, carbonless carbon paper, catheters, lacquer, and adhesives, among many others.

PCBs became a major national issue in the United States with the publication of a study by the University of California oceanographer Robert Risebrough that gained the attention of West Coast newspapers. On February 24, 1969, the *San Francisco Chronicle* published a front-page article reporting on "bay scientist's pollutant warning," which told of a "newly-identified chemical pollutant" that had "arisen on our planet" and that had already seriously threatened the existence of peregrine falcons by weakening their eggs. "The peregrine falcon, a bird of prey that once abounded all over America, is bearing a bitter warning to man," it began. The chemical's "long-term hazards at low levels to the human species are wholly unknown—although in concentrated gaseous form the chemical is highly poisonous, and chemicals closely related to it are known to cause cancer." In the piece, it became clear that the "newly-identified chemical pollutant" was PCB, a close relative of DDT, as we've seen, and the potential "long-term hazards at low levels." The article raised the alarm by pointing out that Risebrough had found evidence that PCBs, like DDT, are "carried widely across the oceans by winds and water currents" and "may affect human food supplies and human lives." "The one certainty now is that they can be found everywhere, that they have invaded the food-producing levels of the oceans, and their presence is rising swiftly."[127]

Although Monsanto initially refused to comment on the article, the public response was swift: letters poured into the *Chronicle* and to Monsanto headquarters itself. One irate Oakland resident wrote to Charles Sommer, president of Monsanto, demanding that the company cease production. "If you care nothing for birds or wildlife, at least consider your fellow man—yourself and your family."[128]

The intensity of the attention forced Monsanto to respond. A week after the article appeared, the company sent a letter to its executives and officials in various parts of the country as well as a press release outlining the "sensational story." In a disingenuous attempt to counter the narrative of the story, Monsanto questioned a "few facts." "These conclusions are puzzling in several aspects," the letter noted, as PCBs "are not easily released to the natural environment." Perhaps "the substance identified by the scientists" was not PCBs but "a compound which only appears to be PCBs due to metabolism of other materials in the marine environment."[129]

By 1969, the year the article on Risebrough's research was published, Monsanto's executives knew, of course, how PCBs were getting into the environment: they had been flooded with complaints and reports of PCBs leaking into streams from their production plants, from cracked drums used in shipping, from leaking equipment in doughnut-frying machines, from cracked casings in navy shipyards, and from vapors emanating from tanks. By the fall of that year, despite the increasing scrutiny that PCBs were receiving and three years after the report by the two Swedish investigators, Monsanto officials acknowledged that they were at a crossroads. The company could either "go out of [the Aroclor] business," "sell the hell out of them as long as we can," or restrict sales to what they called "closed systems," capacitors and transformers that, they claimed, would not leak into the environment.[130] The following year, Monsanto sold more PCBs than at any time in its history, sending millions of pounds into the environment and a lesser amount into our bodies as well.[131]

THE 1970s: A PIVOTAL DECADE

By the late 1960s and early 1970s, Monsanto and other polluting companies realized that many of their previous efforts to allay public concerns about the impact of their industries and products on the nation were not having the success they had hoped for. An assumed link between chemistry, industry, and unalloyed progress on the part of the public could no longer be taken for granted, and press coverage of the presence of PCBs, among other toxic chemicals, in the environment was becoming increasingly critical.[132] They recognized the danger that scientists and civil service officials, armed with regulatory powers and with the megaphone of the federal government through the offices of EPA, OSHA, and other agencies, could tell the nation about these industrial toxins. Merely downplaying the environmental movement as a fringe group of "tree huggers" would not quell public outrage. There were too many environmental groups to write them off with a simple public relations barrage or threat of lawsuits. They could not quell the voices of lawyers willing to bring environmental suits to court, national environmental advocacy groups, civil rights activists concerned with issues of environmental justice, and local organizations worried about pollution of their waterways and toxic waste dumped in their communities.

PCBs were Monsanto's immediate concern as newspapers around the country detailed the local crises their communities were facing, but Monsanto knew that the situation was even worse than the public realized. In 1969, one of Monsanto's consultants estimated that 2 billion pounds of PCBs had been produced since their introduction in the 1930s and that, because of their persistence, 200 million pounds had entered the environment.[133] The toll of PCB pollution along the California coast, in Lake Michigan, along the Florida coast, and in the Gulf of Mexico was mounting, and the death of shrimp, and fish in Anniston, as well as possible toxic contamination in the nation's food industry, was becoming understood.

THE HEALTH CONSEQUENCES OF THE INDUSTRIALIZATION OF AGRICULTURE

For much of world history, agricultural production was largely a local affair. The variabilities of climate, transportation, and the perishability of product made it difficult to move foods from farms to distant markets. Canning fruits and vegetables, drying spices and some foods, and salting and smoking selected meats were early means of extending the useful life of some products, but the true industrialization of foods would await revolutions in transport, refrigeration, and developments in chemistry.

The decades around the beginning of the twentieth century were a turning point in this transformation. The invention of chemical preservatives, new canning techniques, the reliable and consistent refrigeration that came with the introduction of electricity, and the flash freezing of fish and vegetables, developed by Clarence Birdseye in 1912, accompanied the growing organization, industrialization, and concentrations of the food industry. Construction of a transcontinental railway system along with improvements in river transportation could now more efficiently integrate the movement of beef, vegetables, and fruit from rural towns to the growing ports and industrial cities across the country.

By the 1940s, what had once been a labor-intensive, local enterprise in which farmers brought their goods to local towns where families would buy or barter for them had largely vanished. Farms became larger, their agricultural output was less diverse, chemical fertilizers, insecticides, and herbicides were increasingly used, and productivity mushroomed. By the 1950s a few large firms dominated food production—Campbell's food-processing company (whose brands now include soups, V-8 juice, Swanson, Goldfish, and Pepperidge Farm); Kellogg's (makers of a host of breakfast cereals); Nabisco (cookies and snacks); and Borden (which in 1958 established a chemical division and whose dairy division produced jams, cheese, ice cream, milk, and other products).

To take just one example of these transformations, the chicken broiler industry, according to agricultural historians William Boyd and Michael Watts, changed dramatically in the 1950s. At the start of the decade, the industry was characterized by "a variety of specialized independent firms and small independent farmers. . . . By the end of the decade . . . the majority of production had fallen under the control of vertically integrated firms." Since the early 1960s, companies that owned their own hatcheries, feed mills, and processing operations— what economists call "integrated" firms—came to control as much as 90 percent of America's broiler production.[134] The result, Boyd and Watts argue, was that the chicken broiler industry, concentrated in the South, became "one of the most tightly coordinated and institutionally dense commodity systems in U.S. agriculture."[135]

The concentration of the food industry created more food but also more problems. In the 1960s, PCBs were discovered to have leaked into the frying oil of Mrs. Paul's Kitchen products, among them baked goods, and into Kellogg's and Frito Lay chips. In February 1971, the discovery that 180,000 pounds of chicken at Campbell Soup Company plants were tainted by PCBs fed the alarm.[136] Deep in the winter of 1971, representatives of the Food and Drug Administration, Campbell Soup Company, and the Department of Agriculture met to discuss the problem. The tainted chicken had been destined for use in chicken soup. In addition, farmers in upstate New York had discovered tens of thousands of eggs and chickens contaminated with PCBs. One farmer alone had to kill thirty thousand chickens and destroy tens of thousands of eggs. Tests of a sample of the birds found that they contained as much as 40 parts per million PCBs, way over any limit that anyone thought reasonable.[137]

The group was faced with an enormous problem. With no clear understanding of the impact that the mass distribution of PCB-tainted chickens could cause, what were Campbell Soup and other users and distributors of these birds to do? If they simply disposed of the birds in landfills or burned them in incinerators, the entire nation would soon test its chickens and perhaps be forced to destroy them as well. Given that chicken soup and chicken dinners had become a mainstay of the national diet, the economic consequences for distributors, farmers, Campbell's, and other companies that either packaged or used chickens would be enormous, as millions of families would wonder what they might be eating when they opened up cans of soup or broiled a chicken for lunch or dinner.[138]

The discussion went on for many hours before a tentative solution was reached. The chicken fat and skin seemed to contain the highest levels of PCBs, so a new product would be created: skinless chicken parts. "All chickens containing 5 ppm or less in their fat" could be used in the soup and skinless chickens could be sold to consumers. "Those chickens with greater than 5 ppm in their fat would have to go through a salvaging procedure," it was decided. The fat and skin of those birds would have to be ripped off and discarded. The rest of the meat could be sold to the public. The FDA was, according to a Monsanto representative's description of the meeting, "very careful to point out that they are by no means establishing a level of 5 ppm of PCB as an allowable residue" because "as of now, no one is sure exactly how PCB is getting into these chickens."[139]

Two weeks after the meeting, Monsanto learned of one source of PCB-contaminated chickens: it had sold Therminol FR, a PCB-containing fluid used in coils that heated huge vats in which food products were boiled, to a North Carolina company, East Coast Terminal. This company, to the apparent surprise of Monsanto, produced fish meal–based chicken feed and provided it to some of the large chicken growers around the country. Monsanto's "Therminol FR" had leaked into the vats containing the fish meal. Nine drums of PCB fluid had been purchased just two months before the contamination of chickens was discovered, and even more had been purchased in August and December of the previous year.[140] The *Wall Street Journal* reported that over a ten-week period, 16,000 tons of the contaminated fish meal had been distributed nationally. "At the normal blending level of 2 percent fishmeal, the mishap is estimated to have produced some 880,000 tons of contaminated feed." The *Journal* pointed out the vast impact of this leak: "Flocks fed the suspected feed apparently contain millions of birds."[141] In addition, according to an article in *Time* magazine, by mid-August the FDA "disclosed that it had seized more than 75,000 fresh eggs from wholesalers in Norfolk, Va., because the chickens that laid them had eaten feed containing the tainted fishmeal." The FDA tried to assure the public that PCB-contaminated food would not reach them, but, according to *Time*, "it later admitted an official goof: a shipment of sixty thousand eggs had somehow got through federal inspectors, and, presumably into the stomachs of Washington, D.C. residents."[142]

The problem for Monsanto was twofold. First, the company had promised in 1970 that it would stop selling PCBs for any food-related use; second, Monsanto knew that it might be held liable for the damages caused to the companies whose products were affected. During that year Monsanto had been hit with a stream of lawsuits both by people who claimed they had been harmed by PCB exposure and by companies that claimed their reputations and businesses had been damaged by the huge number of newspaper and magazines articles and extensive television coverage devoted to PCBs.[143] After all, by the early 1970s millions of Americans were regularly eating hundreds of millions of pounds of chickens, virtually all of which were being raised in industrial chicken mills (where, incidentally, they were pumped full of hormones and antibiotics to promote their growth and fend off diseases) during their brief three to six weeks of life before they were shipped off for slaughter.

At the federal level, Representative William Ryan (D-NY) introduced legislation in Congress as early as 1970 to ban PCBs, but with Ryan's death from throat cancer in 1972, it died in committee. In the following years, Congress considered legislation to control toxic substances in general and specifically to ban the production of PCBs. In 1975, the EPA held a press conference during which Russell Train, its administrator, pressed for passage of that legislation, pointing out that the EPA believed that "PCBs constitute a significant hazard to human health and the environment." He explained that "there are hundreds of millions of pounds of PCBs out there in the environment—in landfills, soils, and the bottom sediments of rivers, lakes, and estuaries." He lamented, like

Wilhelm Hueper and others before him, that PCBs would "be there for years, like a delayed action time bomb, . . . which we have no way to keep from moving into life systems, including humans."[144] The same day he delivered his devastating critique of Monsanto's product, Train wrote to the company's president saying, "We must, as a society, accept and work toward a goal of totally eliminating the production, importation and use of PCBs as rapidly as possible."[145] Monsanto got the message. In its internal summary of Train's news conference, Monsanto noted Train's image of PCBs as "a delayed action time bomb waiting to go off," and then added his conclusion that "we may have to live with them for the rest of our lives."[146] The Toxic Substances Control Act (TSCA) was passed in 1976 and empowered the EPA to "require reporting, record-keeping and testing . . . and restrictions relating to chemical substances and/or mixtures," and specifically to ban the production of PCBs, which it did, the ban to go into effect in 1979.[147] (In response, Monsanto stopped selling PCBs at the end of August 1977, though it allowed and encouraged some customers to buy extra quantities of PCBs in anticipation of this cutoff.)

At the very time that they were in the process of being banned, PCBs along with some other toxic chemicals were being illegally dumped along highways in various poor communities around the country, legal disposal being far more expensive than surreptitious burial or dumping. In North Carolina, for example, 30,000 gallons of PCB oils were dumped in 1978 along 210 miles of roadways, in what Robert Bullard called "the largest PCB spill ever documented in the United States."[148] Four years later, the state's governor made the decision to bury the pollutant in largely (63.7 percent) African American Warren County, one of the poorest counties in the state. Concerted protests, including sit-ins and blockages of roads by African American activists, made this an important moment in environmental history because it joined together two powerful forces, the environmental and the civil rights movements, and inspired environmental justice movements around the nation.[149] In community after community, local activists focused on the impact of pollutants in their soil and air. In Houston, Texas, in the heart of the oil and chemical industry, the African American community organized to stop a solid waste disposal site that was scheduled to open in a primarily minority neighborhood. All of the previous five solid waste dumps in the city had been sited in African American and Hispanic neighborhoods.[150]

Public attention to chemical pollution continued at other sites across the country as communities—both Black and white—took notice of the impact of PCBs and other toxic materials around and under their homes. In 1978, simultaneous to the revelations in North Carolina, Love Canal gained national attention when residents of this primarily white, working-class community near Niagara Falls, New York, found 22,000 pounds of chemical waste, including PCBs, dioxins, and pesticides, seeping into their basements. The source was barrels of waste buried decades earlier in a 350-acre area by the Hooker Electrochemical Company, a company that since 1903 had produced a wide variety of chlorinated products, including chlorinated lime, caustic soda, and lye, as well as solvents and a host of other products.[151] For weeks public protests and newspaper headlines focused the nation on Hooker's chemical wastes. Physicians, residents, and environmentalists identified epilepsy, miscarriages, asthma, migraines, and birth defects among children who played in puddles of polluted water and adults exposed while doing their laundry in their basements where chemicals from leaking barrels of benzene had seeped through the walls. After months of headlines and protest, New York State fenced off the area and planned to cap portions with plastic and concrete and to drain and treat tainted groundwater and sewer and creek sediment. But it would not be until 2004 that the area and the 260 homes still standing on the site were deemed "safe" for occupancy.[152]

In 1982, PCBs were discovered to have polluted Times Beach, Missouri: furans, a contaminant in PCB production and a feared cause of cancer, and other oils were found to have been used to wet down roads in the area. Following protests and national headlines, in 1985 the entire town had to be abandoned and the residents resettled.[153] Another site of environmental pollution and environmental justice advocacy was the 3-mile-wide by 100-mile-long stretch along the Mississippi River between Baton Rouge and New Orleans, an area deemed "Cancer Alley" because of the horrendous health effects of air, ground, and water pollution emanating from the string of chemical plants and oil refineries along the river. The average exposure per person in Louisiana was 21 pounds of toxic pollutants in 1995, according to the Toxic Release Inventory, a federal voluntary reporting system developed to track industrial pollutants. One of the poorest and most heavily African American communities along "Cancer Alley," Convent, Louisiana, was found to have an incredible burden: the average exposure over a given year was 2,277 pounds per person. In response to the threats posed to their health, communities along the Mississippi mobilized, pressuring legislators, suing polluting companies, and protesting publicly to gain some measure of justice.[154]

By the 1970s and 1980s, widespread concern that an array of synthetic materials could cause cancer or other serious diseases had become a formidable threat to American industry's image and, potentially, to its profits. Americans no longer believed that progress was the most important product of the chemical industry. Indeed, the chemicals that were now ubiquitous were the source of new threats to people's health and happiness. Perception of the threat of disease had itself changed substantially. Broadly speaking, Americans no longer feared the germ with the intensity they had in the late nineteenth century and early twentieth century. Before the AIDS epidemic in the 1980s once again raised the specter of communicable disease, many were largely convinced that infections were issues that science and the pharmaceutical laboratory could address through antibiotics, vaccines, and public health measures. Researchers and investigative reporters had largely turned their attention to threats posed by various synthetic chemicals and other pollutants in the air we breathed and the water we drank, in the walls of our homes, and in our furniture and clothing. Suspected carcinogens were the issues of concern. Formaldehyde, for example, a colorless chemical used in mortuaries as a preservative and elsewhere as a fungicide, germicide, and disinfectant, could be found in plywood, particle board, hardwood paneling, and the "medium density fiberboard" commonly used for the fronts of drawers and cabinets or the tops of furniture. As the material aged, formaldehyde evaporated into the home as a known cancer-producing vapor, which slowly accumulated in bodies. These toxins affected people in cities, suburbs, and rural areas. They afflicted the rich and powerful and the poor and disenfranchised.

Flame retardants were introduced in the 1970s and commonly used on sofas, chairs, carpets, love seats, curtains, baby products, and even TVs. Making common household furniture and objects fire retardant sounded like a good idea, but researchers have linked one of the most common flame retardants, polybrominated diphenyl ethers (pbde), to a wide variety of potentially undesirable health effects, including thyroid disruption, memory and learning problems, delayed mental and physical development, lower IQ, and early onset of puberty.

Other flame retardants, like tris (1,3-dichloro-2-propyl) phosphate, have been linked to cancer. As the CDC has documented in an ongoing study of the accumulation of hazardous materials in our bodies, flame retardants can now be found in the blood of "nearly all" of us.[155] Nor are these particular chemicals anomalies. Lurking in the cabinet under the kitchen sink, for instance, are window cleaners and spot removers that contain known or suspected cancer-causing agents. The same can be said of some cosmetics in makeup cases, plastic water bottles, and microwavable food containers. Since the 1960s we have learned that asbestos may have been in the baby powder that Johnson & Johnson and other companies marketed to millions of parents to prevent diaper rash.[156]

More recently, bisphenol A (BPA), the synthetic chemical used in a variety of plastic consumer products, including some baby bottles, epoxy cements, the lining of tuna fish cans, and even credit card receipts, has been singled out as another everyday toxin increasingly found inside all of us. Recent studies indicate that its effects are as varied as they are distressing. As Sarah Vogel of the Environmental Defense Fund has written, "New research on very-low-dose exposure to BPA suggests an association with adverse health effects, including breast and prostate cancer, obesity, neurobehavioral problems, and reproductive abnormalities."[157] Teflon, or perfluorooctanoic acid (PFOA), the heat-resistant, nonstick coating that has been sold to us as indispensable for pots and pans, is a suspected carcinogen and yet another in the list of substances that may be poisoning us, almost unnoticed.

These synthetic materials are just a few of the thousands now firmly embedded in our lives and our bodies. Most have been put into our air, water, homes, and fields without having been studied for potential health risks. Nor has much attention been given to how they interact in the environments in which we live, let alone our bodies. The groups that produce these miracle substances—like the petrochemical, plastics, and rubber industries, including major companies like Exxon, Dow, and Monsanto—argue that, until we can definitively prove that the chemical products slowly leaching into our bodies are dangerous, we have no "right" to demand of them, and they have no obligation, to remove them from our homes, schools, and workplaces. These corporations argue that the threats being identified are vastly overblown. They have begun campaigns to support those scientists and spokespeople who downplay the dangers and the idea that the problems were of industry's doing. In large measure, industries have denied the existence of serious environmental and health problems when they could; and when the evidence of possible harm was overwhelming, they have tried to shift the blame from the company to the victims of disease. This was certainly the case in lawsuits against the tobacco industry, in which companies argued that it was people's choice to smoke. In environmental contaminant cases, residents of polluted communities were often admonished to clean their houses better. In lawsuits about lead paint damage to children, mothers have been blamed for not keeping their children from touching walls and furniture. Industry rejects the idea that an industry should prove its products safe before exposing the entire population to them. The world of chemistry in the years following World War II has transformed the environment. Now we are left to face the still largely unknown consequences of the production and dissemination of untested processes and products and of cancers, endocrine disruptions, and subtle neonatal and childhood neurological changes. As a nation, we have emerged into a new, unknown world that might harm, even kill us, in new ways.

THE ACCOMPLISHMENTS AND LIMITS OF REFORM IN THE POST–WORLD WAR II ERA

The labor movement, along with the civil rights movement of the 1950s through the 1970s and the environmental movement, was a harbinger of a newly awakened public consciousness of the impact of powerful reactionary forces on our health and well-being. Following the examples of labor and the civil rights movements, women's groups and consumer, gay, and lesbian activists all mobilized around different aspects of the unhealthy and repressive world that shaped their lives. Women's groups organized and pushed for reproductive rights that were recognized in the Supreme Court decision *Roe v. Wade*, a decision that set off a fifty-year effort to overturn it which was accomplished in 2022 by the conservative majority on the Supreme Court and their allies.

The provision of legal abortion ended in many states, with the prospect of another period of deaths and butchering of women during backroom abortions; gay and lesbian groups like the Gay Men's Health Collective successfully mobilized to press governments to devote resources to research treatments for AIDS, which converted AIDS from a death sentence to a chronic condition that allows those with the disease to live a relatively normal life. Major efforts spurred by the disabled community, which took off in the 1960s, have led to greater mainstreaming in public schools and have integrated the disabled more successfully, while still inadequately, into the broader society. Medicare and Medicaid programs, Obamacare, and now the legislation to lower prescription drug prices have had a dramatic impact on senior health. As with other movements that have sought to remedy some of the inequalities that have shaped American history, these efforts have resulted in significant improvements in the lives of millions of Americans.

Yet, simultaneously, every one of these successes, as well as others attained after enormous struggles, have not addressed the fundamental inequalities that are at the basis of so much of American society and the health of its people. The differentials in life span between African Americans, Latinos, Native Americans, the white working-class, and other poor persons and middle-class and upper-class whites is an enduring, tragic feature of American health statistics. Not only have we built a world of chemicals that often unnecessarily compromise our health, but we have built a world where the poor and minorities bear an undue measure in years of life lost and decades of poorer health.

CHAPTER SEVEN

Darkest Before the Dawn?

The close relationship between a nation's physical health and its economic and political health has been a central tenet of statecraft since the rise of the mercantile economy in the eighteenth century. Especially in England, France, Germany, and Austria during this time, health statistics became an important measure of the threats to social cohesion— specifically the inequalities that were becoming ever more threatening in a developing capitalist economy. In the nineteenth century, politicians, doctors, social reformers, and revolutionary thinkers—from William Farr and Otto von Bismarck to Rudolf Virchow, Edwin Chadwick, Karl Marx, and Friedrich Engels—continued to use the physical health of a nation's citizens as a broad gauge of its social and political well-being.[1] Indeed, the arguments they made combined with the data they collected became central to the establishment of various forms of social security and health insurance.

In the twentieth century, policymakers also looked to health statistics that indicated deteriorating population health as a harbinger of social and political disequilibrium. One notable example was a 1981 article entitled "The Health Crisis in the USSR" in the *New York Review of Books* by the demographer Nick Eberstadt, who made some startling assertions.[2] He found that alcoholism, infant mortality, and suicide rates were taking a horrendous toll on Soviet society and concluded that a society plagued by so many markers of poor health was not sustainable as an industrial economy. Coming in the midst of the Cold War, even the most hardened spokespeople from both the Right and the Left found it difficult to believe his conclusion that the Soviet Union was on the verge of collapse. In the weeks and months that followed, there appeared a flurry of furious responses in the letters to the editor of the *Review* and other forums, accusing Eberstadt of grossly exaggerating and misinterpreting the data.[3] Twelve years later, Eberstadt's assertions, not primarily based on political analysis or even economic data, but on health statistics alone, proved eerily prescient as the Soviet Union's economy and political structure collapsed.

Forewarnings that health and the cohesiveness of civil society are intimately interlocked should give us pause today as the impact of Covid-19 on the stability of our own economic and political life has become more apparent. A 2020 Pew Research opinion poll in the midst of the epidemic found that the U.S. population was "more politically divided" over how to handle the epidemic than "other advanced societies," with divisions largely following political party lines.[4] Unsurprisingly, political divisions have been predictive of Covid-19 death rates, with the highest toll largely among Republican-led states whose governors opposed mask mandates or vaccination requirements.[5] But even before Covid-19 struck, there were disturbing trends about mortality in the United States. "Rising Morbidity and Mortality in Midlife Among White Non-Hispanic Americans in the 21st Century," a paper by the Princeton economists Anne Case and Angus Deaton (a Nobel laureate) and published in the *Proceedings of the National Academy of Sciences,* garnered considerable attention when it first appeared in 2015.[6] See figure 7.1.

The paper showed that between 1999 and 2013, middle-aged white American males and females experienced "a marked increase" in mortality, an increase that accounted for at least 96,000 more deaths than what would have been expected if mortality rates had stayed at their 1998 levels. Case and Deaton argued that "this change reversed decades of progress in mortality and was unique to the United States; no other rich country saw a similar turnaround." They noted that if the mortality rates for this group had instead continued to decline over this period at a lower pace, as they had in other industrialized nations, more than 500,000 more American men in this cohort would still have been alive

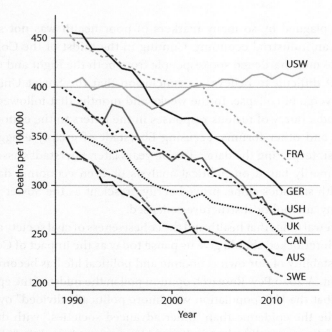

FIGURE 7.1 All-cause mortality, ages 45 to 54, for U.S. white non-Hispanics (USW), U.S. Hispanics (USH), and six comparison countries: France (FRA), Germany (GER), the United Kingdom (UK), Canada (CAN), Australia (AUS), and Sweden (SWE).

in 2015.[7] Mary Bassett, professor at Harvard's Chan School of public health and former commissioner of health for New York State, points to the long history of racism and class inequalities and, especially since the 1980s, what she calls "a particularly predatory form of capitalism [in the United States] that is now damaging [the health of] virtually every group in this country."[8]

The fact of increased mortality among men was troubling enough. What was even more troubling, however, was the fact that these deaths were not due solely to some epidemic catastrophe like Covid-19 or AIDS. Rather, the leading causes of death were suicides, alcohol-related liver disease, poisonings, and drug-related or mental health issues. Accidental or "intent undetermined" poisonings actually took more lives than lung cancer, and the investigators suggested that "suicide appears poised to do so" as well. "Increasing midlife distress" related to unemployment and occupational insecurity appeared to account for the overall rise.

The "at risk" populations were those without a high school degree, those without jobs, individuals experiencing considerable economic and personal stress, and those socially isolated, in physical pain, or in poor health, according to self-reports.[9] This observation was consistent with the growing body of literature documenting the impact of the opioid epidemic and the role of both the Sacklers and the larger pharmaceutical industry in its creation. In 2018, before the Covid-19 epidemic took hold, the *Journal of the American Medical Association (JAMA)* reported a startling 345 percent rise in deaths among America's young adults, two-thirds of whom were men, just in the previous decade and a half. Fully 20 percent of deaths in men between ages fifteen and twenty-four were due to opioids: "Overall, opioid-related deaths resulted in 1,681,359 years of life lost . . . in the United States in 2016, most of which . . . were among men."[10]

The American Lung Association has been publishing an annual "State of the Air" report since the turn of the twenty-first century. Until 2021, it detailed progress in the nation's air quality since passage of the landmark Clean Air Act of 1970. But in its 2021 report, it noted that rising atmospheric temperatures associated with increased greenhouse gases were destroying the quality of the very air people breathe. For the first time in the report's twenty-one-year history, air quality, as measured by increases in ozone concentrations and particulate matter, had declined compared to the preceding year. The report documented that over 40 percent of Americans, 135 million people, lived in areas with "unhealthy levels of ozone or particle pollution." The dangerous air was affecting "people of color" disproportionately: they were over three times more likely than white people to be breathing the most polluted air.[11] Covid-19 only accentuated those trends. A 2022 study by the Centers for Disease Control and Prevention (CDC) of life expectancy in the United States showed that air quality had declined "to its lowest level since 1996." The CDC documented a 2.7-year decline from 2020 to 2022, with the heaviest burden on communities of color, "the biggest two year decline . . . since 1921–1923," following the 1918–1919 influenza epidemics.[12] This leaves us to wonder anew if the world we as a nation have built, with its embedded racism and inequalities of class, will ever really address the structural inequalities that continue to take years of life off of some members of the society compared to others.[13]

The economic downturn during the height of the Covid-19 epidemic reinforced and accentuated trends that had been present for at least a few decades: the decline in opportunities for those without higher education to find meaningful employment; the undercutting of the federal government's ability to insist on safety precautions by Supreme Court decisions limiting OSHA from "interfering" in the workplace by requiring masks; the decline of the union movement and the respectable wages they often guaranteed; the growth of part-time, low-wage jobs; the erosion of job security; the replacement of guaranteed pensions by more risky stock market investments; and the greed of certain industries willing to pollute the very environment if doing so keeps their expenses low and their profits high—all have fed a health crisis most directly but far from exclusively affecting working-class families even in the prime of their lives. Depression, economic insecurity, polluted air and soil, inadequate access and exorbitant cost of health care, "food deserts" in poorer communities where fresh produce is largely unavailable or overpriced, along with climate change—exacerbated floods, fires, and droughts, have together created a mushrooming health crisis. It is no longer a germ, one pollutant, or one natural disaster that we can focus on by developing a new technology or mobilizing disaster relief efforts. The world that we as a nation have built socially, politically, economically, and racially has created an environment where our bodies and even the globe are at risk.

The unsightly toll that the Covid-19 epidemic exacted from communities of color, particularly the African American community, is the cruelest reminder of what are often politely and benignly termed the "inequities" in our social order and the "disparities," as public health academics have politely termed it, in health status. African Americans, disproportionately burdened by diseases and disabilities, have throughout American history had shorter lives than whites. The death rate for African American women giving birth is over two and a half times the rate for white women.[14] Black infants, for example, even in utero the victims of the racism of a health care system that privileges the wealthy, die at twice the rate as white infants; American Indians and Alaskan Natives can, on average, expect to live to 65.2 years and African Americans can, on average, expect to live to 70.8 years, while white people can expect to live into their late 70s.[15]

Although we as a species have created an amazing civilization, the damage wrought by the physical, economic, social, and political worlds we have built is most directly apparent in what has been done to undermine the ecological systems that will determine whether our species flourishes in the future. The earth is an extremely resilient place. Over the centuries, humans have destroyed many of its natural forests, burned its surface, and polluted its waters only to find that, for the most part, the earth recovers. The Hudson River, for example, was once made virtually lifeless as cities and towns used it as a dump for human and animal waste and early manufacturing plants used it as their private sewer. Given enough care and time, the river has been brought back to life. Forests cut down to create fields soon grew again once left to do so. Like Robert Frost, we need only wander through New England's verdant woods, imagining that we are the first to marvel at their beauty, only to notice the remains of rock walls that were built by people who had denuded this land to create fields for grazing and to prepare the soil for sowing. Humans also cut down trees and converted them into charcoal to fuel the small furnaces, kilns, and foundries that dotted the agricultural landscape to manufacture the iron plows and tools needed to farm.

Some believe that the damage done by humans to environments can be reversed, that "nature" will always "recover," if people only stop their destructive behavior. Not surprisingly, such belief in the stability of the natural system has often been played on by corporate actors who seek an intellectual rationale for downplaying or dismissing the damage they have done to the environment, and those in it, for the sake of profit. As we've detailed elsewhere,[16] for nearly half a century, the pollution produced by leaded gasoline in automobiles was justified by scientists at the Kettering Institute who were supported by General Motors and Ethyl Corporation in arguing that lead was "naturally" in all of us, and thus something our bodies could handle. In the 1970s, DuPont and others supported researchers who promoted the "Gaia" hypothesis that posited that the earth was a self-regulating system whose ecology ultimately "adjusted" to human disruption. Along with Exxon Mobil Corporation's sowing of doubt that climate change was caused predominantly by human actions, these arguments were used to legitimate the continued disruptions caused by greenhouse gases and other toxic emissions.[17]

But the comfort derived from believing that nature or great technological breakthroughs will undo damage to the environment has been challenged by reality. For example, during the past 150 years the fossil fuel industries in particular have not only transformed the earth's surface to suit their purposes but have done so in ways that could well be both permanent and existentially threatening.

Similarly, changes in food production have had a deleterious effect on health. For example, antibiotics, hormones, and genetic selection have produced larger chickens with more white meat for distribution around the country and the globe. In 1928, the year Herbert Hoover's campaign slogan was "a chicken in every pot," the average American consumed only 8 ounces of chicken a year. By 1945, the average had increased to 5 pounds a year, and in 1994 the per capita consumption had increased to nearly 70 pounds per year.[18] This increase has created huge health problems that public health is only now beginning to address. As Maryn McKenna, the author of *Big Chicken*, has said, "Because of the consolidation of food production, in which now fewer very large firms are distributing their products over very large spaces, we get very large outbreaks of antibiotic-resistant foodborne illness that can be distributed hundreds and thousands of miles away from where the original farms are." Millions of consumers are vulnerable to a host of pathogens that are now resistant to the antibiotics that would once have been used to treat them.[19] Also, the need for both adults in a family to work full time to support the ever-increasing cost of child care and rent has led to a greater dependence on fast foods.

In addition, corporations have sacrificed public purpose and consumers' health for private gain. During the past few decades, there has been an expansion of what Nick Freudenberg has called "hyperpalatable foods," foods that "provide eaters with greater physical and psychological rewards than traditional foods." He cites former commissioner of the Food and Drug Administration David Kessler, who noted that these foods have been created to trigger " 'supernormal stimuli' via the release of the neurotransmitter dopamine that produces cravings." One consequence of this process has been that, in the United States, people now consume 250 to 300 more calories per day than they did in the 1950s and 1960s. "Nearly half the increase comes from drinking more sugary beverages," a sector of the food economy in which 93 percent of the market is controlled by just three companies. This increased consumption has contributed to a dramatic increase in obesity and diabetes, among other chronic diseases.[20]

Our health has also been greatly impacted by the use of old, and the introduction of new, chemicals into our environment. Chemical plants and smokestacks pollute the air. Now synthetic products are sprayed in homes, on gardens, and throughout neighborhoods; lead covers our walls, plastics are used to wrap food in, and plasticizers are in babies' pacifiers. Because we understand so little about the effects of many of these new synthetic chemicals, we are all unwitting subjects in a huge observational study. Since 1999, the CDC has been monitoring Americans' bodies for the potential presence of 212 chemicals, detailing the variety of pollutants stored in their bones, muscle, blood, and fat.[21] The CDC's explicit goals are "to determine which chemicals are getting into [Americans] and at what concentrations" and what impact these chemicals might have.[22] One broad category of chemicals the CDC has been following, chlorinated hydrocarbons (such as vinyl chloride and polychlorinated hydrocarbons such as PCBs and DDT), can be found in virtually every living thing on earth, from the shrimp that swim in the salt waters of the Gulf of Mexico to the poultry and red meat that have become staples of the American diet.[23] And one subset, PCBs, long identified as the cause of chloracne (systemic skin eruptions), neurological problems, and liver disease, is now "probably carcinogenic to humans" according to the International Agency for Research on Cancer (IARC).[24]

The first CDC list of chemical compounds (1999–2000) included lead, manganese, mercury, and the traditional heavy metal poisons. The latest set of revised tables, published in 2019, is a lexicon of names only a chemist could love. To the original list, seventy-five new chemicals have been added, including phthalates, twenty-nine volatile organic compounds, four environmental phenols, four disinfection byproducts, three "non-dioxin like" PCBs, and twelve perfluorinated compounds. The latest report shows that our bodies now include a chemical soup of new synthetics that evolution could not possibly adapt us to. While previously lead encephalopathy and chronic diseases such as asbestosis or lung cancer were the primary worry, now the worry is about subtle biological changes to our endocrine systems, effects on our neurological development, and other biological changes that have not yet been named as diseases. Scientists do not know what the long-term effects of these chemicals will be, nor do they understand the synergistic effects on complex biological systems of combining so many novel materials in unknown quantities.

The petrochemical, plastics, and rubber industries producing these toxins and toxic products argue that until it can be definitively proven that these chemicals in our bodies are dangerous, they have no obligation to remove them from the market or recall products from homes, schools, and workplaces. They reject the idea that they should prove their products safe before exposing the entire population, despite the fact that in the past they have acknowledged their responsibility to do so. The approach today is different in some other countries. The European Union, for example, employs what public health professionals and activists call the "precautionary principle." New chemicals should pass stringent tests proving their safety *before*, not after, their introduction into our homes and the environment. While many in the public health community in the United States agree that the precautionary principle is needed here, the resistance of industry is immense. When the Toxic Substances Control Act (TSCA) was revised in 2016, it exempted the vast majority of chemicals that were in existence in 1976 when TSCA was first enacted.

In the 1920s, the oil industry argued that until it was proven that lead in gasoline was dangerous to consumers, even though it was known to be a dangerous toxin to workers, the government had no right to demand its removal.[25] This resistance led to sixty years of environmental pollution and continuing serious health issues. Yet, today, we as a society have still not learned from our history; we all too often continue to watch and wait until damage is done before we act. Increasingly, we are all toxic dumps, and there's no remedial superfund to clean up our bodies. We are, to one degree or another, walking, talking biohazards to ourselves, and most of us don't even know it. See figure 7.2.

The Covid-19 pandemic has raised additional troubling ethical, political, and humane concerns. No country, irrespective of its wealth or technological sophistication, has escaped its impact. The pandemic is another instance of creating a world that kills us. Knowledgeable people for decades have been pointing out what happens when populations, especially impoverished populations, expand into various animal

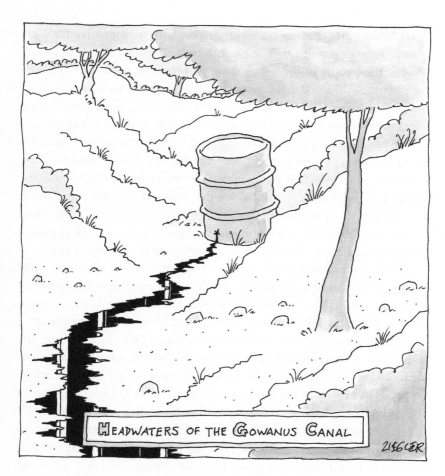

FIGURE 7.2 Jack Ziegler, "Headwaters of the Gowanus Canal," *New Yorker*, December 5, 2016. Courtesy of Jack Ziegler/Cartoonstock.

habitats and when other questionable human practices here and elsewhere remain uncurbed. Laurie Garrett, in *The Coming Plague: Newly Emerging Diseases in a World Out of Balance*, points out that failure to mount a global effort to vaccinate the vast proportion of people in poorer countries makes it likely that the virus will eventually mutate in ways that allow it to evade the protections that vaccines currently afford those in more developed countries.[26] Science may be facing the social limits of its reliance on technologies: with no incentive for companies or richer nations to provide low-cost pharmaceuticals to poorer nations, the people in those countries will become incubators for new and potentially more dangerous variants. And, closer to home, vaccination resistance makes areas of the United States also incubators. Garrett points out that, as of 2022, "of the more than 8 billion doses of vaccines . . . only 26 million [had] gone into arms [of the 56 million people] in South Africa . . . or 0.3 percent of the global supply" of vaccines because of the shortsighted approach of policymakers in the richer countries and the greed of pharmaceutical companies that refused to make their product available inexpensively.[27] Covid-19, like climate change, infectious disease, and industrial pollution, threatens everyone and, as generally happens, has caused disproportionate suffering for people of color.

There are reasons to take heart, however. Two decades ago, while driving through the countryside, wind turbines for generating power were a rare sight. Those of us with children born in the 1980s or 1990s can remember the kids announcing from the backseat that they spotted a windmill across an open field. Hybrids just didn't exist. As recently as the early 2000s, owners of hybrid Priuses would wave to each other when stopped for a traffic light. In 2012 there were no electric cars on the road, but by 2023 there were millions, and in Europe the sales of electric vehicles have now surpassed those of diesel-powered cars.[28] Today, it is commonplace to see solar-paneled houses, street lights, and traffic signals in communities across the land. In the coming decade, hydro, wind, and solar energy sources will replace coal and oil as the major source of electricity in the United States and many portions of the rest of the world. Efforts to capture the power of the oceans and tides may eventually provide limitless clean energy—if we don't run out of time.[29]

We can hope that, going forward, antibiotics, pharmaceuticals, and vaccines will continue to work against disease. Unfortunately, the widespread uses of antibiotics in our food supply, as well as the overprescription of these drugs by providers, is already destroying one of the most important medical advances available. Many bacteria have developed resistance to the armamentarium of antibiotics developed since World War II. Over fifteen years ago, the CDC issued its suggestions to hospitals on "Multidrug-Resistant Organisms (MDRO) Management."[30]

Since then hospitals around the world have been on high alert for out-breaks of MRSA (Methicillin-resistant *Staphylococcus aureus*) and a host of bacteria that show resistance to commonly used antibacterial, antiviral, and antiparasitic agents.

Meanwhile, many movements in the United States and the world are pushing to preserve a livable planet and to ameliorate if not elim-inate the inequalities we have discussed in this book. Despite various attempts to pull back from the Paris Agreement on greenhouse gas reductions and despite attempts by some who still "promise" to bring back coal and to lower the standards for emissions from cars and trucks (the Corporate Average Fuel Economy—CAFE—Standards), many state and local governments have stood firm in their attempts to address cli-mate change, even adopting California's strict air pollution controls. Numerous cities around the country have mayors and administrators who have vowed to lower traffic congestion, support bike lanes and com-munity biking, create green spaces, switch to electric municipal buses and other vehicles, and require more climate-friendly building retro-fits. When the EPA during the Trump administration announced that it would not mandate the use of efficient LED lighting, even light bulb manufacturers protested.[31] Young people around the world have mobi-lized, staging huge rallies in their nation's capitals demanding that those in power reverse the policies that hasten the looming environmental catastrophe and adopt more sustainable policies.

It is important to remember, however, that efforts at reform gen-erally meet with resistance from those whose financial interests are affected by them. On the federal level, for example, regulatory agencies such as the EPA, OSHA, and the Mine Safety and Health Administra-tion (MSHA) in their efforts to control pollution have run into numer-ous roadblocks from Congress and the Supreme Court, roadblocks that may make progressive efforts seem hopeless. In 2022, the Supreme Court issued a decision in *West Virginia v. Environmental Protection Agency* that limited the federal regulatory agency's ability and authority to "reduce carbon dioxide from power plants." The 6–3 ruling by the conservative members of the Court severely curtails the ability of the Environmental Protection Agency to limit emissions from coal-burning power plants. In what the *New York Times* called a "crucial moment" in the "Republican Drive to Tilt Courts Against Climate Action," it noted that this case was the "product of a coordinated, multi-year strategy by Republican attorneys general, conservative legal activists and their funders, several with ties to the oil and coal industries, to use the judicial system to rewrite environmental law, weakening the executive branch's ability to tackle global warming."[32] The majority decision left the EPA unable to regulate air pollution without clear congressional authorization.[33] The implications of this decision go well beyond West Virginia. The decision may provide the basis, according to the *Times*, for dismantling the governmental apparatus used to regulate polluting industries that had been put in place over the course of the last half of the twentieth century. If the Supreme Court applied this doctrine across the board, the EPA, OSHA, the FDA, and the Consumer Products Safety Commission would be unable to enact or enforce either new regulations or older, long-standing ones: regulations that limit the amount of lead in gasoline and paint, limit the exposure of workers to asbestos, and limit the emissions of methane and other greenhouse gases that threaten the world as we know it.

Given the present opposition to regulation, OSHA has scaled back attempts to set new standards or enforce old ones. Sharon Lerner, a journalist for *ProPublica* who has been tracking changes at OSHA and the EPA over the years, notes that OSHA has been "paralyzed by industry lawsuits from decades ago" and "has all but given up on trying to set a truly protective threshold" for thousands of chemicals. "The agency has only updated standards for three chemicals in the past 25 years," she points out, and "each took more than a decade to complete." David Michaels, OSHA's director throughout the Obama years, says legal challenges so tied his hands that he decided to put the following disclaimer on the agency's website: "OSHA recognizes that many of its permissible exposure limits (PELs) are outdated and inadequate for ensuring protection of worker health." This remarkable admission of defeat remains today on the official site of the very U.S. agency that is devoted to protecting worker health.[34] "You can't lie and say you're offering protection when you're not," Michaels told Lerner. "It seemed much more effective to say, 'Don't follow our standards.'"[35]

Despite the assault on federal efforts to protect both workers and the environment, a series of local initiatives, court cases, and regulatory decisions give some cause for hope. What can't be accomplished in Washington at the federal level may have to be addressed through local court cases and decisions at the community level. California has been at the forefront of efforts to control environmental pollutants. For example, in 2013 it established emission standards for cars that have had a national impact as they were adopted by other states, leading car manufacturers interested in the huge California market to improve their cars' fuel efficiency and to push their efforts to develop hybrids and electric vehicles. The California Safer Food Packaging and Cookware Act, which took effect in 2023, banned the use of PFAS (per- and poly-fluoroalkyl substances), sometimes called "forever" chemicals because of their persistence in the environment, food packaging, and cookware such as Teflon.[36] New York, Maryland, and Washington are among the states that have banned fracking. (Vermont also banned fracking, but it has no known "frackable" natural gas deposits.) These local decisions are having a profound impact on debates about environmentalism and health, both community and individual. Even without federal or state legislation, for example, asbestos is rarely used in consumer items anymore; primary lead smelting has virtually ceased in the United States; and recently, efforts to regulate and clean up the mess left by decades of lead pollution have met some success. Of course, many states may not enact similar laws, so the regulation of pollution, at best, can end up as a kind of patchwork affair.

Perhaps the most direct challenge to the host of environmental threats that are foisted on us by various polluting industries comes from local communities, particularly communities of color, who have merged environmentalism and civil rights. *Environmental justice*, a term coined by Robert Bullard, has brought to light the unequal impact of certain decisions on poor communities. Garbage dumps, for example, are located disproportionately in or near communities of color. Polluting industries locate themselves in poor areas. A general observation of Bullard's about the impact of pollution is equally applicable to the impact of climate change due to greenhouse gas emissions: that the communities that contribute least to the problem are nonetheless those that suffer most. Coastal nations in the Pacific, Asia, and South America are clearly among the most vulnerable to rising oceans and heat waves; resulting waterborne diseases are likely to affect African nations more than the wealthy nations in Europe or North America; and lead miners and residents in the surrounding communities in Peru undoubtedly suffer from the mineral's extraction and smelting much more than do those in wealthier nations who use lead in cell phones and other electronic devices. Mass migrations from drought-stricken or flood-prone areas of the earth are overwhelmingly of the world's poorest.[37]

Local environmental justice efforts are beginning to gain traction in some regions. In Appalachia, a prolonged and important court battle is being waged over mountaintop removal (MTR), the process of coal extraction that has damaged huge swaths of Virginia, West Virginia, Tennessee, and Kentucky. Beginning in the 1980s and accelerating throughout the 1990s as mine shafts were abandoned, mountaintop removal emerged as Appalachia's most profitable, and destructive, method of removing coal from beneath the bedrock of mountains. In the past thirty years it is estimated that this process has seriously damaged over five hundred mountains in the region. One study found that 1–1.2 million acres of the Appalachian range have been surface-mined and that at least five hundred mountains have been defiled, some resulting in over 600 feet of bedrock removed and dumped in a single site elsewhere. "Only twenty-six locations (6.3 percent of the total)," for example, "host some form of verifiable post-mining economic development," according to the study.[38] The heavy diesel equipment with its polluting exhaust, the huge quantities of debris dumped in local watersheds, and the scars created by the use of explosives loaded with ammonium nitrate are the visual insults. In addition, the processing of the coal ore thus recovered releases arsenic, barium, mercury, lead, and chromium into the wells and water supplies of those living nearby.[39]

Health data reflect the lasting effects of such mining on residents' health and well-being. Recent studies drawn from the National Center for Health Statistics data of 1.8 million live births showed that the incidence of "circulatory/respiratory, central nervous system, musculoskeletal, gastrointestinal, urogenital," and "other" birth defects was significantly higher than the national average among those living in mountaintop mining areas.[40] What was once primarily a battle over CO_2 emissions, national air quality, and local water pollution has expanded dramatically. An extraordinary interactive website reveals county by county the growing increase in mortality and the general health disparities that exist in counties of West Virginia. In one 2012 study, it was documented that counties in West Virginia experiencing mountaintop removal had "nearly double" the cancer rates of nearby counties "with no mountaintop removal."[41]

Not surprisingly, given the rich history of local struggles against the coal interests, new forms of resistance from local groups have emerged. Legal battles have replaced pitched battles between union members and company enforcers as statewide groups like the Tennessee-based Organizing for Community Empowerment, the West Virginia Highlands Conservancy and Coal River Mountain Watch, the Southern Appalachian Mountain Stewards, and the Ohio Valley Environmental Coalition organize demonstrations and lawsuits. Needless to say, coal companies have been active in opposing every attempt by local groups, the EPA, or other federal agencies to constrain mining activities.

As climate change alters the ecologies in which pathogens and vectors propagate, the world will undoubtedly confront diseases for which governments and people are not prepared. We may, for example, even see the resurgence of diseases that have not had a major impact in the United States for more than a century. As global temperatures rise and the mosquito moves into newly warmer habitats, yellow fever, caused by the *Aedes aegypti* mosquito, or malaria, caused by the parasite carried by mosquitoes, may reappear.[42] As National Public Radio summarized the November 2023 National Climate Assessment, the congressional report on the effects of climate change on the U.S. population:

> The health costs of climate change have gone from theoretical to personal for many Americans. The most obvious risk? Extreme weather, particularly heat. . . . Heat waves have become hotter, longer, and more dangerous, and they're hitting areas that aren't ready for them—like the "record-shattering" heat dome that descended on the Pacific Northwest in 2021 and caused hundreds of deaths.
>
> But it's not just heat. Wildfire smoke can send people thousands of miles from the fires to hospitals with respiratory problems and heart disease complications. Hurricanes can disrupt people's access to healthcare: when a clinic is flooded or people are displaced, for example, kidney patients can't get dialysis treatment.
>
> In most cases, the people who bear the brunt of the disasters are those already at risk: poor communities, communities of color,

women, people with disabilities, and other marginalized groups. Temperatures in formerly redlined neighborhoods in cities across the country can soar nearly 15 degrees Fahrenheit hotter than wealthier areas just blocks away, putting residents at much higher risk of heat exposure.[43]

In its simplest terms, humans are fundamentally altering the ecology within which disease silently and quickly moves across borders by air and boat travel, animal or insect.[44]

The existential problem of human survival in the face of climate change is outlined in numerous, frequently updated reports. In a report on the October 2022 United Nations (UN) meeting on climate change, a grim picture of the future emerged. In an article headlined "World Close to 'Irreversible' Climate Breakdown," the *Guardian* quoted "the UN environment agency's report [that] found there was 'no credible pathway to 1.5C in place.'" It concluded that the "woefully inadequate" progress on cutting carbon emissions "means the only way to limit the worst impacts of the climate crisis is a rapid transformation of societies," a goal seemingly impossible in light of the unprecedented profits that the petrochemical companies are reaping. "Current pledges for action by 2030, even if delivered in full, would mean a rise in global heating of about 2.5C, a level that would condemn the world to catastrophic climate breakdown, according to the UN's climate agency."[45] In a previous report, the UN secretary general, Antonio Guterres, declared that "unless governments everywhere reassess their energy policies, the world will be uninhabitable." He went to add that "this is not a fiction or exaggeration. It is what science tells us will result."[46]

Because of decades of inaction and stalling on the part of companies and governments around the world, what was once an effort that would have required a decades-long international effort has emerged as a crisis with startling immediacy. Climate disruption is no longer a problem just for future generations; it is clear that it is happening now.[47] While the number of all-electric cars is expanding and the cost of the batteries used to power them is dropping dramatically, fossil fuel use on a world scale is continuing to rise. In the United States, which accounts for the largest per capita percentage of greenhouse gas emissions, efforts to reduce emissions remain contentious. While nowhere near enough, the Biden administration has set much in motion, including the Inflation Reduction Act, which provided over $400 billion for renewable energy. Even so, worldwide, the gas-guzzling SUV has emerged as the hottest-selling automobile on the market. In 2000, only 18 percent of cars sold throughout the world were SUVs; in 2019, 42 percent were.[48] Even the move from coal to what has been marketed as "natural" gas has clouded our understanding that natural gas is itself a major contributor to CO_2 emissions. In Asia hundreds of coal-powered plants still operate and many more are being built, portending decades of future pollution. Globally, greenhouse gas emissions have grown by 1.5 percent a year, despite the growth in green technologies and pledges of reductions in country after country.[49]

The climate crisis is being felt in both industrialized and less industrialized societies now. In North America, wildfires have raged in Canada and Hawaii, and California is preparing for year-round fire seasons. Extensive droughts in the West, followed by extraordinary rainfall and flooding and ever more severe hurricanes and tornadoes, auger a stark future for expanding cities, especially along the coasts and in the sunbelt. Regular flooding in Miami, more powerful hurricanes in the Gulf, and disabling storms in New York are but a few weather events that can be linked to rising sea levels and warming ocean waters. A 2019 world assessment soporifically headlined "New Elevation Data Triple Estimates of Global Vulnerability to Sea-Level Rise and Coastal Flooding" contains hair-raising graphics showing that South Vietnam "could all but disappear" by midcentury, along with portions of Thailand, including Bangkok, and major cities such as Jakarta, Indonesia; Mumbai, India; coastal Bangladesh; the Pearl River Delta in China; Alexandria, Egypt; and other locales with populations of over 150 million people.[50]

A few still close their eyes to the devastating impact of climate change around the world and to the all-too-clear graphic predictions of what may occur in the next two or three decades. Even though climate change is no longer a subject of debate but is now a reality, the petrochemical and oil industries and their political allies oppose even the most basic efforts to document the impacts of climate change. In some states, oil and gas companies are no longer even required to report methane emissions. Hydrofluorocarbons, the greenhouse gas, were phased out of use in light duty vehicles in 2015 because they were identified as a potent cause of warming,[51] but they continued to be used in refrigerators and air conditioners until the U.S. Senate in late 2022 ratified "an international agreement to phase them out."[52] At the national level, senators like Sheldon Whitehouse have constantly reminded the American people of the need to gain control over the huge interests that are profiting from climate change denial. Whitehouse has delivered over two hundred speeches to the Senate trying to awaken senators to their responsibility to literally save the planet.[53]

The lack of regulation and the resistance to regulation are not only changing our climate in the long term but also affecting our health in the short term. The *Lancet*'s Commission on Pollution and Health declared in 2018 that "pollution [of all sorts] is the largest environmental cause of disease and death in the world today, responsible for an estimated 9 million premature deaths . . .—16 percent of all deaths worldwide." The report detailed that 92 percent of deaths were in low- and middle-income countries and that "children are most affected."[54]

Whether the forces promoting effective action to forestall further global warming will prevail is not at all clear. But there's a further puzzle here: Why is there not a collective will to confront threats to the health of us all? How did domestic politics in the United States get to a point where society cannot adequately address even the most basic threats? During the Covid-19 pandemic, huge cross-sections of the American population refused to be vaccinated or to wear masks. Is our collective interest in shaping the environment so limited that we can't even mobilize to address obvious and immediate threats? Are the economic interests of polluting industries so powerful and shortsighted that their executives put their own children and grandchildren at risk? How do we regulate industries in a country where a sizable number of people see government regulation as an ultimate evil? Are coastal communities in the United States and the rest of the world just not "worth saving"? Are the lives of people of Bangladesh worth less than the lives of residents of Miami or Newport Beach? Some think so. It may also be that dealing adequately with global warming and related crises would mean radical changes in people's normal lives, changes that many cannot or do not want to imagine. They hope, perhaps, that the looming disaster will not affect them in their own or children's lifetime.

For much of recent history, Americans have put their faith in technologies that would ameliorate the worst effects of the arrangements that lay at the heart of disease, death, and suffering. In the decades following the Civil War, America invested in huge infrastructural projects to provide pure water, to remove human and animal waste, and to enact housing regulations that demanded that tenement rooms have access to outside air. These reforms undoubtedly cut down on the incidence of epidemic and infectious diseases like cholera, typhoid, and tuberculosis. In the twentieth century, the development of pharmaceuticals, specifically antibiotics and vaccines, immeasurably improved the health of infants and adults alike. The development of antiretrovirals, drugs that interfere in the ability of certain viruses to replicate, addressed the HIV epidemic of the 1980s and 1990s and led many to imagine that the laboratory and science itself would ultimately prove a defense in all future epidemics.

Such reliance on medical technologies may ultimately prove hopelessly inadequate, however. The steady stream of terrifying infectious diseases that have been identified, from Ebola to SARS and MERS, along with the growing body of evidence that viruses and bacteria are developing resistance to our armamentarium of drugs, should be a warning about potentially catastrophic futures unless remedial action is taken. The development of vaccines for Covid-19 is indicative of the power of the laboratory to protect us in some crises, but it is also a warning that one day some variant or entirely new threat may not respond to our biomedical interventions.[55] Statistics gathered in 2022 tell us that about 1 out of every 300 Americans has died from the variants of Covid-19. Should any of us be surprised when a new variant—or an entirely new bacteria immune to our antimicrobials, or a virus for which our truly magical scientific enterprise is ineffective—emerges somewhere in the world and shows up in our midst? What will Americans do then? Our faith in the laboratory to protect us may prove correct or not.

But one thing we could do is address the social inequalities that leave essential workers vulnerable to infections when they deliver food, provide care in hospitals, or aid us in our homes. We could pay them adequately so that they have the health insurance and social benefits that the middle class enjoys. Should we not address the fact that American society has placed the burden of maintaining our society largely on the poor and people of color?

There is a deeply disturbing answer that some may give explicitly, many others implicitly: Why bother changing the social relations that perpetuate suffering when the problem does not appear to be a problem for those in power or their families? Communities in the paths of wildfires and people whose homes are destroyed by hurricanes or tornadoes are abstractions to many who are unaffected. Right now the "affected" of southern Asia and Africa seem far away, as do the migrants from fleeing ecological disasters. Even poisonings in our own country from lead-bearing water pipes seem like abstractions to those not themselves directly affected. Perhaps those living in isolated gated communities may believe they will never personally feel the impact of the changes imposed on the environment.[56] That so many may not feel empathy for others or not feel that they themselves are vulnerable is truly a terrifying idea, but one that may help to explain the willful ignorance and resistance to change that are evident today. It is the nature of so many environmentally caused diseases that they take so long to manifest themselves. Hence, we can more easily ignore their causes and avoid addressing the profound political, economic, and social changes that are required to address them, even when they shorten our own lives.

Some have seen the suffering of others who disproportionately bear the burden of the Covid-19 epidemic as a "cost" that others "need" to pay for a "return" to "normalcy." We have already seen that in the past some accept that our economy is and will be built on the backs of working people and people of color. "I'm not saying anything is perfect," Trump announced when "only" 72,000 people had died of Covid-19 (as of February 2023, over 1 million Americans had died of Covid).[57] "Will some people be affected badly? Yes," he answered. "But we have to get our country open, and we have to get it open soon."[58] In the current assumption that we are in the process of returning to a "normal" world, one can see an obliviousness to the fact that wealth, access to health care, and even life span are not equitable.

Ultimately, all the political and economic analyses aside, the truly terrifying conclusion of this long history may come down to a simple truth uttered by David Michaels. During a television interview about the 6–3 decision of the Supreme Court to deny the Biden administration's OSHA mandate that required workers in corporations with more than one hundred employees to wear masks and be vaccinated, Michaels bluntly said referring to the Court's majority, "They really don't want to stop this pandemic. I believe in my heart that they don't care."[59] Michaels's fear is not limited to the Supreme Court nor only to the impact of Covid-19 on the workforce. Women as well have been put at risk by the Court's decision in Dobbs v. Jackson Women's Health Organization, overturning of Roe v. Wade and state restrictions on access to the abortion pill. At the heart of our political, social, and economic system and the analyses that seek to justify the suffering of others lies the question: Do we care? Do we care to create a world that sustains rather than diminishes life?

All over the country there are local activist groups resisting the notion that Americans are incapable of caring for each other and especially the most vulnerable. Thankfully, many still believe that decent conditions of life for all, along with access to decent care, yield the basis for a truly healthy society. Throughout U.S. history there have been movements that refused to accept a status quo rooted in privilege and power: the abolitionist movement fought against the entrenched slave system whose conditions caused disease and death; and labor and reformist movements of the early twentieth century challenged the primacy of social Darwinism and the cynical belief that the wealthiest and powerful "deserved" their status and good health and had no responsibility to even support regulations to protect everyone else. During the New Deal, when chronic disease was killing and disabling the "slaves of the depression," members of Congress, spurred on by labor unions and other citizen groups, passed legislation that took a large portion of the elderly out of poverty; and in the 1960s, Fannie Lou Hamer and a generation of young civil rights activists refused to accept a segregated system that denied African Americans access to jobs, hospital care, and even physicians and forced the government to wage a war on poverty. While today's world seems bleak, headed toward climate disaster and the resulting displacement and death of millions, we might take solace from the old proverb that "it's always darkest before the dawn." We have to remember that we as a nation, we as a species, created this dark moment and we have the ability to change it.

Notes

INTRODUCTION: "SICK AND TIRED OF BEING SICK AND TIRED"

1. Fannie Lou Hamer, "Sick and Tired of Being Sick and Tired," Archives of Women's Political Communication, December 19, 2019 (speech at CME Church, Harlem, New York, organized by the Mississippi Democratic Party's Congressional Challenge, December 20, 1964), https://awpc.cattcenter.iastate .edu/2019/08/09/im-sick-and-tired-of-being-sick-and-tired-dec-20-1964/, accessed March 31, 2021.

2. Jack Geiger, "Jack Geiger and the Lessons of Pholela, South Africa" (interview for National Library of Medicine exhibit), Against the Odds, 2008, https://www.nlm .nih.gov/exhibition/againsttheodds/podcast/audiotour.html#s5, accessed June 3, 2022.

3. Hamer, "Sick and Tired."

4. Studs Terkel, *Working: People Talk About What They Do All Day and How They Feel About What They Do* (New York: Avon, 1972), xiii.

5. Crystal Eastman, *Work-Accidents and the Law* (New York: Russell Sage, 1910), 12–13.

6. See, for example, Nancy Krieger, "Measures of Racism, Sexism, Heterosexism, and Gender Binarism for Health Equity Research: From Structural Injustice to Embodied Harm—an Ecosocial Analysis," *Annual Review of Public Health* 41, no. 1 (April 2020): 37–62; Paula Braveman, Nancy Krieger, and John Lynch, "Health Inequalities and Social Inequalities in Health," *Bulletin of the World Health Organization* 78, no. 2 (2000): 232–233.

7. M. T. Bassett, J. T. Chen, and N. Krieger, "Variation in Racial/Ethnic Disparities in COVID-19 Mortality by Age in the United States: A Cross-Sectional Study," *PLOS Medicine* 17, no. 10 (October 2020): e1003402.

8. "A Poor People's Pandemic Report," https://sdsn.maps.arcgis.com/apps /dashboards/5f63359b4889476380d12b1cb5299f3d; "Health Equity Considerations and Racial and Ethnic Minority Groups," Centers for Disease Control and Prevention (CDC), July 24, 2020, https://www.cdc.gov/coronavirus/2019-ncov /community/health-equity/race-ethnicity.html; "Impact of Racism on Our Nation's Health," CDC, https://www.cdc.gov/healthequity/racism-disparities /impact-of-racism.html, accessed June 3, 2022.

9. "A Poor People's Pandemic Report: Mapping the Intersections of Poverty, Race and COVID-19," April 2022, https://www.poorpeoplescampaign.org/wp-content /uploads/2022/04/ExecutiveSummary_7.pdf, accessed June 3, 2022. By the end of the third year of the epidemic, rates were highest among whites.

10. United States Public Health Service, *Proceedings of a Conference to Determine Whether or Not There Is a Public Health Question in the Manufacture, Distribution, or Use of Tetraethyl Lead Gasoline*, Public Health Bulletin no. 158 (Washington, DC: Government Printing Office, 1925), 4, 69, 105–107.

11. See Gerald Markowitz and David Rosner, *Lead Wars: The Politics of Science and the Fate of America's Children* (Berkeley: University of California Press, 2014), for an expansive discussion of lead poisoning.

12. Marian Nestle, *Food Politics: How the Food Industry Influences Nutrition and Health* (Berkeley: University of California Press, 2003); Marian Nestle, *Unsavory Truth: How Food Companies Skew the Science of What to Eat* (New York: Basic Books, 2018).

13. One need only look at the ever-expanding range of public health concerns to see the growing scope and evolving definition of what constitutes public health. The World Health Organization's post–World War II definition that health "is a state of complete physical, mental and social well-being" has come in for numerous critiques as too broad and amorphous. Yet today, even that definition has been broadened to include prison reform, economic injustice, environmental racism, and gender and racial inequalities.

14. The view that disease is a primary actor in changing world history has a long tradition. See, for example, Hans Zinsser, *Rats, Lice and History* (Boston: Atlantic Monthly/Little, Brown, 1935), which is a classic history of typhus that opens with a preface discussing "the influence of [epidemic disease] upon the fate of nations"; see also William McNeill's now-classic *Plagues and People* (New York: Doubleday, 1977), which begins by explaining that smallpox and European diseases were more important in the conquest of the Aztecs and Incas than was gun powder.

15. An early example of this influential approach is McNeill's *Plagues and People*. See also Jared Diamond, *Guns, Germs, and Steel: The Fates of Human Society* (New York: Norton, 1999).

16. Siddhartha Sanghi and Amy Smaldone, "The Evolution of the Racial Gap in U.S. Life Expectancy," Federal Reserve Bank of St. Louis, January 27, 2022, https://www.stlouisfed.org/en/on-the-economy/2022/january/evolution -racial-gap-us-life-expectancy#:~:text=Because%20of%20systemic %20differences%20in,fewer%20years%20othan%20white%20Americans, accessed July 14, 2023.

17. R. Easterlin, *Growth Triumphant: The Twenty-First Century in Historical Perspective* (Ann Arbor: University of Michigan Press, 1996), quoted in S. R. Johansson and Alice Kasakoff, "Mortality History and the Misleading Mean," *Historical Methods* 33, no. 2 (Spring 2000): 56–58.

18. Nancy Krieger, Christian Testa, Jarvis Chen, William Hanage, and Alecia McGregor, "Relationship of Political Ideology of US Federal and State Elected Officials and Key COVID Pandemic Outcomes Following Vaccine Rollout to Adults: April 2021–March 2022," *Lancet Regional Health—Americas* 16 (December 2022): 100384, https://www.sciencedirect.com/science/article/pii /S2667193X22002010, accessed December 13. 2022; Akilah Johnson and Sabrina Malhi, "U.S. Life Expectancy Down for Second-Straight Year, Fueled by Covid-19," *Washington Post*, August 31, 2022, https://www.washingtonpost.com /health/2022/08/31/life-expectancy-drops-again/, accessed December 17, 2022; Akilah Johnson, "Can Politics Kill You? Research Says the Answer Increasingly Is Yes," *Washington Post*, December 16, 2022, https://www .washingtonpost.com/health/2022/12/16/politics-health-relationship/, accessed December 17, 2022. More recently, there appears to have been a slight rise once again.

19. Nancy Krieger, David H. Rehkopf, Jarvis T. Chen, Pamela D. Waterman, Enrico Marcelli, and Malinda Kennedy, "The Fall and Rise of US Inequities in Premature Mortality: 1960–2002," *PLOS Medicine* 5, no. 2 (February 2008), https:// doi.org/10.1371/journal.pmed.0050046, accessed December 15, 2022; see also Sanghi and Smaldone, "The Evolution of the Racial Gap."

20. Krieger et al., "The Fall and Rise of US Inequities."

21. See Charles Rosenberg, *Framing Disease: Studies in Cultural History* (New Brunswick, NJ: Rutgers University Press, 1992); Stephen Kunitz, *Disease and Social Diversity: The European Impact on the Health of Non-Europeans* (New York: Oxford University Press, 1994); and Susan Reverby and David Rosner, *Health Care in America: Essays in Social History* (Philadelphia: Temple University Press, 1979). Historians of medicine embraced the new paradigm with an enthusiasm that, for some decades, subsumed disease history in a separate,

cloistered intellectual world, a community more identified with the history of science than with social or even political history. Indeed, the history of medicine, as the field was immediately defined, was located in medical schools themselves, often with a distinct agenda of reinforcing the unicausal ideals of the profession. Other PhD programs were generally located in history of science, not history, departments. See Nancy Tomes, *The Gospel of Germs: Men, Women, and the Microbe in American Life* (Cambridge, MA: Harvard University Press, 1999), for the ways in which older and newer ideas intersected.

22. See Elizabeth Fee, *Disease and Discovery: A History of the Johns Hopkins School of Hygiene and Public Health, 1916–1939* (Baltimore, MD: Johns Hopkins University Press, 1987), p.19.

23. Gerald Markowitz and David Rosner, "Doctors in Crisis: A Study of the Use of Medical Education Reform to Establish Modern Professional Elitism in Medicine," *American Quarterly* 25, no. 1 (March 1973): 83–107.

24. Stephan Kunitz, "Explanations and Ideologies of Mortality Patterns," *Population and Development Review* 13, no. 3 (September 1987): 379–408.

25. René Dubos and Jean Dubos, *The White Plague: Tuberculosis, Man, and Society* (New Brunswick, NJ: Rutgers University Press, 1987), 122.

26. J. E. Gordon, "The Twentieth Century: Yesterday, Today, and Tomorrow (1920–)," in *The History of American Epidemiology*, ed. F. H. Top (St. Louis, MO: Mosby, 1952), quoted in Kunitz, "Explanations," 383.

27. George Davey Smith and Ezra Susser, "Zena Stein, Mervyn Susser and Epidemiology: Observation, Causation and Action," *International Journal of Epidemiology* 31, no. 1 (2002): 34–37.

28. Centers for Disease Control and Prevention (CDC), *Our Risk of Infectious Diseases Is Increasing Because of Climate Change*, https://www.cdc.gov/ncezid/pdf/climate-change-and-infectious-diseases-H.pdf, accessed June 3, 2022.

29. CDC, *Our Risk of Infectious Diseases Is Increasing*.

1. DISEASE AND EXPLOITATION DURING THE COLONIAL AND REVOLUTIONARY ERAS

1. William Bradford, *Of Plymouth Plantation*, ed. Harvey Wish (New York: Capricorn, 1962), 164–165. Written between 1630 and 1650 and rediscovered in 1855.

2. Figures cited in Alan C. Swedlund, "Contagion, Conflict, and Captivity in Interior New England: Native American and European Contacts in the Middle Connecticut River Valley of Massachusetts, 1616–2004," in *Beyond Germs: Native Depopulation in North America*, ed. Catherine M. Cameron, Paul Kelton, and Alan C. Swedlund (Tucson: University of Arizona Press, 2015), 152.

3. Bradford, *Of Plymouth Plantation*, 164–165.

4. Sporadic earlier contact with Europeans had occurred along the coast for decades before the Pilgrims arrived in 1620 and may have introduced some diseases to the population. Some scholars have argued that this earlier contact had devastated Indigenous communities even before the Pilgrims arrived.

5. Swedlund, "Contagion, Conflict, and Captivity," 154. Swedlund argues that the basic process of destruction of native peoples by colonists and early Americans of European extraction occurred through this process of social disruption. (Later white colonists used guns more extensively.)

6. Herbert Klein, *A Population History of the United States*, 2nd ed. (New York: Cambridge University Press, 2012), 21; see discussions of the changing demographic estimates and their ideological and methodological arguments in John Daniels, "The Indian Population of North America in 1492," *William and Mary Quarterly* 49, no. 2 (April 1992): 298–320. A recent critical evaluation of the arguments over the impact of disease as a culprit in the decimation of certain Native American populations is Catherine Cameron, Paul Kelton, and Alan Swedlund, eds., *Beyond Germs: Native Depopulation in North America* (Tucson: University of Arizona Press, 2015).

7. Michael Crawford, *The Origins of Native Americans: Evidence from Anthropological Genetics* (New York: Cambridge University Press, 1998), 39; see also Alexander Koch, Chris Brierly, Mark Maslin, and Simon Lewis, "Earth System Impacts of the European Arrival and Great Dying in the Americas After 1492," *Quaternary Science Reviews* 207 (March 2019): 13–36; and Klein, *A Population History*, 20. Klein reports that there were "half a million on the Atlantic Coast, about 450,000 in the Southwest and under 400,000 along the Pacific Coast."

8. William Cronon, *Changes in the Land: Indians, Colonists, and the Ecology of New England* (New York: Hill and Wang, 1983), 42.

9. Klein, *A Population History*. For some reviews and examples of the long historical, demographic, and methodological debates about population size and death rates, see William M. Denevan, "Estimating the Aboriginal Population of Latin America in 1492: Methodological Synthesis," in *Latin America: Search for Geographic Explanations* (Austin: University of Texas Press, 1976), 5: 125–132; Virginia P. Miller, "Aboriginal Micmac Population: A Review of the Evidence," *Ethnohistory* 23, no. 2 (Spring 1976): 117–127; Jeffrey R. Zorn, "Estimating the Population Size of Ancient Settlements: Methods, Problems, Solutions, and a Case Study," *Bulletin of the American Schools of Oriental Research* 295 (August 1994): 31–48; Ann F. Ramenofsky, Alicia K. Wilbur, and Anne C. Stone, "Native American Disease History: Past, Present and Future Directions," *World Archeology*, 35, no. 2 (October 2003): 241–257; and Russell Thornton, "Native American Demographic and Tribal Survival into the Twenty-First Century," *American Studies* 46, no. 3 (September 2005): 23–38.

10. Klein, *A Population History*, 509. A recent piece in the *Journal of American History* neatly traces the long historiographic discussion of the "virgin soil" hypotheses. See Tai S. Edwards and Paul Kelton, "Germs, Genocides, and America's Indigenous Peoples," *Journal of American History* 107, no. 1 (June 2020): 52–76.

11. David Jones, "Death, Uncertainty, and Rhetoric," in Cameron, Kelton, and Swedlund, *Beyond Germs*, 19–49, for an excellent review of the debates over disease and depopulation.

12. Cronon, *Changes in the Land*, 38. For detailed accounts of the varied cultures that populated the continent and their fate at the hands of colonizers, see Roxanne Dunbar-Ortiz, *An Indigenous Peoples' History of the United States* (Boston: Beacon, 2014); and Andres Resendez, *The Other Slavery: The Uncovered Story of Indian Enslavement in America* (New York: Houghton Mifflin Harcourt, 2016).

13. Cronon, *Changes in the Land*, 42.

14. Dunbar-Ortiz, *An Indigenous Peoples' History*, 45.

15. Klein, *A Population History*; Cronon, *Changes in the Land*, 40.

16. Cronon, *Changes in the Land*, 39.

17. Cronon, *Changes in the Land*, 42.

18. Paul Kelton, *Epidemics and Enslavement: Biological Catastrophe in the Native Southeast, 1492–1715* (Lincoln: University of Nebraska Press, 2007), 11–13. See also Debra L. Martin and Alan H. Goodman, "Health Conditions Before Columbus: Paleopathology of Native North Americans," *Western Journal of Medicine*, 176, no. 1 (January 2002): 65–68; Clark Larsen, "In the Wake of Columbus," Supplement, *American Journal of Physical Anthropology* 37, no. S19 (1994): 109–154; and Swedlund, "Contagion, Conflict, and Captivity," 146–173.

19. Viruses such as smallpox, measles, yellow fever, chickenpox, and influenza, along with some bacterial diseases such as anthrax, whooping cough, and typhus and some parasites like malaria and schistosomiasis, are generally thought to have plagued native populations in the colonial period. See Ramenofsky, Wilbur, and Stone, "Native American Disease History."

20. Jones, "Death, Uncertainty, and Rhetoric," 9.

21. George R. Milner, "Population Decline and Cultural Change in the American Midcontinent," in Cameron, Kelton, and Swedlund, *Beyond Germs*, 6.

22. Milner, "Population Decline and Cultural Change," 6.

23. Bradford, *Of Plymouth Plantation*, 164–165.

24. Patricia Scott Deetz and James Deetz, "Population of Plymouth Town, Colony and County, 1620–1690," 2000, http://www.histarch.illinois.edu/plymouth/townpop .html#:~:text=Population%201650&text=78%20estimates%20that%20in%20 1650,population%20of%20about%201500%20persons, accessed November 11, 2022.

25. Bradford, *Of Plymouth Plantation*, 164–165.

26. *Of Plymouth Plantation*, 164–165.

27. Swedlund, "Contagion, Conflict, and Captivity," 161.

28. Terry L. Anderson and Robert Paul Thomas, "White Population, Labor Force and Extensive Growth of the New England Economy in the Seventeenth Century," *Journal of Economic History* 33, no. 3 (September 1973): 634–667.

29. Swedlund, "Contagion, Conflict, and Captivity," 154.

30. Swedlund, "Contagion, Conflict, and Captivity," 157.

31. Swedlund, "Contagion, Conflict, and Captivity," 157.

32. Society of Colonial Wars in the State of Connecticut, "1675—King Philip's War," colonialwarsct.org/1675.htm.

33. Swedlund, "Contagion, Conflict, and Captivity," 150.

34. Swedlund, "Contagion, Conflict, and Captivity," 161.

35. Swedlund, "Contagion, Conflict, and Captivity," 159.

36. Rueben G. Thwaites, *The Jesuit Relations and Allied Documents* (Cleveland, OH: Burrrows Brothers, 1899), 35: 89, quoted in Milner, "Population Decline and Cultural Change," 65.

37. Paul Kelton, "Slave Raids and Smallpox, 1659–1700," in *Epidemics and Enslavement*, 101–159.

38. Kelton, *Epidemics and Enslavement*, 158, 102–103.

39. Jones, "Death, Uncertainty, and Rhetoric," 16.

40. Daniel K. Richter, "War and Culture: The Iroquois Experience," *William and Mary Quarterly* 40, no. 4 (October 1983): 538; David Jones, "Virgin Soils Revisited," *William and Mary Quarterly* 60, no. 4 (October 2003): 703–742; Dunbar-Ortiz, *An Indigenous Peoples' History*, 40; Kelly Evonne Hopkins, "A New Landscape: Changing Iroquois Settlement Patterns, Subsistence Strategies, and Environmental Use, 1630–1783" (PhD diss., University of California, Davis, 2010), 20–21. Jones states, "Other factors of the environment, defined broadly, also have profound effects on immunity. A population's physical, social, economic, and political environments all interact to create patterns of vulnerability, regardless of its genetic substrate" (Jones, "Virgin Soil Revisited," 735). For similar arguments, see Giovanni Berlinguer, "The Interchange of Disease and Health Between the Old and New Worlds," *International Journal of Health Services* 23, no. 4 (1993): 706; Jeffrey Ostler, *Surviving Genocide: Native Nations and the United States from the American Revolution to Bleeding Kansas* (New Haven, CT: Yale University Press, 2009); and David E. Stannard, *American Holocaust: The Conquest of the New World* (New York: Oxford University Press, 1993). Others have made similar arguments regarding the ill health of Native Americans in the nineteenth century. See Jennifer Seltz, "Complicating Colonial Narratives: Medical Encounters Around the Salish Sea, 1853–1878,"

in *Precarious Prescriptions: Contested Histories of Race and Health in North America*, ed. Laurie B. Green, John McKiernan-Gonzalez, and Martin Summers (Minneapolis: University of Minnesota Press, 2014), 23–42.

41. Alan Taylor, *American Colonies* (New York: Penguin, 2001), 197.

42. Cameron, Kelton, and Swedlund, *Beyond Germs*, 3.

43. Swedlund, "Contagion, Conflict, and Captivity," 154.

44. See Claudio Saunt, *Unworthy Republic: The Dispossession of Native Americans and the Road to Indian Territory* (New York: Norton, 2020), for a full accounting of resistance and dispossession.

45. Michael Witgen, *An Infinity of Nations: How the Native New World Shaped Early North America* (Philadelphia: University of Pennsylvania Press, 2012); Daniel Richter, *Facing East from Indian Country: A Native History of Early America* (Cambridge, MA: Harvard University Press, 2003).

46. Philip Greven, *Four Generations: Population, Land, and Family in Colonial Andover, Massachusetts* (Ithaca, NY: Cornell University Press, 1970), 124, 26.

47. Klein, *A Population History*, 47.

48. Greven, *Four Generations*, 124.

49. Ben Mutschler, *The Province of Affliction: Illness and the Making of Early New England* (Chicago: University of Chicago Press, 2020).

50. Daniel Defoe, *A Journal of the Plague Year . . . in 1665* (London: 1722), available at Project Gutenberg EBook: https://www.gutenberg.org/files/376/376-h/376-h.htm, accessed December 12, 2020.

51. "Anon. to Rev. Boyd," quoted in James Henretta, *Evolution of American Society, 1700–1815* (New York: D. C. Heath, 1973), 7.

52. Klein, *A Population History*, 49. By the mid-eighteenth century, colonial whites were 7 centimeters taller than their English counterparts.

53. K. L. Sokoloff, "The Heights of Americans in Three Centuries: Some Economic and Demographic Implications," in *The Biological Standard of Living on Three Continents*, ed. J. Komlos (Boulder, CO: Westview, 1995), 133–150; K. L. Sokoloff and G. C. Villaflor, "The Early Achievement of Modern Stature in America," *Social Science History* 6, no. 4 (1982): 453–481; R. H. Steckel, "The Health and Mortality of Women and Children, 1850–1860," *Journal of Economic History* 48, no. 2 (1988): 333–345.

54. Taylor, *American Colonies*, 170–172; Arlington Historical Society, "Daniel Reed (1666–1741) and Colonial New England Farms," https://arlingtonhistorical.org/daniel-reed-1666-1741-and-colonial-new-england-farms/, accessed November 14, 2022.

55. I. H. comment on John Smith, "A True Relation, To the Courteous Reader, 1608," in *Narratives of Early Virginia, 1606–1625*, ed. Lyon Gardiner Tyler (New York: Scribner's, 1907), 32.

56. Smith, "A True Relation," 33. Similar accounts of first encounters reinforce this narrative, in the West Indies and elsewhere. George Percy in 1607 recounted his landing in Dominico, West Indies: "a very faire Iland, the Trees full of sweet fruit ns good smels." While the native people were at first wary, they soon "came to our ships with their Canoas, bringing us many kindes of sundry fruites, as Pines, Potatoes, Plantons, Tobacco, and other fruits, and Roane Cloth abundance." Percy recounted a similar unfolding elsewhere. Upon reaching the Chesapeake, initial hesitancy quickly became feasts in welcoming native communities. "Observations by Master George Percy, 1607," in *Narratives of Early Virginia*, 6.

57. John Pory to Sir Dudley Carleton, "Letter of John Pory, 1619," in *Narratives of Early Virginia*, 283.

58. Edmund Morgan, *American Slavery, American Freedom* (New York: Norton, 1975), 158.

59. Edmund Morgan, "The Labor Problem in Jamestown, 1607–18," *American Historical Review* 76, no. 3 (June 1971): 595.

60. Wyndham B. Blanton, "Epidemics, Real and Imaginary, and Other Factors Influencing Seventeenth Century Virginia's Population," *Bulletin of the History of Medicine* 31, no. 5 (September/October 1957): 454–462.

61. Karen Ordahl Kupperman, "Apathy and Death in Early Jamestown," *Journal of American History* 66, no. 1 (June 1979): 24.

62. Morgan, *American Slavery, American Freedom*, 159.

63. Daniel Blake Smith, "Mortality and Family in the Colonial Chesapeake," *Journal of Interdisciplinary History* 8, no. 3 (Winter 1978): 415.

64. Klein, *A Population History*, 38–39.

65. Smith, "Mortality and Family," 413–414.

66. Morgan, *American Slavery, American Freedom*, 159.

67. Morgan, *American Slavery, American Freedom*, 158-179.

68. Kupperman, "Apathy and Death," 25.

69. Morgan, "The Labor Problem in Jamestown," 595.

70. I. H. comment on Smith, "A True Relation," 32.

71. Nicole Hannah-Jones, *The 1619 Project: A New Origin Story* (New York: One World, 2021).

72. Anna Suranyi, *Indentured Servitude: Unfree Labour and Citizenship in the British Colonies* (Montreal: McGill-Queen's University Press, 2021).

73. David W. Galenson, *White Servitude in Colonial America* (New York: Cambridge University Press, 1981); David W. Galenson, "The Rise and Fall of Indentured Servitude in the Americas: An Economic Analysis," *Journal of Economic History* 44, no. 1 (March 1984): 1–26; Suranyi, *Indentured Servitude*, 17. Suranyi estimates that "more than half of all indentured servants went to the

Chesapeake colonies of Virginia and Maryland, while 6 per cent travelled to Pennsylvania, 2 per cent to other mainland colonies, and about 35 per cent to the colonies in the Caribbean. . . . During the same period, over 1 million enslaved Africans were brought across the ocean [between 1607 and 1776]."

74. Taylor, *American Colonies*, 142-143; Suranyi, *Indentured Servitude*, 17.

75. Aaron O'Neill, "Estimated Annual Number of Slaves Who Embarked on Ships in Africa and Disembarked in Mainland North America from 1628 to 1860," Statista, https://www.statista.com/statistics/1196042/slaves-brought -africa-to-us-1628-1860/, accessed March 23, 2022. "Trans-Atlantic Slave Trade—Database," Slave Voyages, https://www.slavevoyages.org/voyage/database, accessed March 23, 2022.

76. Jennifer Morgan, *Laboring Women: Reproduction and Gender in New World Slavery* (Philadelphia: University of Pennsylvania Press, 2004), 3; See also David Eltis, *The Rise of African Slavery in the Americas* (Cambridge: Cambridge University Press, 2000), 96–97. With the growing investment in southern cotton production, prices for slaves rose substantially. See Herbert Klein, *The Atlantic Slave Trade*, 2nd ed. (Cambridge: Cambridge University Press, 2012), 46.

77. "The African Slave Trade," *De Bow's Review and Industrial Resources, Statistics, Etc., 1855*, n.s. 18, no. 1 (January 1855): 16.

78. Jay Coughtry, *The Notorious Triangle: Rhode Island and the African Slave Trade, 1700–1807* (Philadelphia: Temple University Press, 1981), 6. Coughtry explains the development of eighteenth-century Rhode Island slave traders in some detail, exploring the ecology of Rhode Island and the difficulties of agricultural production throughout the eighteenth century. As a result of these conditions, Rhode Island turned to the ocean, shipping, and slave trading.

79. Klein, *A Population History*, 38; "Trans-Atlantic Slave Trade—Database."

80. Coughtry, *The Notorious Triangle*, 7.

81. Coughtry, *The Notorious Triangle*, 53–54.

82. Coughtry, *The Notorious Triangle*, 148.

83. Coughtry, *The Notorious Triangle*.

84. Richard B. Sheridan, "The Guinea Surgeons on the Middle Passage: The Provision of Medical Services in the British Slave Trade," *International Journal of African Historical Studies* 14, no. 4 (1981): 602; see also Coughtry, *The Notorious Triangle*.

85. Coughtry, *The Notorious Triangle*.

86. Coughtry, *The Notorious Triangle*, 145–146.

87. Coughtry, *The Notorious Triangle*, 146.

88. Dr. Collins, *Practical Rules for the Management and Medical Treatment of Negro Slaves in the Sugar Colonies* (London: J. Barfield, 1803), 52–53.

89. *The Interesting Narrative of the Life of Olaudah Equiano, or Gustave Vassa, the African* (London: 1789), 71–75. See Tom Zoellner, *Island on Fire: The Revolt That Ended Slavery in the British Empire* (Cambridge, MA: Harvard University Press, 2020), for a systematic review of British cruelty in Jamaica.

90. Collins, *Practical Rules*, 55.

91. Collins, *Practical Rules*, 55.

92. Peter Wood, *Black Majority: Negroes in Colonial South Carolina from 1670 Through the Stono Rebellion* (New York: Norton, 1974), 64–65.

93. Edward Baptist, *The Half Has Never Been Told: Slavery and the Making of American Capitalism* (New York: Basic Books, 2014), 310. See also Tristan Stubbs, *Masters of Violence: The Plantation Overseers of Eighteenth-Century Virginia, South Carolina, and Georgia* (Columbia: University of South Carolina Press, 2018), 9–11.

94. Wood, *Black Majority*, 150.

95. Stubbs, *Masters of Violence*.

96. Wood, *Black Majority*, 64, 76.

97. Quoted in Wood, *Black Majority*, 79.

98. Slaves were the engine of the plantation economy, and their owners carefully read and used this popular handbook by "Dr. Collins"; see Collins, *Practical Rules*. See also Richard D. deShazo, Robert Smith, and Leigh Baldwin Skipworth, "Black Physicians and the Struggle for Civil Rights: Lessons from the Mississippi Experience: Part 1: The Forces for and Against Change," *American Journal of Medicine* 127, no. 10 (October 2014): 920–925.

99. Collins, *Practical Rules*, 51–52.

100. Collins, *Practical Rules*, 58.

101. Collins, *Practical Rules*, 60.

102. Collins, *Practical Rules*, 60.

103. Collins, *Practical Rules*, 87.

104. Collins, *Practical Rules*, 87.

105. Collins, *Practical Rules*, 87–88.

106. Collins, *Practical Rules*, 89.

107. Collins, *Practical Rules*, 89–90.

108. Rana A. Hogarth, *Medicalizing Blackness: Making Racial Difference in the Atlantic World, 1780–1840* (Chapel Hill: University of North Carolina Press, 2017). See also Zoellner, *Island on Fire*, for vivid descriptions of the depravity of British sugar planters in the years before the end of slavery and the social chaos it promoted.

109. Hogarth, *Medicalizing Blackness*. See also Rana Hogarth, "Of Black Skin and Biopower: Lessons from the Eighteenth Century," *American Quarterly* 71, no. 3 (September 2019): 837–847; Rana Hogarth, "The Myth of Innate Racial Differences Between White and Black People's Bodies: Lessons from the 1793 Yellow

Fever Epidemic in Philadelphia, Pennsylvania," *American Journal of Public Health* 109, no. 10 (October 2019): 1339–1341; Rana Hogarth, "A Contemporary Black Perspective on the 1793 Yellow Fever Epidemic in Philadelphia," *American Journal of Public Health* 109, no. 10 (October 2019): 1337–1338; "A Narrative of the Proceedings of the Black People During the Late Awful Calamity in Philadelphia in the Year 1793," *American Journal of Public Health* 109, no. 10 (October 2019): 1336–1337; Martin S. Pernick, "Politics, Parties, and Pestilence: Epidemic Yellow Fever in Philadelphia and the Rise of the First Party System," *William and Mary Quarterly*, 29 (October 1972), 559-586.

110. Benjamin Franklin, "Observations Concerning the Increase of Mankind," 1751, National Archives, Founders Online, https://founders.archives.gov/documents /Franklin/01-04-02-0080.

111. Franklin, "Observations Concerning the Increase of Mankind."

112. Franklin, "Observations Concerning the Increase of Mankind." Franklin incorporated racist and nativist arguments about the dangers of the dilution of the English "stock" of America both by the migration of other Europeans of "swarthy Complexions" and by the slave trade and its movement of Africans to the American South. He worried that "the number of purely white People in the World is proportionately very small. All Africa is black or tawny. Asia chiefly tawny. America (exclusive of the new Comers) wholly so. And in Europe, the Spaniards, Italians, French, Russians and Swedes, are generally of what we call a swarthy Complexion; as are the Germans also, the Saxons only excepted, who with the English, make the principal Body of White People on the Face of the Earth. I could wish their Numbers were increased. And while we are, as I may call it, *Scouring our Planet*, by clearing America of Woods, and so making this Side of our Globe reflect a brighter Light to the Eyes of Inhabitants in Mars or Venus, why should we in the Sight of Superior Beings, darken its People? why increase the Sons of Africa, by Planting them in America, where we have so fair an Opportunity, by excluding all Blacks and Tawneys, of increasing the lovely White and Red? But perhaps I am partial to the Complexion of my Country, for such Kind of Partiality is natural to Mankind."

113. Henretta, *Evolution of American Society*, 15.

114. Sophia died the year Boylston's letter was written.

115. Zabdiel Boylston, *An Historical Account of the Small-Pox Inoculated in New-England . . . Princess of Wales* (London: S. Chandler, 1726; reprinted Boston: S. Gerrish, 1730), iv, 38, https://curiosity.lib.harvard.edu/contagion/catalog /36-990046038020203941, accessed March 22, 2024.

116. Boylston, *An Historical Account*, iv.

117. Boylston, *An Historical Account*, 38–40. "Bark" may refer to a herbal treatment or the relative innocuousness of the symptoms.

118. Laurel Thatcher Ulrich, *A Midwife's Tale; The Life of Martha Ballard, Based on Her Diary, 1785–1812* (New York: Vintage, 1990), 45, 172–173. She points out that "in some eighteenth-century London and Dublin hospitals maternal mortality ranged from 30 to 200 (!) per thousand births, compared with 5 per 1000 for Martha [Ballard]."

119. "From Thomas Jefferson to David Humphreys, 11 September 1793," National Archives, Founders Online, https://founders.archives.gov/documents/Jefferson /01-27-02-0088, accessed November 14, 2022. See also Martin Pernick, "Politics, Parties, and Pestilence: Epidemic Yellow Fever in Philadelphia and the Rise of the First Party System," *William and Mary Quarterly* 29, no. 4 (October 1972): 559–586.

120. Noah Webster, *A Brief History of Epidemic and Pestilential Diseases* (Hartford: Hudson and Godwin, 1799), 1: 291, Available at: https://collections.nlm .nih.gov/bookviewer?PID=nlm:nlmuid-2576058RX2-mvpart, Accessed: March 22, 2024.

121. Webster, *A Brief History*, 294–295.

122. Webster, *A Brief History*, 311–314.

123. George Rosen, "Noah Webster—Historical Epidemiologist," *Journal of the History of Medicine and Allied Sciences* 20, no. 2 (April 1965): 110.

124. Sven Beckert, *Empire of Cotton: A Global History* (New York: Alfred Knopf, 2014).

2. LIFE AND DEATH IN ANTEBELLUM AMERICA

1. Joshua Freeman, *Behemoth: A History of the Factory and the Making of the Modern World* (New York: Norton, 2018), xii. Many historians and contemporary observers have documented the extraordinary history of the Industrial Revolution. See E. P. Thomson, *The Making of the English Working Class* (New York: Vintage, 1966); Eric Hobsbawm, *Industry and Empire: From 1750 to the Present Day* (London: Penguin, 1999); Eric Hobsbawm, *The Age of Revolution, 1789–1848* (New York: New American Library, 1980); and Eric Hobsbawm, *Primitive Rebels: Studies in Archaic Forms of Social Movement in the 19th and 20th Centuries* (Manchester, UK: Manchester University Press, 1971), among many others.

2. Gergely Baics, *Feeding Gotham: The Political Economy and Geography of Food in New York, 1790–1860* (Princeton, NJ: Princeton University Press, 2016). Baics argues that the early market system was highly regulated, at least in the urban Northeast, and that government regulation of the distribution system of local marketplaces licensed by the city was dismantled as populations rose and markets developed in widely dispersed areas of the growing nineteenth -century city.

3. Dora Costa, "Height, Wealth, and Disease Among the Native-Born in the Rural, Antebellum North," *Social Science History* 17, no. 3 (Autumn 1993): 358.

4. In his review of the available statistical materials in nineteenth-century America, David Hacker argues: "All three genealogy-based studies suggest a significant increase in mortality in the antebellum era, especially in the three decades between 1830 and 1860." See J. David Hacker, "Decennial Life Tables for the White Population of the United States, 1790–1900," *Historical Methods* 43, no. 2 (April 2010): 8, https://www.ncbi.nlm.nih.gov/pmc/articles/PMC2885717/pdf/nihms205286.pdf, accessed February 18, 2021. This general point about the declining longevity of white Americans is reiterated by Dora Costa, "Health and the Economy in the United States, from 1750 to the Present," *Journal of Economic Literature* 53, no. 3 (September 2015): 503: "A white American ten-year old boy born in the early 1880s could expect to live to age 48 and to grow to 169 cm, a short, stunted life compared to his counterparts born at the time of the American Revolution or after the 1920s."

5. Yellow fever initially and primarily affected the mosquito-infested marshlands of rice cultivation in the South but soon traveled along the waterways and eastern seaboard as the commercial economy expanded.

6. Herbert Klein, *A Population History of the United States*, 2nd ed. (New York: Cambridge University Press, 2012), 48–50.

7. Tom Dublin, "Rural Putting-Out Work in Early Nineteenth-Century New England: Women and the Transition to Capitalism in the Countryside," *New England Quarterly* 64, no. 4 (December 1991): 531–573.

8. W. Cudworth, *Condition of the Industrial Classes of Bradford & District* (Bradford, 1887), as quoted in E. P. Thompson, *The Making of the English Working Class* (New York: Vintage, 1966), 283–284.

9. Andreas Malm, *Fossil Capital: The Rise of Steam Power and the Roots of Global Warming* (London: Verso, 2016), 244–245.

10. Malm, *Fossil Capital*, 242, 247–248.

11. Frederick Engels, *The Condition of the Working Class in England*, trans. W. O. Henderson and W. H. Chaloner (Stanford: Stanford University Press, 1968), 110; originally published 1844.

12. Engels, *The Condition*, 108–109.

13. See the literature on the perception of the American industrial system as an alternative to the more exploitative and harsher British system: Leo Marx, *The Machine in the Garden: Technology and the Pastoral Ideal in America* (New York: Oxford University Press, 1965); Jacob E. Cooke, "Tench Coxe, Alexander Hamilton, and the Encouragement of American Manufactures," *William and Mary Quarterly* 32, no. 3 (July 1975): 369–392.

14. Charles Dickens, *American Notes for General Circulation* (London: Chapman and Hall, 1913), https://www.gutenberg.org/files/675/675-h/675-h.htm#footnote1, accessed August 22, 2020.

15. Dickens, *American Notes*.

16. Dicken, *American Notes*.

17. Dickens, *American Notes*.

18. Dickens, *American Notes*.

19. Dickens, *American Notes*.

20. David Crockett, *An Account of Col. Crockett's Tour to the North and Down East, in the Year of Our Lord 1834* (Philadelphia: Carey and Hart, 1835), 80, 96, https://www.loc.gov/resource/gdcmassbookdig.accountofcolcrocoocrock /?st=gallery&c=80 Accessed: March 22, 2024.

21. Crockett, *An Account*.

22. Anthony Trollope, "Cambridge and Lowell," in *North America*, vol. 1 (London: Chapman and Hall, 1862), 383, republished online at https://www .gutenberg.org/files/1865/1865-h/1865-h.htm.

23. Trollope, "Cambridge and Lowell," 383. Alexis de Tocqueville visited Manchester, a much larger city that presented him with a vivid contrast: "Thirty or forty factories rise on the tops of the hills. . . . Their six stories tower. . . . The wretched dwellings of the poor are scattered haphazard around them. Round them stretches land uncultivated. . . . The soil has been taken away, scratched and torn up in a thousand places. . . . Heaps of dung, rubble from buildings, putrid, stagnant pools are found here and there among the houses and over the bumpy, pitted surfaces of the public places. . . . [W]ho could describe the interiors of these quarters set apart, home of vice and poverty, which surround the huge palaces of industry and clasp them in their hideous folds. . . . Narrow, twisting roads lead down to it . . . lined with one-story houses whose ill-fitting planks and broken windows show them up, even from a distance, as the last refuge a man might find between poverty and death. . . . Below some of their miserable dwellings is a row of cellars to which a sunken corridor leads. Twelve to fifteen human beings are crowded pell-mell into each of these damp, repulsive holes. The fetid, muddy waters, stained with a thousand colours by the factories they pass, . . . wander slowly round this refuge of poverty. . . . A sort of black smoke covers the city. The sun seen through it is a disc without rays. Under this half daylight 300,000 human beings are ceaselessly at work. . . . From this foul drain the greatest stream of human industry flows out to fertilize the whole world. From this filthy sewer pure gold flows. Here humanity attains its most complete development and its most brutish; here civilisation works its miracles, and civilised man is turned back almost into a savage." See Alexis de

Tocqueville, *Journeys to England and Ireland* (New Haven, CT: Yale University Press, 1958), 104–107, http://www.pitt.edu/~syd/toq.html, accessed July 20, 2020.

24. Alexis de Tocqueville, "That Aristocracy May Be Engendered by Manufactures," chapter 20 in *Democracy in America*, book 2, section 2, republished online at https://www.gutenberg.org/files/816/816-h/816-h.htm#link2HCH0040, accessed August 22, 2020. See also Freeman, *Behemoth*, 59.

25. Freeman, *Behemoth*.

26. Quoted by David A. Zonderman, *Aspirations and Anxieties: New England Workers and the Mechanized Factory System, 1815–1850* (New York: Oxford University Press, 1992), 76.

27. Zonderman, *Aspirations and Anxieties*, 82.

28. Freeman, *Behemoth*.

29. United States Census Bureau, *Bicentennial Edition: Historical Statistics of the United States, Colonial Times to 1970* (Washington, DC: Government Printing Office, 1975), chapter A: Population, table entitled "Annual Population Estimates for the United States: 1790 to 1970," 8, https://www.census.gov/library/publications/1975/compendia/hist_stats_colonial-1970.html, accessed November 17, 2022.

30. Klein, *A Population History*, 102; table 4.2.

31. See Ben Mutschler, *The Province of Affliction: Illness and the Making of Early New England* (Chicago: University of Chicago Press, 2020).

32. Catharine E. Beecher, *Letters to the People on Health and Happiness* (New York: Harper, 1855), 7, https://collections.nlm.nih.gov/catalog/nlm:nlmuid-61360570R-bk; see also Martha Verbrugge, "The Social Meaning of Personal Health: The Ladies' Physiological Institute of Boston and Vicinity in the 1850s," in *Health Care in America: Essays in Social History*, ed. Susan Reverby and David Rosner (Philadelphia: Temple University Press, 1979), 45–66.

33. Beecher, *Letters to the People*, 8–9.

34. Beecher, *Letters to the People*, 9.

35. Beecher, *Letters to the People*, 9.

36. Beecher, *Letters to the People*, 10.

37. Beecher, *Letters to the People*, 111.

38. Beecher, *Letters to the People*, 10.

39. Beecher, *Letters to the People*, 89, 98.

40. Beecher, *Letters to the People*, 7.

41. Beecher, *Letters to the People*. For statistics, see United States Census Bureau, p.93; *Bicentennial Edition: Historical Statistics*, chapter C: Migration, table entitled "Immigrants, by Country: 1820 to 1970," 105–109; see also United States Census Bureau, "Fast Facts," https://www.census.gov/history/www/through_the_decades/fast_facts/.

42. Beecher, *Letters to the People*, 93.

43. Beecher, *Letters to the People*, 93.

44. George R. Grant, "The Meteorology, Sanitary Condition, Prevailing Disease, and Mortuary Statistics of Memphis, Tennessee, in 1852," *American Journal of the Medical Sciences* 51 (July 1853): 108, Available at: https://www.google .com/books/edition/The_American_Journal_of_the_Medical_Scie /KgQHAAAAcAAJ?hl=en&gbpv=1&dq=George+Grant+The+%22Meteorology, %22+Sanitary+Condition,+Prevailing+Disease,+and+Mortuary+Statistics +of+Memphis&pg=PA94&printsec=frontcover, Accessed: March 22, 2024.

45. Costa, "Height, Wealth, and Disease among the Native Born," Social Science History 17 (Autumn, 1993), 358.

46. Hacker, "Decennial Life Tables," 45–79.

47. Richard Harrison Shryock, "The Health of the American People: An Historical Survey," *Proceedings of the American Philosophical Society* 90, no. 4 (September 1946): 252.

48. Scott Carson, "Height of Female Americans in the Nineteenth Century and the Antebellum Puzzle," *Economics and Human Biology* 9, no. 2 (March 2011): 157–164.

49. Costa, "Health and the Economy," 516–517; Costa, "Height, Wealth, and Disease," 376. See also Farley Grubb, "Withering Heights: Did Indentured Servants Shrink from an Encounter with Malthus? A Comment on Komlos," *Economic History Review*, n.s., 52, no. 4 (1999): 714–729, http://www.jstor.org /stable/2599325; Michael R. Haines, "Growing Incomes, Shrinking People— Can Economic Development Be Hazardous to Your Health? Historical Evidence for the United States, England, and the Netherlands in the Nineteenth Century," *Social Science History* 28, no. 2 (2004): 249–270, http://www.jstor .org/stable/40267842; and Michael R. Haines, Lee A. Craig, and Thomas Weiss, "The Short and the Dead: Nutrition, Mortality, and the 'Antebellum Puzzle' in the United States," *Journal of Economic History* 63, no. 2 (2003): 382–413, http:// www.jstor.org/stable/3132441.

50. Costa, "Height, Wealth, and Disease," 376. See also Grubb, "Withering Heights"; Haines, "Growing Incomes, Shrinking People"; Haines, Craig, and Weiss, "The Short and the Dead"; and Carson, "Height of Female Americans."

51. Howard Bodenhorn, "A Troublesome Caste: Height and Nutrition of Antebellum Virginia's Rural Free Blacks," *Journal of Economic History* 59, no. 4 (1999): 993, 994: Bodenhorn argues that in Maryland and Virginia, at least, free Blacks were "better fed, better housed, better clothed, and better shod than Virginia's slaves [and therefore] grew somewhat taller than slave coevals, and fell only slightly short of the white[s]." He points out that "white Virginians did their best to keep blacks from disturbing a two-tiered southern social

order by restricting their occupational choices, by denying them educations, by denying them ownership of certain types of property and by limiting their economic mobility in numerous ways. Yet Virginia's free blacks found work, developed skills, acquired property, and provided for themselves and their families. By contemporary standards, most fed, clothed, and housed themselves adequately. Some earned and saved enough to purchase loved ones from bondage. A fortunate few even acquired a semblance of middle class respectability."

52. *War capitalism* is the term Sven Beckert uses to describe the growing power of European states in imposing their will on other nations. He argues that it is the more accurate term to describe Europe's domination of trade throughout Asia and Africa, as well as the Americas, in the period generally identified by other historians as the age of "mercantilism." See Sven Beckert, *Empire of Cotton: A Global History* (New York: Vintage, 2015).

53. Beckert, *Empire of Cotton*, chap. 1.

54. Beckert, *Empire of Cotton*, chap. 1.

55. Beckert, *Empire of Cotton*, chap. 1, See also: Sven Beckert, "Emancipation and Empire: Reconstructing the Worldwide Web of Cotton Production in the Age of the American Civil War," *American Historical Review* 109, no. 5 (December 2004): 1405-1438.

56. Beckert, "Emancipation and Empire," 1408–1409.

57. "Cotton Financing," *Federal Reserve Bulletin* (Washington, DC: Government Printing Office, May 1923), 567, chrome-extension://efaidnbmnnnibpcajpcglcle findmkaj/https://fraser.stlouisfed.org/files/docs/publications/FRB/1920s /frb_051923.pdf, accessed July 18, 2023.

58. Beckert, *Empire of Cotton*, 201.

59. For a riveting description of the expropriation of native lands and the forced movement of slaves from the eastern shore to the southern and western cotton fields, see Claudio Saunt, *Unworthy Republic: The Dispossession of Native Americans and the Road to Indian Territory* (New York: Norton, 2020); and for the forced movement of African Americans to the cotton South, see Edward Baptist, *The Half Has Never Been Told: Slavery and the Making of American Capitalism* (New York: Basic Books, 2014).

60. Baptist, *The Half Has Never Been Told*; Richard H. Steckel, "The African American Population of the United States, 1790–1920," in *A Population History of North America*, ed. Michael R. Haines and Richard H. Steckel (Cambridge: Cambridge University Press, 2000), 440; Jenny Bourne, "Slavery in the United States," Economic History Association, https://eh.net/encyclopedia /slavery-in-the-united-states/.

61. "Liverpool's Abercromby Square and the Confederacy During the U.S. Civil War," LDHI, https://ldhi.library.cofc.edu/exhibits/show/liverpools-abercromby -square/britain-and-us-civil-war/impact-cotton-trade, accessed April 18, 2022.

62. Gavin Wright, *Slavery and American Economic Development* (Baton Rouge: Louisiana State University Press, 2006), 57.

63. Wright, *Slavery and American Economic Development*, 60; see also Roger L. Ransom, "Economics of the Civil War," Economic History Association, https:// eh.net/encyclopedia/the-economics-of-the-civil-war/; Samuel Williamson and Louis Cain, "Measuring Slavery in 2020 Dollars," MeasuringWorth.com, https:// www.measuringworth.com/slavery.php, accessed April 2022; Eric Foner, personal communication, April 15, 2021.

64. Blight's estimate does not include the farms, the land, and other aspects of the economy.

65. Rana A. Hogarth, *Medicalizing Blackness: Making Racial Difference in the Atlantic World, 1780–1840* (Chapel Hill: University of North Carolina Press, 2017). See also Rana Hogarth, "Of Black Skin and Biopower: Lessons from the Eighteenth Century," *American Quarterly* 71, no. 3 (September 2019): 837–847; Rana Hogarth, "The Myth of Innate Racial Differences Between White and Black People's Bodies: Lessons from the 1793 Yellow Fever Epidemic in Philadelphia, Pennsylvania," *American Journal of Public Health* 109, no. 10 (October 2019): 1339–1341; Rana Hogarth, "A Contemporary Black Perspective on the 1793 Yellow Fever Epidemic in Philadelphia," *American Journal of Public Health* 109, no. 10 (October 2019): 1337–1338; and Absalom Jones and Richard Allen, "A Narrative of the Proceedings of the Black People During the Late Awful Calamity in Philadelphia in the Year 1793," *American Journal of Public Health* 109, no. 10 (October 2019): 1336–1337.

66. Khalil Gibran Muhammad, "The Sugar That Saturates the American Diet Has a Barbaric History as the 'White Gold' That Fueled Slavery," *New York Times Magazine*, August 14, 2019, https://www.nytimes.com/interactive/2019/08/14 /magazine/sugar-slave-trade-slavery.html.

67. Michael Tadman, "The Demographic Cost of Sugar: Debates on Slave Societies and Natural Increase in the Americas," *American Historical Review* 105, no. 5 (December 2000): 1547, 1554. The historian Khalil Muhammad quotes Solomon Northrup's memoir, *Twelve Years a Slave* (Chapel Hill: University of North Carolina Press, 2011), 118; originally published 1841, about the intense work that occurred during the sugar harvest season: "On cane plantations in sugar time, there is no distinction as to the days of the week." See Muhammad, "The Sugar That Saturates."

68. See Saunt, *Unworthy Republic*, 124–128, 137, 251–254, 275–281. Quote at 38.

69. See Saunt, *Unworthy Republic*, 280: Saunt notes that if you include "deaths in the holding camps as well as miscarriages, infertility, and other causes of reduced birth rate," the toll could be as large as 3,500. .

70. See Saunt, *Unworthy Republic*, 312. During this period a few native peoples remained and were partially integrated into the cotton economy, with some owning African Americans. It was not only cotton that led white settlers to force native communities off their traditional lands. In Illinois, for example, the Sauk, Meskwaki, and Winnebago nations had established thriving communities built on corn, beans, and squash as well as on lead mining. In the eighteenth century, lead was used for local religious ceremonies and as a pigment for paint. With the expansion of white settlements, the demand for lead increased as well, for use in lead shot and other munitions, transforming the value of lead and attracting a swarm of prospectors eager to take part in the profits. By the 1820s, whites were forcing the native peoples out of their Illinois homes, across the Mississippi River into what is now Iowa. In 1832, in what is now called the Black Hawk War, the local Sauks in Iowa crossed the Mississippi to regain territory in Illinois. They were met by U.S. troops and militia organized by the federal government, and a broader war resulted that led to massive deaths and starvation for the native population. Saunt quotes a local paper that "urged the governor to 'carry on a war of extermination until there shall be no Indian (with his scalp on) left in the northern part of Illinois.'" Indeed, over the next couple of decades, Indians on the eastern banks of the Mississippi were forced to Oklahoma, Kansas, and other western territories. See Saunt, *Unworthy Republic*, 143–145.

71. See U.S. Constitution, Article 1, Section 2, Clause 3: "Representatives and direct Taxes shall be apportioned among the several States which may be included within this Union, according to their respective Numbers, which shall be determined by adding to the whole Number of free Persons, including those bound to Service for a Term of Years, and excluding Indians not taxed, three fifths of all other Persons."

72. U.S. Constitution, Article IV, Section 2, Clause 3: "No Person held to Service or Labour in one State, under the Laws thereof, escaping into another, shall, in Consequence of any Law or Regulation therein, be discharged from such Service or Labour, but shall be delivered up on Claim of the Party to whom such Service or Labour may be due."

73. John Clegg, "Capitalism and Slavery," *Critical Historical Studies* 2, no. 2 (September 2015): 281. Clegg notes that this is not a radically new observation but was remarked upon by Karl Marx, who "famously argued that 'without slavery you have no cotton; without cotton you have no modern industry'" (Clegg, "Capitalism and Slavery," 283).

74. James Oakes, "Capitalism and Slavery and the Civil War" (review essay), *International Labor and Working-Class History* 89 (Spring 2016): 198.

75. Steckel, "The African American Population," 453–461.

76. D. B. Harris, *A Statistical Inquiry into the Condition of the People of Colour of the City and Districts of Philadelphia* (Philadelphia, 1849), quoted in Christian Warren, "Northern Chills, Southern Fevers: Race-Specific Mortality in American Cities, 1730–1900," *Journal of Southern History* 63, no. 1 (February 1997): 39.

77. Steckel, "The African American Population," 453–461.

78. Various sources estimate the total number of millionaires in the United States as between nineteen and fifty; see Oakes, "Capitalism and Slavery and the Civil War," 200.

79. Oakes, "Capitalism and Slavery and the Civil War," 200.

80. Walter Johnson, *River of Dark Dreams: Slavery and Empire in the Cotton Kingdom* (Cambridge, MA: Harvard University Press, 2013), 186, 178.

81. "The American Cotton Planter," editorial in *The American Cotton Planter* 1 (1853): 20–23, identified by Johnson, *River of Dark Dreams*, in his notes.

82. "The American Cotton Planter," 21.

83. Robert Gallman, "Self-Sufficiency in the Cotton Economy of the Antebellum South," *Agricultural History* 44, no. 1 (January 1970): 5–23.

84. Johnson, *River of Dark Dreams*, 186, 178–179.

85. Eugene Genovese, "Commentary: A Historian's View," *Agricultural History* 44, no. 1 (January 1970): 143–147. There is a long historiographic discussion of agricultural production of the South and particularly of the impact of cotton lands in the Mississippi valley and west. Much of it centers on the impact on domestic growing of foods and the diets of enslaved peoples. See the special issue of *Agricultural History* 44, no. 1 (January 1970), "The Structure of the Cotton Economy of the Antebellum South," for a variety of essays on the economic structure of southern agriculture. Also, more recently, see Johnson, *River of Dark Dreams*, which describes the importation of foods from the Upper Midwest down the Mississippi River because the value of land for cotton growing prevented its use for crops or livestock, especially hogs. James Oakes, in a long review of the book, takes issue with this point, arguing that it had long been disproven that the South was "food deprived." He points to the issue of *Agricultural History* here identified as a source of articles indicating that the South was food sufficient. See Oakes, "Capitalism and Slavery and the Civil War," 195–220. Suffice it to say that, whether food was imported or was grown on the plantation, different grades of meat and varieties of vegetables were undoubtedly distributed to master and slave. For economists' critique of Beckert, Baptist, and Johnson, see Alan L. Olmstead and Paul W. Rhode, "Cotton, Slavery, and the New History of Capitalism," *Explorations in Economic History* 67 (January 2018): 1–17.

86. Eugene Genovese, *The Political Economy of Slavery* (New York: Pantheon, 1965), 44. Whatever other objections might be made to Genovese's arguments about slavery as "paternalistic" or "pre-industrial," his observations about the exploitative nature of the plantation system provide important insights, especially regarding slave diet, health, and the cruelty of the institution.

87. Genovese, *The Political Economy of Slavery*, 96.

88. Genovese, *The Political Economy of Slavery*, 45.

89. Harry Marks, "Epidemiologists Explain Pellagra: Gender, Race, and Political Economy in the Work of Edgar Sydenstricker," *Journal of the History of Medicine and Allied Sciences* 58, no. 1 (January 2003): 34–55.

90. Tyson Gibbs, Kathleen Cargill, Leslie Sue Lieberman, and Elizabeth Reitz, "Nutrition in a Slave Population: An Anthropological Examination," *Medical Anthropology* 4, no. 2 (Spring 1980): 175.

91. Northrup, *Twelve Years a Slave*, 118.

92. Charles Ball, *Fifty Years in Chains, or, The Life of an American Slave* (Indianapolis, IN: Asher, 1859), 11, https://docsouth.unc.edu/fpn/ball/ball.html, accessed August 31, 2020.

93. Ball, *Fifty Years in Chains*, 17.

94. Ball, *Fifty Years in Chains*, 12. Throughout the story we learn the personal meaning of what cliometricians (economic historians who use statistical analysis of large-scale numerical data) objectify to gain a more panoramic view: the sexual mistreatment and rape of women, the selling of children, and the whippings that were the physical means and psychological tool that maintained the slave order.

95. Patricia Lambert, "Infectious Disease Among Enslaved African Americans at Eaton's Estate, Warren County, North Carolina, ca. 1830–1850," Supplement 2, *Memórias do Instituto Oswaldo Cruz* 101 (December 2006): 107–117.

96. Lambert, "Infectious Disease," 109; see, for example, Richard Sutch, "The Treatment Received by American Slaves: A Critical Review of the Evidence Presented in *Time on the Cross*," *Explorations in Economic History* 12, no. 4 (October 1975): 335–438; and Richard Sutch, "The Care and Feeding of Slaves," in *Reckoning with Slavery*, ed. Paul A. David, Herbert G. Gutman, Richard Sutch, Peter Temin, and Gavin Wright, 231–301 (New York: Oxford University Press, 1976).

97. Steckel, "The African American Population," 449.

98. Richard H. Steckel, "A Peculiar Population: The Nutrition, Health, and Mortality of American Slaves from Childhood to Maturity," *Journal of Economic History* 46, no. 3 (September 1986): 721–741.

99. Steckel, "The African American Population," 450.

100. Steckel, "A Peculiar Population"; Steckel, "The African American Population," 450.

101. Steckel, "The African American Population," 450–451.

102. Steckel, "A Peculiar Population."

103. Scott Alan Carson, "The Effect of Geography and Vitamin D on African American Stature in the Nineteenth Century: Evidence from Prison Records," *Journal of Economic History* 68, no. 3 (September 2008): 812–831. Others point to the increase in height of African Americans following emancipation, while others argue that changing height was a problem not with slavery or racism alone, before and after emancipation, but with changing agricultural practices that affected white and Black alike. Still other economic historians are focused on the methodological weaknesses of the data—should June or January estimates of meat consumption inform the conclusion, should region and specific time period be closely studied to make fine distinctions?—rather than the social meaning of inadequate diet. Others cite the decline of specific measures such as overall meat consumption in the nineteenth century, in efforts to identify in the bones of slaves the calcium and other vitamin deficiencies that led to diseases like pellagra. See, for example, the continuing debate over sources and interpretations of diet and height in the economic history literature in the two decades following the publication of Robert Fogel and Stanley Engerman, *Time on the Cross: The Economics of American Negro Slavery* (Boston: Little, Brown, 1974): John Komlos, "Toward an Anthropometric History of African-Americans: The Case of the Free Blacks in Antebellum Maryland," in *Strategic Factors in Nineteenth Century American Economic History: A Volume to Honor Robert W. Fogel,* ed. Claudia Goldin and Hugh Rockoff, 297–329 (Chicago: University of Chicago Press, 1992); Robert Gallman, "Dietary Change in Antebellum America," *Journal of Economic History* 56, no. 1 (March 1996): 193–201; John Komlos, "Anomalies in Economic History: Toward a Resolution of the 'Antebellum Puzzle,'" *Journal of Economic History* 56, no. 1 (1996): 202–214; John Komlos, "Shrinking in a Growing Economy? The Mystery of Physical Stature During the Industrial Revolution," *Journal of Economic History* 58, no. 3 (September 1998): 779–802; John Komlos, "On the Biological Standard of Living of African-Americans: The Case of Civil War Soldiers," in *The Biological Standard of Living in Comparative Perspective,* ed. John Komlos and Jorg Baten, 236–248 (Stuttgart: Franz Steiner Verlag, 1998); John Komlos and Bjorn Alecke, "The Economics of Antebellum Slave Heights Reconsidered," *Journal of Interdisciplinary History* 26, no. 3 (1996): 437–457; Sophia Dent, "Interindividual Differences in Embodied Marginalization: Osteological and Stable Isotope Analyses of Antebellum Enslaved Individuals," *American Journal of Human Biology* 29, no. 4 (July/August 2017): 1–16, https://doi.org/10.1002/ajhb.23021, accessed August 7, 2020; Kenneth F. Kiple and Virginia H. Kiple, "Black Tongue and Black Men: Pellagra and Slavery in the Antebellum South," *Journal of Southern History* 43, no. 3 (August 1977): 411–428.

104. The debate over the parameters to be used extend far back into the literature. It appears that method has overtaken logic in some of the discussions, with often poor data substituting for logic. Finely tuned studies seek to identify a host of variables from region, time period, specific crop, and plantation size to create a refined, if suspect, look at diet and health in the slave South. Some argue that "the conditions of slaves can be studied more accurately if the data resources related to slave diet are divided into ecozones, i.e., coastal versus interior, and then examined using the available climatic, agricultural, archeological, zooar-cheological, historical and epidemiological information specific to that zone. This information could then be combined with appropriate ergonomic and physiological data to develop a holistic picture of the adequacy of slave diet for a particular ecozone, within a particular time frame." See Gibbs, Cargill, Lieberman, and Reitz, "Nutrition in a Slave Population," 176.

105. Genovese, *The Political Economy of Slavery*, 94–95.

106. Kenneth Stampp, *The Peculiar Institution: Slavery in the Ante-Bellum South* (New York: Vintage, 1956), 302.

107. Saunt, *Unworthy Republic*, 146.

108. Stampp, *The Peculiar Institution*, 302–306.

109. Stampp, *The Peculiar Institution*, 306.

110. Richard Shryock, "Medical Practice in the Old South," *South Atlantic Quarterly* 29, no. 2 (April 1930): 174–175. Shryock was arguing with what was then a prominent view that slaves were generally well fed and well cared for in the pre–Civil War plantations. In his piece he sarcastically took on the economic argument some historians used to downplay the horror of the slave system, that it was in the self-interest of slave owners to care for their property: "In a word, the a priori argument for slave health, in terms of a property interest, has only a partial validity—men have been known to neglect even their livestock."

111. By a Country Practitioner, "Sterility Among the Negroes: A Case," *New Orleans Medical News and Hospital Gazette* 3 (1856–1857): 392,

112. Stampp, *The Peculiar Institution*, 317–318. See also Todd Savitt, *Medicine and Slavery: The Diseases and Health Care of Blacks in Antebellum Virginia* (Urbana: University of Illinois Press, 2002).

113. Stampp, *The Peculiar Institution*, 289.

114. Stampp, *The Peculiar Institution*, 290–292.

115. Stampp, *The Peculiar Institution*, 294.

116. See, for example, L. L. Wall, "The Medical Ethics of Dr. J. Marion Sims: A Fresh Look at the Historical Record," *Journal of Medical Ethics* 32, no. 6 (June 2006): 346–350. See also Harriet A. Washington, *Medical Apartheid* (New York: Vintage, 2008).

117. Louis Hughes, *Thirty Years a Slave, from Bondage to Freedom* (New York: Negro Universities Press, 1959), 187. Originally published in 1897.

118. Margaret Humphreys, *Yellow Fever and the South* (New Brunswick, NJ: Rutgers University Press, 1992), 47–48.

119. Humphreys, *Yellow Fever and the South*, 50.

120. *Report of the Sanitary Commission of New Orleans on the Epidemic Yellow Fever of 1853* (New Orleans, LA: Picayune Office, 1854), 504–505, as quoted in Urmi Engineer Willoughby, *Yellow Fever, Race, and Ecology in Nineteenth-Century New Orleans* (Baton Rouge: Louisiana State University Press, 2017), 67.

121. Humphreys, *Yellow Fever and the South*, 6.

122. Willoughby, *Yellow Fever, Race, and Ecology*, 12.

123. Willoughby, *Yellow Fever, Race, and Ecology*, 32.

3. "THE SURGING TIDE OF BUSINESS . . . YIELDING UP THE BONES OF THE DEAD": OVERWORK, POOR NUTRITION, UNHYGIENIC HOMES, AND A HAZARDOUS WORKPLACE

1. Clay McShane, *Down the Asphalt Path: The Automobile and the American City* (New York: Columbia University Press, 1994), 41–45.

2. Elizabeth Blackmar, *Manhattan for Rent, 1785–1850* (Ithaca, NY: Cornell University Press, 1989).

3. Dora Costa, "Health and the Economy in the United States, from 1750 to the Present," *Journal of Economic Literature* 53, no. 3 (September 2015): 503.

4. Gergely Baics, *Feeding Gotham: The Political Economy and Geography of Food in New York, 1790–1860* (Princeton, NJ: Princeton University Press, 2016).

5. Jeffrey Williamson and Peter Lindert, "Unequal Gains: American Growth and Inequality Since 1700," Centre for Economic Policy Research, https://cepr.org/voxeu/columns/unequal-gains-american-growth-and-inequality-1700#:~:text=A%20long%20steep%20rise%20in,have%20witnessed%20since%20the%201970s, accessed December 22, 2022: "A long steep rise in US inequality took place between 1800 and 1860, matching the widening income gaps we have witnessed since the 1970s."

6. Costa, "Health and the Economy," 503; see also J. David Hacker, "Decennial Life Tables for the White Population of the United States, 1790–1900," *Historical Methods* 43, no. 2 (April 2010): 8, https://www.ncbi.nlm.nih.gov/pmc/articles/PMC2885717/pdf/nihms205286.pdf, accessed February 18, 2021.

7. E. Franklin Frazier, *The Negro in the United States* (New York: Macmillan, 1957), 569.

8. Massachusetts Bureau of Statistics of Labor, *Fourth Annual Report* (Boston: Wright and Potter, 1873), 34, https://catalog.hathitrust.org/Record/012508034, accessed March 23, 2024.

9. United States Census Bureau, *Bicentennial Edition: Historical Statistics of the United States, Colonial Times to 1970* (Washington, DC: Government Printing Office, 1975), chapter C: Migration, table entitled "Immigrants, by Country: 1820 to 1970," 106, https://www.census.gov/library/publications/1975/compendia/hist_stats_colonial-1970.html.

10. "The Children's Hospital—What 'Fireside' Thinks About It," *Evening Transcript* (Boston), January 22, 1879. This article was first uncovered by Morris Vogel, *The Invention of the Modern Hospital: Boston 1870–1930* (Chicago: University of Chicago Press, 1980).

11. Massachusetts Bureau of Statistics of Labor, *Fourth Annual Report*, 285.

12. Massachusetts Bureau of Statistics of Labor, *Fourth Annual Report*, 29.

13. Massachusetts Bureau of Statistics of Labor, *Fourth Annual Report*, 7–8. One person who received the report wrote that the bureau contained some "startling and ghastly" descriptions of working-class life that included "harrowing sights of squalor and wretchedness" (24).

14. Massachusetts Bureau of Statistics of Labor, *Fourth Annual Report*, 25.

15. Massachusetts Bureau of Statistics of Labor, *Fourth Annual Report*, 25.

16. Massachusetts Bureau of Statistics of Labor, *Fourth Annual Report*, 501–502.

17. Massachusetts Bureau of Statistics of Labor, *Sixth Annual Report* (Boston: Wright and Potter, 1875), vii, https://www.google.com/books/edition/Annual_Report_of_the_Bureau_of_Statistic/TPcbAQAAIAAJ?hl=en&gbpv=1&dq=Massachusetts+Bureau+of+Statistics+sixth+annual+report&pg=PA328&printsec=frontcover, accessed August 26, 2020.

18. Massachusetts Bureau of Statistics of Labor, *Sixth Annual Report*, 392. https://www.google.com/books/edition/Public_Documents_of_Massachusetts/5sIWAAAAYAAJ?hl=en&gbpv=1&dq=%E2%80%9Callowed+to+run+wherever+they+can+make+their+way.%E2%80%9D&pg=RA1-PA392&printsec=frontcover

19. Massachusetts Bureau of Statistics of Labor, *Sixth Annual Report*, 392.

20. Joshua L. Rosenbloom and Gregory W. Stutes, *Reexamining the Distribution of Wealth in 1870*, Working Paper 11482 (Cambridge: National Bureau of Economic Research, June 2005), nber.org/system/files/working_papers/w11482/w11482.pdf, accessed April 11, 2022.

21. Massachusetts Bureau of Statistics of Labor, *Sixth Annual Report*, 384–392.

22. Massachusetts Bureau of Statistics of Labor, *Sixth Annual Report*, 68.

23. Massachusetts Bureau of Statistics of Labor, *Sixth Annual Report*, 68–69.

24. Massachusetts Bureau of Statistics of Labor, *Sixth Annual Report*, 68–69.

25. Massachusetts Bureau of Statistics of Labor, *Sixth Annual Report*, 70–71.

26. Massachusetts Bureau of Statistics of Labor, *Sixth Annual Report*, 71.

27. Massachusetts Bureau of Statistics of Labor, *Sixth Annual Report*, 72.

28. See David Montgomery, *The Fall of the House of Labor: The Workplace, the State, and American Labor Activism, 1865–1925* (New York: Cambridge University Press, 1989); and David Rosner and Gerald Markowitz, *Deadly Dust: Silicosis and the Politics of Industrial Disease* (Princeton, NJ: Princeton University Press, 1991).

29. "The Children's Hospital—What 'Fireside' Thinks About It."

30. *Annual Report of the Bureau of Statistics of Labor, 1870–1871*, Senate of the General Court of Massachusetts, no. 120, 150, March 1, 1870, to March 1, 1871 (Boston: Wright and Potter, 1871), 518, https://babel.hathitrust.org/cgi/pt?id=uc1.c024783287&view=1up&seq=526&q1=health

31. *Annual Report*, 519.

32. *Annual Report*, 520–521.

33. *Annual Report*, 521–525.

34. *Annual Report*, 519.

35. *Annual Report*, 519–520.

36. *Annual Report*, 528.

37. *Annual Report*, 529.

38. Commonwealth of Massachusetts, House of Representatives, "1877 House Bill 0355: An Act Relating to the Inspection of Factories and Public Buildings," State of Massachusetts Digital Collections, https://archives.lib.state.ma.us/items/081247aa-2d3b-4cea-800b-6058eb8c65fe. See: chrome-extension://efaidnbmnnnibpcajpcglclefindmkaj/https://archives.lib.state.ma.us/server/api/core/bitstreams/38e61a1c-3e09-4cc2-b911-647edb88c4f8/content

39. Citizens' Association of New York, Council of Hygiene and Public Health, *Report of the Council of Hygiene and Public Health of the Citizens' Association of New York upon the Sanitary Condition of the City* (New York: D. Appleton, 1865), 77; available at National Library of Medicine Digital Collections, https://collections.nlm.nih.gov/catalog/nlm:nlmuid-63120960R-bk.

40. See Clay McShane, Joel Tarr, and Harriet Ritvo, *The Horse in the City: Living Machines in the Nineteenth Century* (Baltimore, MD: Johns Hopkins University Press, 2007); and McShane, *Down the Asphalt Path*, for detailed accounts of the impact of the horse on nineteenth-century urban life.

41. Citizens' Association, *Report . . . upon the Sanitary Condition of the City*, 80; Elizabeth Blackmar, "Accountability for Public Health: Regulating the Housing Market in Nineteenth-Century New York," in *Hives of Sickness: Epidemics and Public Health in New York City*, ed. David Rosner, 42–64 (New Brunswick, NJ: Rutgers University Press, 1995); Blackmar, *Manhattan for Rent*.

42. John Duffy, *A History of Public Health in New York City, 1866–1966* (New York: Russell Sage, 1974), 20.

43. "New York Urbanized Area: Population and Density from 1800 (Provisional)," *Demographia* (before 1950 drawn from census data and from 1950 to 2000 drawn from U.S. Census Bureau), demographia.com/db-nyuza1800.htm, accessed January 4, 2023.

44. Blackmar, "Accountability for Public Health"; Blackmar, *Manhattan for Rent.*

45. Elizabeth Cromley, *Alone Together: A History of New York's Early Apartments* (Ithaca, NY: Cornell University Press, 1990), 13; Blackmar, *Manhattan for Rent*, 13.

46. Cromley, *Alone Together*, 13; Blackmar, *Manhattan for Rent*, 13.

47. Cromley, *Alone Together*, 13; Blackmar, *Manhattan for Rent.*

48. Citizens' Association, *Report . . . upon the Sanitary Condition of the City.* In 1859, the Citizens' Committee organized a subcommittee to agitate for the establishment of a new permanent administrative body capable of responding to the city's environmental crisis. Shortly thereafter, during the Civil War, the Citizens' Association organized a Special Council of Hygiene and Public Health, whose first agenda item was to document the horrifying changes in living conditions that had overtaken much of the city in the preceding few decades. To do so, the council organized a district-by-district, block-to-block inspection of living conditions in Manhattan.

49. "Introductory Statement by the Council of the Citizens' Association," in Citizens' Association, *Report . . . upon the Sanitary Condition of the City*, xii, xiv.

50. Citizens' Association, *Report . . . upon the Sanitary Condition of the City*, xxxiv–cxliii.

51. Mortality data were collected and presented in a way that highlighted the city's apparent decline.

52. Gretchen Condran, "Changing Patterns of Epidemic Disease," in Rosner, *Hives of Sickness*, 30–32.

53. Citizens' Association, *Report . . . upon the Sanitary Condition of the City*, xi. See also Charles Rosenberg, *The Cholera Years* (Chicago: University of Chicago Press, 1964).

54. Condran, "Changing Patterns of Epidemic Disease," 27–41.

55. "Introductory Statement," xv.

56. "Introductory Statement," xv.

57. Citizens' Association, *Report . . . upon the Sanitary Condition of the City*, 37.

58. Citizens' Association, *Report . . . upon the Sanitary Condition of the City*, 89.

59. Citizens' Association, *Report . . . upon the Sanitary Condition of the City*, 89–90.

60. Citizens' Association, *Report . . . upon the Sanitary Condition of the City*, 36.

61. Citizens' Association, *Report . . . upon the Sanitary Conditions of the City*, 89–90.

62. Nayan Shah, *Contagious Divides: Epidemics and Race in San Francisco's Chinatown* (Berkeley: University of California Press, 2001). See also Mae Ngai, *Impossible Subjects: Illegal Aliens and the Making of Modern America* (Princeton, NJ: Princeton University Press, 2003); and Mae Ngai, *The Chinese Question: The Gold Rushes and Global Politics* (New York: Norton, 2021).

63. Susan Craddock, *City of Plagues: Disease, Poverty, and Deviance in San Francisco* (Minneapolis: University of Minnesota Press, 2000), 204–207.

64. Shah, *Contagious Divides*, 129–133; Natalia Molina, *Fit to Be Citizens? Public Health and Race in Los Angeles, 1879–1939* (Berkeley: University of California Press, 2006).

65. Shah, *Contagious Divides*, 129–133.

66. Shah, *Contagious Divides*, 129–133.

67. *Municipal Report, 1869–1870*, 233, quoted in Craddock, *City of Plagues*, 73.

68. Natalia Molina, *How Race Is Made in America: Immigration, Citizenship, and the Historical Power of Racial Scripts* (Berkeley: University of California Press, 2014), 91–103; Craddock, *City of Plagues*, 4.

69. John Griscom, *The Sanitary Condition of the Laboring Population of New York: with Suggestions for Its Improvement: A Discourse (with Additions) Delivered on the 30th December, 1844, at the Repository of the American Institute* (New York: Harper, 1845), https://collections.nlm.nih.gov/catalog/nlm:nlmuid -63140820R-bk, accessed January 4, 2023. This report followed two years after Chadwick produced his similarly titled report in the United Kingdom.

70. See "Bibliographic Notices," in John Griscom, "The Sanitary Condition of the Labouring Population of New York. . . . Delivered on the 30th December, 1844," *American Journal of the Medical Sciences* (April 1845): 400, https:// www.google.com/books/edition/The_American_Journal_of_the_Medical _Scie/RC9kYYo9w_QC?hl=en&gbpv=1&dq=Griscom+%22Teach+them +how+to+live,+so+as+to+avoid+diseases+and+be+more+comfortable %22&pg=RA1-PA400&printsec=frontcover, accessed January 9, 2023.

71. H. N. Hoople, "Economics of the Practice of Medicine," *Brooklyn Medical Journal* 17 (June 1903): 271–272, quoted in David Rosner, "Health Care for the 'Truly Needy,'" *Health and Society* 60, no. 1 (1982): 371.

72. Myron Raymond Chartier, "The Social Views of Dwight L. Moody and Their Relation to the Workingman of 1860–1900," *Fort Hays Studies Series* 40 (1969), https://scholars.fhsu.edu/fort_hays_studies_series/40?utm_source=scholars .fhsu.edu%2Ffort_hays_studies_series%2F40&utm_medium=PDF&utm_campaign =PDFCoverPages, accessed July 19, 2023.

73. Vogel, *The Invention of the Modern Hospital*; Rosner, "Health Care for the 'Truly Needy.'"

74. David Rosner, *A Once Charitable Enterprise* (New York: Cambridge University Press, 1982).

75. A few institutions can be seen as forerunners of modern voluntary hospitals. Massachusetts Hospital in Boston, Pennsylvania General in Philadelphia, and New York Hospital in New York City were set up in the eighteenth century. But these were the exceptions, not the rule, in a pre-urban America. See Charles Rosenberg, *The Care of Strangers: The Rise of America's Hospital System* (Baltimore, MD: Johns Hopkins University Press, 1995); Rosner, *A Once Charitable Enterprise*; and Vogel, *The Invention of the Modern Hospital.*

76. Rosner, "Health Care for the 'Truly Needy,'" 365.

77. Robert Hunter, *Poverty* (New York: Macmillan, 1904), 76–77.

78. Hunter, *Poverty* 84.

79. Methodist Episcopal Hospital (Brooklyn, New York), Annual Report 1896.

80. Methodist Episcopal Hospital (Brooklyn, New York), Annual Report, 1890.

81. Methodist Episcopal Hospital (Brooklyn, New York), Annual Report, 1887.

82. John S. Billings, Bureau of the Census, *Vital Statistics of New York and Brooklyn Covering a Period of Six Years Ending May 31, 1890* (Washington, DC: Government Printing Office, 1894), 66.

83. See Duffy, *A History of Public Health*, xxi.

84. Department of Health of the City of New York, *Annual Report of the Board of Health of the Department of Health of the City of New York for the Year Ending December 31, 1890* (New York: Martin B. Brown, 1891), 13, www.tlcarchive.org /images/search/archive/1890_011_033.pdf, accessed January 4, 2023. Teachers would not be employed without proof of vaccination.

85. Department of Health, *Annual Report*, 15.

86. Department of Health, *Annual Report*, 23. Department of Health of the City of New York, *Annual Report of the Board of Health of the Department of Health of the City of New York*, 1912, "General Sanitary Inspection Report," 34: By the turn of the century, dead animals were now regularly picked up off the streets. In 1912, the Department of Health removed 113,911 dead cats and dogs, 19,044 dead horses, and 1,118 dead calves, as well as thousands of donkeys, mules, cattle, and pigs. In addition, the Health Department removed 3,725,928 pounds of offal, the innards of the animals slaughtered in the city's meatpacking district. chrome-extension://efaidnbmnnnibpcajpcglclefindmkaj/http://www.tlcarchive .org/images/search/archive/1912_026_034.pdf.

87. New York City, Department of Health, "Vital Statistics Report," in *Annual Report*, 120, chrome-extension://efaidnbmnnnibpcajpcglclefindmkaj/http://www.tlcarchive .org/images/search/archive/1912_113_262.pdf, accessed December 28, 2022.

88. U.S. Department of Labor, Bureau of Labor Statistics, *History of Wages in the United States*, Table G-1, Laborers 1840–1900 (Washington, DC: Government Printing Office, 1934), 255.

89. Rosner, *Hives of Sickness*, 12.

90. Judith Leavitt, "'Typhoid Mary' Strikes Back: Bacteriological Theory and Practice in Early Twentieth-Century Public Health," *ISIS* 83, no. 4 (1992): 608–629; Nancy Tomes, *The Gospel of Germs: Men, Women, and the Microbe in American Life* (Cambridge, MA: Harvard University Press, 1998).

91. See Jane Addams, *Twenty Years at Hull House* (New York: Macmillan, 1912); and Lillian Wald, *The House on Henry Street* (New York: H. Holt, 1915).

92. René Dubos and Jean Dubos, *The White Plague: Tuberculosis, Man, and Society* (New Brunswick, NJ: Rutgers University Press, 1987).

93. Heini Hakosalo, "Lust for Life: Coping with Tuberculosis in Late Nineteenth-Century Europe," *Medical History* 64, no. 4 (October 2020): 523; Lotta Larsson, "Dealing with Death: The Romanticizing of Tuberculosis in Three Victorian Novels" (degree project in English literature, Lund University, Fall 2018), chrome-extension://efaidnbmnnnibpcajpcglclefindmkaj/viewer.html?pdfurl=https%3A%2F%2Flup.lub.lu.se%2Fluur%2Fdownload%3Ffunc%3DdownloadFile%26recordOId%3D8973158%26fileOId%3D8973159&clen=818771&pdffilename=Dealing_with_Death_The_Romanticising_of_Tuberc.pdf.

94. Dubos and Dubos, *The White Plague*, 10, 69. For an expanded discussion of tuberculosis, see Rosner and Markowitz, *Deadly Dust*, chap. 1.

95. John Harley Warner, *The Therapeutic Perspective: Medical Practice, Knowledge, and Identity in America, 1820–1885* (Princeton, NJ: Princeton University Press, 1997), 58.

96. Rosner, *Hives of Sickness*, 11; Frederick Hoffman, *Mortality from Respiratory Diseases in Dusty Trades (Inorganic Dusts)*, Bulletin of the United States Bureau of Labor Statistics No. 231 (Washington, DC: Government Printing Office, 1918), 329, 335.

97. "Tuberculosis in Europe and North America, 1800–1922," Harvard Library: Contagion—Historical Views of Diseases and Epidemics, https://curiosity.lib.harvard.edu/contagion/feature/tuberculosis-in-europe-and-north-america-1800-1922, accessed July 19, 2023.

98. Correspondence, "Cause and Treatment of Consumption," *Scientific American* 90, no. 21 (May 21, 1904): 403. George Rosen, *The History of Miners' Diseases: A Medical and Social Interpretation* (New York: Schuman's, 1943). The discovery by Koch of the tuberculosis bacillus led to the expectation of a "cure" for consumption.

99. Elizabeth Fee, *Disease and Discovery: A History of the Johns Hopkins School of Hygiene and Public Health, 1916–1939* (Baltimore, MD: Johns Hopkins University Press, 1987), 19; see also Barbara Rosenkrantz, *Public Health and the State: Changing Views in Massachusetts, 1842–1936* (Cambridge, MA: Harvard University Press, 1972), especially chaps. 3, 4, and 5.

100. Paul de Kruif, *The Microbe Hunters* (New York: Harcourt, Brace, 1926).

101. George Homan, "The Danger of Dust as a Cause of Tuberculosis," *Journal of the American Medical Association* 48, no. 12 (March 23, 1907): 1013. William Sedgewick is quoted in Fee, *Disease and Discovery*, 19, as saying that "before 1880 we knew nothing; after 1890 we knew it all; it was a glorious ten years."

102. S. A. Knopf, "Our Duties Toward the Consumptive Poor," *Charities* 6 (February 2, 1901): 76.

103. Heneage Gibbes, "Is The Unity of Phthisis an Established Fact?," *Boston Medical and Surgical Journal* 123 (December 25, 1890): 608.

104. "Consumption Widespread," *Charities* 3 (June 17, 1899): 9.

105. See Francis Albert Rollo Russell, "The Atmosphere in Relation to Human Life and Health," quoted in Hoffman, *Mortality from Respiratory Diseases*, 13.

106. George W. Comstock, " Commentary: The First Framingham Study—a Pioneer in Community-Based Participatory Research," *International Journal of Epidemiology* 34 (2005), 1188–1190. See modern analyses of the importance of this study: "Equal, but Different? Ecological, Individual and Instrumental Approaches to Understand Determinants of Health," *International Journal of Epidemiology* 34 (2005), 1179–1180; Susser M., Stein Z., "Commentary: Donald Budd Armstrong (1886-1968) - Pioneering Tuberculosis Prevention in General Practice," *International Journal of Epidemiology* 34 (2005),1191-1193.

107. Samuel Roberts, *Infectious Fear: Politics, Disease, and the Health Effects of Segregation* (Chapel Hill: University of North Carolina Press, 2009), 24, chrome-extension://efaidnbmnnnibpcajpcglclefindmkaj/viewer.html ?pdfurl=http%3A%2F%2Ftlcarchive.org%2Fimages%2Fsearch%2Farchive %2F1912_026_034.pdf&clen=747311&chunk=true, accessed April 21, 2022.

108. New York Board of Health, *Annual Report of the Department of Health of the City of New York for the Years 1910–1911*, (New York: New York Printing Company, 1913), 31–33.

109. Clay McShane and Joel Tarr, *The Horse in the City: Living Machines in the Nineteenth Century* (Baltimore, MD: Johns Hopkins University Press, 2011), 16.

110. New York Board of Health, *Annual Report*, 11.

111. "Life Expectancy (from Birth) in the United States, from 1860 to 2020," *Statista*, https://www.statista.com/statistics/1040079/life-expectancy-united-states -all-time/.

112. Michael R. Haines, "The Urban Mortality Transition in the United States, 1800–1940," *Annales de Démographie Historique* 1, no. 101 (2001): 33–64.

113. W. E. B. Du Bois, *The Philadelphia Negro: A Social Study* (Philadelphia: University of Pennsylvania Press, 1896).

114. Du Bois, *The Philadelphia Negro*, 153.

115. Du Bois, *The Philadelphia Negro*, 150–151.

116. Du Bois, *The Philadelphia Negro*, 151.

117. Du Bois, *The Philadelphia Negro*, 156.

118. Du Bois, *The Philadelphia Negro*, 152.

119. Du Bois, *The Philadelphia Negro*, 156.

120. Du Bois, *The Philadelphia Negro*, 161–162.

121. Du Bois, *The Philadelphia Negro*, 163.

122. Roberts, *Infectious Fear*, 68.

123. Roberts, *Infectious Fear*, 57–58.

124. George Edmund Haynes, *The Negro at Work in New York City: A Study in Economic Progress* (New York: Columbia University Press, 1912), 37.

125. New York Board of Health, *Annual Report*, 12.

126. New York Board of Health, *Annual Report*, 31–33, quoted in Rosner, *Hives of Sickness*, 17.

4. RESETTING THE GROUND RULES FOR INEQUALITY: LABOR, LAW, AND HEALTH AFTER THE CIVIL WAR

1. Robert Steinfeld, *The Invention of Free Labor: The Employment Relation in English and American Law and Culture, 1350–1870* (Chapel Hill: University of North Carolina Press, 1991), 8.

2. James Henry Hammond, "Speech of Hon. James H. Hammond, of South Carolina, On the Admission of Kansas, Under the Lecompton Constitution: Delivered in the Senate of the United States, March 4, 1858," Washington, DC, 1858, https://www.americanantiquarian.org/Manuscripts/cottonisking.html https://www.americanantiquarian.org/Manuscripts/cottonisking.html, accessed January 10, 2023. This is often called the "Cotton Is King" speech.

3. For comprehensive discussions of the repression that followed Radical Reconstruction, see Eric Foner, *Reconstruction: America's Unfinished Revolution, 1863–1877* (New York: Harper and Row, 1988); Eric Foner, *Slavery and Freedom in Nineteenth-Century America* (New York: Oxford University Press, 1994); and Eric Foner, *Nothing but Freedom: Emancipation and Its Legacy* (Baton Rouge: Louisiana State University Press, 1984).

4. William Darity Jr. and A. Kirsten Mullen, *From Here to Equality: Reparations for Black Americans in the Twentieth Century* (Chapel Hill: University of North Carolina Press, 2020).

5. Foner, *Reconstruction*, 152. See also, Nicole Hannah-Jones, *The 1619 Project: A New Origin Story* (New York: One World, 2021), chap. 2.

6. Jim Downs, *Sick from Freedom: African American Illness and Suffering During the Civil War and Reconstruction* (New York: Oxford University Press, 2012), 144–145.

7. Downs, *Sick from Freedom*, 148, 155.

8. U.S. Department of Commerce, Bureau of the Census, *Historical Statistics of the United States: Colonial Times to 1957* (Washington, DC: Government Printing Office, 1960), 74.

9. James Henry Hammond, "The Mudsill Theory," speech to the U.S. Senate, March 4, 1858, https://www.pbs.org/wgbh/aia/part4/4h3439t.html, accessed October 22, 2020.

10. Farwell v. Boston and Worcester Railroad Corp., 4 Metcalf 49 (1842), https://play.google.com/books/reader?id=hGY9AAAAIAAJ&as_brr=3&printsec=frontcover&pg=GBS.PA3, accessed October 29, 2020.

11. Department of the Interior, Bureau of Mines, *Coal-Mine Fatalities in the United States 1870–1914*, Bulletin 115 (Washington, DC: Government Printing Office, 1916), 8; Mark Aldrich, *Death Rode the Rails: American Railroad Accidents and Safety, 1828–1965* (Baltimore, MD: Johns Hopkins University Press, 2006), 311–312.

12. Farwell v. Boston and Worcester Railroad Corp., Appendix, 6; John Witt, *The Accidental Republic: Crippled Workingmen, Destitute Widows, and the Remaking of American Law* (Cambridge, MA: Harvard University Press, 2006), argues that *Farwell* represented a reaffirmation of the prevailing attitude in the early republic that skilled workers controlled the workplace.

13. Farwell v. Boston and Worcester Railroad Corp.

14. Steinfeld, *The Invention of Free Labor*, 9.

15. "Inspecting Bakeries in the State: Much Uncleanliness Discovered by the Deputy Factory Inspectors," *New York Times*, July 25, 1895, p.6.

16. "Inspecting Bakeries in the State: Much Uncleanliness Discovered by the Deputy Factory Inspectors," *New York Times*, July 25, 1895, p.6.

17. "A Strike for Clean Bread," *The Survey* 24 (June 18, 1910): 483–488; "Investigations Have Disclosed the Fact That Unhealthy and Poisonous Bread Is Made in Non-Union Bake Shops," *Woman's Label League Journal* (June 1913): 13. U.S. Department of Commerce, *Historical Statistics*, 72.

18. Lochner v. New York, 198 U.S. 45 (1906), 197 - 198; argued February 23, 24, 1905, decided April 17, 1906, Available at: http://supreme.justia.com/cases/federal/us/198/45/case.html, Accessed: March 20, 2024. This decision was in spite of the conditions of the New York bakeries, conditions that had provoked ten years of strikes and labor disputes from the 1890s on. Books have been written on this case, largely interpreting the conflicting constitutional principles

ostensibly embodied in the Fourteenth Amendment's due process clause, which protected the individual from the arbitrary power of the state. This amendment, initially meant to protect freed slaves, has, ironically, been used to assert the "rights" of workmen to work long hours in unhealthy conditions. It has been interpreted in various decisions to mean that the "liberty" of contract trumps the regulatory "intrusion" of the state into management-labor disputes. Most legal scholars have attacked it, some arguing that it was the most reactionary Court decision other than *Plessy v. Ferguson* and *Dred Scott*. More recently, articles and books have appeared maintaining that *Lochner* was a "reasoned" decision based on ample precedent. See David Bernstein, *Rehabilitating Lochner: Defending Individual Rights Against Progressive Reform* (Chicago: University of Chicago Press, 2011).

19. The term *wage slave* first began to appear in the years around the Civil War, with its usage skyrocketing after the 1880s. See "wage slavery" in Google Books N-Gram Viewer, https://books.google.com/ngrams/graph?content=wage+slavery &year_start=1800&year_end=2000&corpus=15&smoothing=3&share =&direct_url=t1%3B%2Cwage%20slavery%3B%2Cco#t1%3B%2Cwage %20slavery%3B%2Cco, accessed December 7, 2019. The term *wage slave* continued to be used well into the twentieth century to capture the evolving exploitation of the new factory system. See Gerald Markowitz and David Rosner, eds., *Slaves of the Depression: Workers' Letters About Life on the Job* (Ithaca, NY: Cornell University Press, 1987). See also the contrast the South drew with northern labor, specifically what was considered northern hypocrisy in the use of the term *free labor*: "Pauperism is prevented by slavery. The idea is absurd, no doubt, in the apprehension of many at the north, who think that slaves are, as a matter of course, paupers. Nothing can be more untrue. Every slave has an inalienable claim in law upon his owner for support for the whole of life. He cannot be thrust into an almshouse, he cannot become a vagrant, he cannot beg his living, he cannot be wholly neglected when he is old and decrepit." "A Northerner's Experiences—Slavery," *DeBow's Review*, n.s., 18 (January 1855): 573.

20. Holly J. McCammon, "Protection for Whom? Maximum Hours Laws and Women's Employment in the United States, 1880–1920," *Work and Occupation* 23, no. 2 (May 1996): 132.

21. As quoted in Alice Kessler-Harris, *Out to Work: A History of Wage-Earning Women in the United States* (New York: Oxford University Press, 1982), 186.

22. Lochner v. New York, 197.

23. Lochner v. New York, 198.

24. Lochner v. New York, 198.

25. Lochner v. New York, 198.

26. Lochner v. New York, 198.

27. Lochner v. New York, 198.

28. Lochner v. New York, 197–198. This "right" was guaranteed "except as controlled by the State in the legitimate exercise of its police power."

29. Lochner v. New York, 198.

30. Lochner v. New York.

31. Legal Information Institute, Muller v. Oregon (1908), https://www.law.cornell.edu/wex/muller_v_oregon_(1908).

32. Lochner v. New York, 198.

33. Lochner v. New York, 198: "Nearly twenty states limited assumption of risk and others restricted contributory negligence."

34. Melvin Urofsky, "State Courts and Protective Legislation During the Progressive Era: A Reevaluation," *Journal of American History* 72, no. 1 (June 1985): 84, quoted in Theda Skocpol, *Protecting Soldiers and Mothers: The Political Origins of Social Policy in the United States* (Cambridge, MA: Harvard University Press, 1992), 289.

35. Kessler-Harris, *Out to Work*, 194–195. Male unions lobbied for banning women from "swing shifts," the short stretch of five or six hours that transitioned between the day and night shifts.

36. Kessler-Harris, *Out to Work*, 188, 212–213.

37. Quoted in Marc Aldrich, *Safety First: Technology, Labor, and Business in the Building of American Work Safety, 1870–1939* (Baltimore, MD: Johns Hopkins University Press, 1997), 76–79. See Aldrich's appendices for railroad, mine, and manufacturing injury and fatality rates. Estimates for the early 1900s vary considerably. For example, see S. E. Roberts, T. Carter, H. D. Smith, A. John, and J. G. Williams, "Forgotten Fatalities: British Military, Mining and Maritime Accidents Since 1900," *Occupational Medicine* 71, nos. 6–7 (August/October 2021): 277–283, https://academic.oup.com/occmed/article/71/6-7/277/6355603, accessed July 21, 2023.

38. Lawrence M. Freedman and Jack Ladinsky, "Social Change and the Law of Accidents," in *American Law and the Constitutional Order: Historical Perspectives*, ed. Lawrence M. Friedman and Harry N. Scheiber (Cambridge, MA: Harvard University Press, 1978), 273, cited in Skocpol, *Protecting Soldiers and Mothers*, 289.

39. Kessler-Harris, *Out to Work*, 184.

40. Florence Kelley, "Minimum-Wage Laws," *Journal of Political Economy* 20 (December 1912): 1005–1006, quoted in Skocpol, *Protecting Soldiers and Mothers*, 407–408.

41. Skocpol, *Protecting Soldiers and Mothers*, 423. In 1923 the Supreme Court, in *Atkins v. Children's Hospital*, struck down the District of Columbia's minimum

wage law largely based on the argument that it interfered in the free market between labor and management.

42. Thomas Piketty, *Capital in the Twenty-First Century*, tr. Arthur Goldhammer (Cambridge, MA: Harvard University Press, 2017).

43. Piketty, *Capital*, 9.

44. Jacob Riis, *How the Other Half Lives* (New York: Hill and Wang, 1890), 10.

45. After all, "the law," observes the legal historian Karen Orren, "was unambiguously favorable to masters over employees, and masters were usually businessmen." See Karen Orren, "The Laws of Industrial Organization, 1870–1920," in *The Cambridge History of Law in America*, ed. Michael Grossberg (Cambridge: Cambridge University Press, 2008), 565.

46. Anthony Bale, "Compensation Crisis: The Value and Meaning of Work-Related Injuries and Illnesses in the United States, 1842–1932" (PhD diss., Brandeis University, 1986).

47. Anthony Bale, "America's First Compensation Crisis: Conflict over the Value and Meaning of Workplace Injuries Under the Employers' Liability System," in *Dying for Work: Workers' Safety and Health in Twentieth-Century America*, ed. D. Rosner and G. Markowitz, 34–52 (Bloomington: Indiana University Press, 1987); Bale, "Compensation Crisis"; Anthony Bale, "The American Compensation Phenomenon," *International Journal of Health Services* 20, no. 2 (1990): 253–275.

48. Crystal Eastman, *Work-Accidents and the Law* (New York: Russell Sage, 1910). This was one of six volumes detailing the life of working people in Pittsburgh. See Paul Kellogg, ed., *The Pittsburgh Survey; Findings in Six Volumes* (New York: Russell Sage, 1909–1914). Scores of reformers, artists, academics, and writers—from Lewis Hines through John R. Commons and Elizabeth Butler—joined Kellogg, John Fitch, and others in producing a detailed portrait of working-class and immigrant life in a city dominated by Carnegie and Mellon's U.S. Steel Company. See Maurine W. Greenwald and Margo Anderson, *Pittsburgh Surveyed: Social Science and Social Reform in the Early Twentieth Century* (Pittsburgh, PA: University of Pittsburgh Press, 1996).

49. "A Strike for Clean Bread," 483–488.

50. "Investigations Have Disclosed," 13.

51. "The Consumers League Label and Its Offspring," *The Survey* 32 (August 8, 1914): 478. The National Consumers League saw such protective legislation for women and children as an opening wedge that could ultimately lead to improved conditions for men as well. See Skocpol, *Protecting Soldiers and Mothers*, 395.

52. Mary H. Loines, Chairman of the Brooklyn Auxiliary of the Consumers League of the City of New York, to Hon. Robert F. Wagner, December 12, 1912, in New

York State, *Second Report of the Factory Investigating Commission* (Albany, NY: J. B. Lyons, 1913), 2: 1330–1331.

53. Frances Perkins quoted in New York State, *Second Report of the Factory Investigating Commission* (Albany, NY: J. B. Lyons, 1913),1576-1577. The Consumers League defined its mandate as extending beyond the shop floor and into what was one of the only white-collar employment opportunities for women, the department store, a symbol and cornerstone of the new modern consumer economy. See William Leach, *Land of Desire: Merchants, Power, and the Rise of a New American Culture* (New York: Pantheon, 1993). At the turn of the century, the league hired Florence Kelley as its director. Kelley, who had lived at Hull House and worked as a factory inspector in Illinois along with Alice Hamilton, "led the organization into a campaign for legislation to regulate department store conditions and to prescribe sanitation and safety measures on the shop floor." See Kessler-Harris, *Out to Work*, 166.

54. "Joint Sanitary Standards in the Cloak, Suit and Skirt Industry," *The Survey* 26 (August 19, 1911): 734.

55. Upton Sinclair, "What Life Means to Me," *Cosmopolitan* 41 (October 1906): 594; Arlene Finger Kantor, "Upton Sinclair and the Pure Food and Drugs Act of 1906," *American Journal of Public Health* 66, no. 12 (December 1976): 1202–1205; Deborah Blum, *The Poison Squad: One Chemist's Single-Minded Crusade for Food Safety at the Turn of the Twentieth Century* (New York: Penguin, 2018).

56. "Bakers and Employers Plan to End Strike," *New York Times*, August 12, 1905, 4, https://timesmachine.nytimes.com/timesmachine/1905/08/12/119119760.html ?pageNumber=4, accessed December 15, 2020.

57. Bureau of Labor Statistics, *Report of the Bureau of Statistics of Labor* 21 (March 1891): 107, https://babel.hathitrust.org/cgi/pt?id=chi.56419611&view =1up&seq=7, accessed September 11, 2020.

58. Bureau of Labor Statistics, *Report*, 107–108.

59. Bureau of Labor Statistics, *Report*, 107–108.

60. Bureau of Labor Statistics, *Report*, 107–108.

61. Bureau of Labor Statistics, *Report*, 107–108.

62. Bureau of Labor Statistics, *Report*, 107.

63. David Rosner and Gerald Markowitz, "Safety and Health During the Progressive Era," in *Sickness and Health in America*, 3rd ed., ed. J. Leavitt and R. Numbers (Madison: University of Wisconsin Press, 1997), 507–521.

64. T. W. Schereshewsky, "Industrial Hygiene," *Public Health Reports* 30 (October 1, 1915): 2928; "Editorial: Our Public Health Service," *American Journal of Public Health* 29 (September 1939): 1044–1045; W. S. Bean, "The Role of the Federal Government in Promoting Industrial Hygiene," *American Journal of Public Health* 15 (July 1925): 626.

5. GASPING FOR BREATH: DISCOVERING NEW INEQUALITIES

1. A. J. Arnold, *"Ex Luce Lucellum"? Innovation, Class Interests and Economic Returns in the Nineteenth Century Match Trade*, Paper 04/06, Business School of Exeter University.

2. T. E. Thorpe, Thomas Oliver, and George Cunningham, *Reports . . . on the Use of Phosphorus in the Manufacture of Lucifer Matches* (London: Her Majesty's Stationery Office, 1899), https://archive.org/details/b2804003x/mode/2up, accessed December 25, 2020.

3. Thorpe, Oliver, and Cunningham, *Reports . . . on the Use of Phosphorus*, 96; Susan Isaac, " 'Phossy Jaw' and the Matchgirls: A Nineteenth-Century Industrial Disease," Royal College of Surgeons of England, September 28, 2018, https:// www.rcseng.ac.uk/library-and-publications/library/blog/phossy-jaw-and-the -matchgirls/, accessed January 19, 2023.

4. Thorpe, Oliver, and Cunningham, *Reports . . . on the Use of Phosphorus*, 83.

5. M. F. Crass, "A History of the Match Industry, Part 1," *Journal of Chemical Education* 18, no. 3 (March 1941): 116–121.

6. " 'Phossy Jaw' Bill, Demanded by Humanity, Pigeonholed," *Oklahoma News*, February 21, 1912, 4.

7. "Queer Legislation, Why Legislate Against 'Lump Jaw' in Cattle and Not Against 'Phossy Jaw' in Human Beings?," *Evansville Press*, February 21, 1912, 4.

8. " 'Phossy Jaw' Bill"; see also John Andrews, of the American Association for Labor Legislation, "The Phossy Jaw Bill," letter to the editor, *Brooklyn Daily Eagle*, April 25, 1912, 26, for a discussion, in the absence of the constitutional power to ban poisons in a free market economy, of the use of taxation as a method for discouraging their use.

9. "Poison—Dr. Jacobs Praises Diamond Match Co.—Phosphorous Poisoning Largely Disappeared," *Akron Daily Democrat*, February 12, 1901, 6.

10. "Poison."

11. "Victims of 'Phossy Jaw' Help Match Trust Pile Up Millions," *Labor World* (Duluth), January 28, 1911, 1.

12. R. Alton Lee, "The Eradication of Phossy Jaw: A Unique Development of Federal Police Power," *The Historian* 29, no. 1 (November 1966): 1–21.

13. Thomas Piketty, *Capital in the Twenty-First Century* (Cambridge, MA: Harvard University Press, 2014), 291, 348.

14. Economic historians continue to analyze the many factors that led to the inequalities that emerged, some arguing that the accumulation of wealth in the hands of the few was, in the long run, beneficial. The argument goes that the wealthy save more than the poor, thereby allowing for future socially beneficial

investments not possible without concentration of capital in the hands of a few. Others have looked at this argument as a rationale for an inequality that is unjustified by its social costs. Regardless of the outcome of what has become a highly ideological debate, there is little argument that by the outbreak of World War I disparities of wealth less than but on the order of what existed in belle époque Europe had emerged, particularly in the industrializing East. As Piketty notes, by the early twentieth century the wealth "gap with old Europe remained, but it had shrunk by half in one century. . . . If we limit our gaze to the East Coast, the gap is smaller still." The catastrophes of World War 1, economic depression, and World War II would alter the story materially. See Piketty, *Capital*, chap. 4.

15. See Samuel Preston and Michael Haines, *Fatal Years: Child Mortality in Late Nineteenth-Century America* (Princeton, NJ: Princeton University Press, 1991), for demographers' take on the mortality of children. The Preston and Haines book set off a flurry over their conclusions as to what social, medical, public health, and personal factors affected the fluctuations in mortality rates and what appeared to be a general decline in mortality rates at the end of the nineteenth and beginning of the twentieth centuries. Gretchen Condran, "What *Fatal Years* Tells Us That We Did Not Already Know," *Bulletin of the History of Medicine* 68, no. 1 (Spring 1994): 95–104.

16. F. T. Gretton, "Hill Farm Mine Explosion," Historic Pittsburgh, https://historicpittsburgh.org/islandora/object/pitt:MSP328.B001.F08.I01; "Eleven Lives Lost," *New York Times*, May 23, 1891, cited in United States Mine Rescue Association, "Pratt No. 1 Shaft Explosion," *Mine Disasters in the United States*, https://usminedisasters.miningquiz.com/saxsewell/pratt.htm; Bob Doucette, "Krebs to Honor 100 Slain Miners," *The Oklahoman*, May 24, 2002, https://www.oklahoman.com/story/news/2002/05/24/krebs-to-honor-100-slain-miners/62093697007/#:~:text=On%20Jan.,sacrifices%20of%20those%20who%20died; Mine Safety and Health Administration, "Fraterville Mine Disaster: 120 Years Later," https://www.msha.gov/fraterville-mine-disaster-120-years-later; Deb Kiner, "Coal Mine Accidents in Pa. Have Killed Hundreds of Miners," *Patriot-News*, July 31, 2018, https://www.pennlive.com/life/2018/07/coal_mine_accidents_in_pa_have.html; United States Mine Rescue Association, "Virginia City Mine Explosion," *Mine Disasters in the United States*, https://usminedisasters.miningquiz.com/saxsewell/virginia_city.htm; "Four Hundred Dead in Mine Explosion," *Washington Times* (Washington, DC), December 6, 1907, 13, in Library of Congress, "Monongah Mine Disaster: Topics in Chronicling America," https://guides.loc.gov/chronicling-america-monongah-mine-disaster/selected-articles; United States Mine Rescue Association, "Pittsburg Coal Company Darr Mine Explosion," *Mine Disasters in the United States*, https://usminedisasters.miningquiz.com/saxsewell/darr.htm; "Scores

Killed by Awful Explosion in Alabama Mine," *Los Angeles Herald*, December 17, 1907, California Digital Newspaper Collection, https://cdnc.ucr.edu/?a=d&d=LAH19071217.2.2&e=-------en--20--1--txt-txIN--------; "Significant Illinois Fires: Cherry Mine Disaster," Illinois Library, https://guides.library.illinois.edu/c.php?g=416856&p=2840930; "Apr. 8, 1911: Banner Mine Explosion," Zinn Education Project, https://www.zinnedproject.org/news/tdih/banner-mine-explosion/.

17. "Four Hundred Dead in Mine Explosion."

18. William Attaway, *Blood on the Forge* (New York: Monthly Review Press, 1987), originally published 1941; John Claborn, "From Black Marxism to Industrial Ecosystem: Racial and Ecological Crisis in William Attaway's *Blood on the Forge*," in *Civil Rights and the Environment in African-American Literature, 1895–1941* (London: Bloomsbury Academic, 2017), 133–164 accessed December 26, 2020.

19. Bernardo Ramazzini, *De Morbis Artificum Diatriba* (Diseases of Workers), rev. and tr. Wilmer Cave Wright (Chicago: University of Chicago Press, 1940), originally published 1713; Charles Turner Thackrah, *The Effects of Arts, Trades and Professions on Health and Longevity* (London, 1832), available at: https://wellcomecollection.org/works/pp7msgx5/items?canvas=7.

20. United States Department of Commerce and Labor, *Bulletin of the Bureau of Labor*, No. 85 (Washington, DC: Government Printing Office, 1909), 40, https://books.google.com/books?id=ITexyP8MPYgC&pg=PA40&lpg=PA40&dq=The+Jawbones+Slowly+Decompose+and+Pass+Away+in+The+Form+of+Nauseating+Pus&source=bl&ots=Af2mDamCRJ&sig=ACfU3U11Q6wGYaGgbiuKzUjCBWjhhrgeog&hl=en&sa=X&ved=2ahUKEwixj-KOg7L3AhUOhYkEHbSiBxcQ6AF6BAgCEAM#v=onepage&q=The%20Jawbones%20Slowly%20Decompose%20and%20Pass%20Away%20in%20The%20Form%20of%20Nauseating%20Pus&f=false, accessed April 25, 2022.

21. Alice Hamilton, *Industrial Poisons in the United States* (New York: Macmillan, 1929), 9.

22. Claudia Clark, *Radium Girls: Women and Industrial Health Reform, 1910–1935* (Chapel Hill: University of North Carolina Press, 1997), 23–24.

23. Claudia Clark's work offers the most complete discussion of the legal and political ramifications of a lawsuit for which five women were awarded $10,000 each for their pain and suffering. "Radium Doom Settlements Up Tomorrow," *New York Daily News*, June 3, 1928, 3.

24. "An Address to the Tuberculosis Committee and to Unionists," *Charities and the Commons* 15 (January 20, 1906): 528.

25. E. Mayo, "The Work That Kills," *The Outlook* 99 (September 23, 1911): 205.

26. O. Nelson, *Twentieth Annual Report of the Chief Factory Inspector of Illinois*, July 1, 1912–June 30, 1913 (Springfield, Illinois, 1913); New York State, *Second*

Report of the Factory Investigating Commission 1913), 3: 662–711; State of New York, "The Diseases of the Bakers," *Preliminary Report of the Factory Investigating Commission* (1913), 1: 225–233; "How to Prevent Consumption," *The International Wood-Worker* 16 (May 1906): 137–139; S. Harrison, "Second National Conference on Industrial Diseases," *Survey* 28 (June 15, 1912): 448–451; F. Hoffman, "Industrial Diseases in America," *American Labor Legislation Review* 1 (June 1911): 35–39; F. Hoffman, "Legal Protection from Injurious Dusts," *American Labor Legislation Review* 1 (June 1911): 110–112; F. L. Hoffman, *Problem and Extent of Industrial Diseases, First National Conference on Industrial Diseases*: American Association of Labor Legislation, Publication No. 10 (Chicago, 1910), 35–51.

27. C.-E. A. Winslow, "Occupational Disease and Economic Waste," *Atlantic* 103 (May 1909): 679.

28. In the second decade of the twentieth century, a series of reports and studies were published by the U.S. Public Health Service and state departments of health and labor documenting the problem of dust, tuberculosis, and their relationship to work: United States Treasury Department, Public Health Service, *Tuberculosis Among Industrial Workers*, Public Health Bulletin No. 73 (Washington, DC: Government Printing Office, March 1916); United States Department of Labor, Working Conditions Service, *Preliminary Report on Mortality from Tuberculosis in Dusty Trades* (Washington, DC: Government Printing Office, 1919); Pennsylvania Labor and Industry Department, "The Hazards to Health from Industrial Dusts," *Monthly Bulletin* 3 (February 1916): 4–9; G. L. Apfelbach, "The Dusty Trades," *Twenty-Fourth Annual Report of the Chief State Factory Inspector of Illinois*, July 1, 1916–June 30, 1917 (Springfield, 1917) 75–77; R. Northrup, "Development in the Removal of Dust, Fumes and Gases," in *Proceedings of the Industrial Safety Congress of New York State* (The [Industrial Safety] Congress 1919), 4: 206–218; United States Department of Labor, Bureau of Labor Statistics, *Causes of Death by Occupation*, Bulletin No. 207, (Washington: GPO, March 1917).

29. It is interesting to note how quickly the influenza epidemic vanished from the American consciousness. In the words of John Cosby, it was "America's Forgotten Pandemic," in part because of the decreasing attention to infectious diseases as the century progressed, a topic only to be unearthed again by historians late in the twentieth century and early in the twenty-first as other infectious diseases such as the swine flu in the 1970s, AIDS in the 1980s and 1990s, and most recently Covid-19 in the 2020s brought attention to this history. Alfred Crosby, *America's Forgotten Pandemic: The Influenza of 1918* (New York: Cambridge University Press, 1989); Centers for Disease Control and Prevention, "History of 1918 Flu Pandemic," https://www.cdc.gov/flu/pandemic-resources/1918-commemoration/1918-pandemic-history.htm,

accessed March 2, 2023. See also Howard Markel, *When Germs Travel: Six Major Epidemics That Have Invaded America and the Fears They Have Unleashed* (New York: Vintage, 2005), as well as his numerous other writings on the 1918 epidemic specifically.

30. Graham Taylor, "The Industrial Viewpoint," *Charities and the Commons* 16 (May 5, 1906): 206.

31. John B. Andrews, "Occupational Diseases and Legislative Remedies," *American Journal of Public Health* 4 (March 1914): 179–184.

32. "Consumption Widespread," *Charities* 3 (June 17, 1899): 9.

33. Taylor, "The Industrial Viewpoint," 205.

34. See F. Hoffman, *The Mortality from Consumption in Dusty Trades*, United States Bureau of Labor, Bulletin No. 79 (Washington, DC: Government Printing Office, 1908), 633–875.

35. Albert Bolles, *Industrial History of the United States*, quoted in C. P. McCord, "Grindstones," *Hygeia* 18 (August 1940): 744.

36. Ludwig Teleky, *History of Factory and Mine Hygiene*, (New York: Columbia University Press, 1948)199.

37. Thomas Oliver, *Dangerous Trades* (London: E.P. Dutton, 1902), p. 272.

38. Script for *Stop Silicosis*, National Archives, Record Group 100, Motion Picture Division, 84–91.

39. David Montgomery, *The Fall of the House of Labor: The Workplace, the State, and American Labor Activism* (Cambridge: Cambridge University Press, 1987).

40. "Official Correspondence," *Granite Cutters' Journal* 31 (February 1908).

41. Frederick L. Hoffman, *The Problem of Dust Phthisis in the Granite-Stone Industry*, U.S. Department of Labor, Bureau of Labor Statistics, Bulletin No. 293 (Washington DC: Government Printing Office, 1922), 6.

42. Elizabeth Fee, *Disease and Discovery: A History of the Johns Hopkins School of Hygiene and Public Health, 1916–1939* (Baltimore, MD: Johns Hopkins University Press, 1987), 20–21.

43. See David Rosner and Gerald Markowitz, *Deadly Dust: Silicosis and the Politics of Occupational Disease in Twentieth-Century America* (Princeton, NJ: Princeton University Press, 1991), 13–48, for a full account of the naming of the disease.

44. P. Demers, "Labor and the Social Relations of the Granite Industry in Barre," unpublished paper, Goddard College, 1974, 54–63.

45. "Official Correspondence," *Granite Cutters' Journal* 34 (June 1910): 9.

46. Rosner and Markowitz, *Deadly Dust*, 210.

47. E. R. Hayhurst, *Industrial Health Hazards and Occupational Diseases in Ohio* (Columbus: Ohio State Board of Health, 1915), 18. For an earlier study, see E. R. Hayhurst, *Consumption and Preventable Deaths in American Occupations* (Columbus, OH: F. J. Heer, 1914), 10.

48. Jim Hare, "The Dawn of the Auto Industry in Elmira," *Star Gazette*, September 22, 2017, https://www.gannett-cdn.com/-mm-/c781fab1806d0fa346e7afdd242a2 ac22225fdff/c=0-275-1517-1132/local/-/media/2017/09/21/CNYGroup/Bing hamton/636416008341539495-Wllys-Morrow-Overland-truck-ca.-1920-600 -dpi-.jpg?width=1320&height=746&fit=crop&format=pjpg&auto=webp.

49. See Alfred Sloan, *My Years with General Motors* (New York: Doubleday & Co., 1963), 163; and Lewis Hacker, "In These Years the Company Went Into High Gear," *New York Times* [Book Review], January 19, 1964, 3.

50. William Kovarik, "Henry Ford, Charles Kettering and the Fuel of the Future," *Automotive History Review* (Spring 1998): 7–27, https://environmentalhistory. org/people/henry-ford-charles-kettering-and-the-fuel-of-the-future/, accessed April 26, 2022.

51. William Mansfield Clark to A. M. Stimson, October 11, 1922, National Archives, Record Group 90, United States Public Health Service, Washington, DC; A. P. Sloan Jr., "My Years with General Motors," in *America in the Twenties*, ed. Paul Goodman and Frank Gatell (New York: Holt, Rinehart and Winston, 1972), 34–50; C. F. Kettering, *The New Necessity* (Baltimore, MD: Williams and Wilkins, 1932), 73–79; J. C. Robert, *Ethyl* (Charlottesville: University of Virginia Press, 1983).

52. William Mansfield Clark, Memorandum to Assistant Surgeon General, A. M. Stimson (through the Acting Director, Hygienic Laboratory), October 11, 1922, National Archives, Record Group 90, U.S. Public Health Service; N. Roberts to Surgeon General, November 13, 1922, National Archives, Record Group 443, National Institutes of Health. See General Records, 0425T Box 23, for further statements on the fears of tetraethyl lead contamination.

53. H. S. Cumming, Memorandum to P. S. DuPont, December 20, 1922, National Archives, Record Group 90, U.S. Public Health Service; Thomas Midgley Jr. to H. S. Cumming, December 30, 1922, National Archives, Record Group 90, U.S. Public Health Service; G. W. McCoy, Memorandum to Surgeon General, November 23, 1922, National Archives, Record Group 90.

54. "Odd Gas Kills One, Makes Four Insane; Stricken at Work in Standard's Experiment Laboratory in Elizabeth, N.J." *New York Times*, October 27, 1924, 1. "

55. "Another Man Dies From Insanity Gas," *New York Times*, October 28, 1924, 1.

56. "Bar Ethyl Gasoline as 5th Victim Dies,"*New York Times*, October 31, 1924, 1.

57. "Third Victim Dies from Poison Gas," *New York Times*, October 29, 1924, 23.

58. New York State Department of Health, "Health News," February 2, 1925, National Archives, Record Group 90, General Files, 1924–1935, 1340–216, Tetraethyl Lead.

59. "Public Health Service Calls Conference on Leaded Gasoline," *New York Times*, May 1, 1925, 1.

60. U.S. Public Health Service, *Proceedings of a Conference to Determine Whether or Not There Is a Public Health Question in the Manufacture, Distribution or Use of Tetraethyl Lead Gasoline*, Public Health Bulletin No. 158 (Washington DC: Government Printing Office, 1925), 4, 69, 105–107.

61. U.S. Public Health Service, *Proceedings of a Conference*. Howard went on to raise the question of how to resolve the problems inherent in the public health dangers of tetraethyl lead. See T. Midgley, "Tetraethyl Lead Poison Hazards," *Industrial and Engineering Chemistry* 17 (August 1925): 827–828.

62. "Demands Fair Play for Ethyl Gasoline," *New York Times*, May 7, 1925, 10.

63. "Demands Fair Play for Ethyl Gasoline," *New York Times*, May 7, 1925, 10.

64. Y. Henderson to R. R. Sayers, January 20, 1925, National Archives, Record Group 70, 101869, File 725. Henderson pointed out the known dangers of lead to printers, painters, and other industrial workers: "I read your paper on 'Exhaust Gases from Engines Using Ethyl Gasoline' with much interest. I note that you compare the risk to that which is faced by painters. I think this comparison is very well taken, for practically all painters suffer, at one time or another, and in some cases repeatedly, from lead poisoning." See also Grace M. Burnham, Director, Workers' Health Bureau, to the Editor, *New York Times*, July 6, 1925: "If the expectations of Standard Oil officials that 15,000,000,000 gallons would be sold in the next year proves true, it would mean that 50,000 tons of lead would be distributed over the streets of the country." See also: U.S. Public Health Service, *Proceedings of a Conference*, 62, 63.

65. U.S. Public Health Service, *Proceedings of a Conference*, 108, 96; Henderson to Sayers.

66. U.S. Public Health Service, *Proceedings of a Conference*, 79.

67. U.S. Public Health Service, *Proceedings of a Conference*, 98; Alice Hamilton, "What Price Safety: Tetra-Ethyl Lead Reveals a Flaw in Our Defences," *The Survey Mid-Monthly* 54 (June 15, 1925): 333; *New York World*, May 22, 1925, 1.

68. Hamilton, "What Price Safety," 333–334.

69. For further elaboration of the committee members' positions, see "Conference of Tetraethyl Lead," *Automotive Industries* 52 (May 7, 1925): 835; "Tetraethyl Lead Sales Are Suspended," *National Petroleum News* 17 (May 27, 1925): 37; and "Ethyl Gasoline Given Clean Bill Thus Far," editorial, *American Journal of Public Health* 16 (1926): 295–296.

70. *New York Times*, January 20, 1926, 13; Charles E.-A. Winslow, professor of public health at Yale, wrote handwritten comments on the draft of the committee's report He wanted a specific statement that "a more extensive study was not possible in view of the limited time allowed to the committee" (Winslow MSS, Box 101, Folder 1805, Yale University Archive); see also other committee members' responses to the draft, Folders 1800 and 1801. For a copy of this report,

see Treasury Department, U.S. Public Health Service, *The Use of Tetraethyl Lead Gasoline in Its Relation to Public Health*, Public Health Bulletin No. 163 (Washington, DC: Government Printing Office, 1926).

71. Jerome O. Nriagu, "The Rise and Fall of Leaded Gasoline," *Science of the Total Environment* 92 (March 1990): 16, https://www.sciencedirect.com/science/article/abs/pii/0048969790903180, accessed June 8, 2022.

72. Robert A. Kehoe et al., *A Study of the Health Hazards Associated with the Distribution and Use of Ethyl Gasoline* (Cincinnati, OH: Eichberg Laboratory of Physiology, 1928).

73. Martin Cherniack, *The Hawk's Nest Incident: America's Worst Industrial Disaster* (New Haven, CT: Yale University Press, 1986).

74. Cherniack, *The Hawk's Nest Incident*, 27.

75. Cherniack, *The Hawk's Nest Incident*, 32.

76. "Village of the Living Dead," *Literary Digest*, January 25, 1936, 6.

77. C. E. Verne, "Zinc's Record Breaking Year," *American Zinc and Lead Journal* 2 (June 1916): 4. On the geological structure of the community and the technical means of early mining, our discussion draws from Arrell M. Gibson, *Wilderness Bonanza: The Tri-State District of Missouri, Kansas, and Oklahoma* (Norman: University of Oklahoma Press, 1972). Between 1905 and 1929, zinc production rose from 204,000 to 724,000 short tons and lead production from 388,000 to over 650,000 short tons. U.S. Department of Commerce, Bureau of the Census, *Historical Statistics of the United States: Colonial Times to 1957* (Washington, DC: Government Printing Office, 1960), 369; *The Story of the Tri-State Mining District* (Joplin, MO, Privately Published Souvenir Booklet, 1931), 31, 35, 7.

78. A. J. Lanza and Edwin Higgins, eds. *Pulmonary Disease Among Miners in the Joplin District, Missouri, and Its Relation to Rock Dust in the Mines: A Preliminary Report*, U.S. Bureau of Mines, Technical Paper, No. 105 (Washington, D.C.: GPO, 1915), 9, 40, 10. See also George S. Rice, "Historical Review of Silicosis," in Higgins et al., *Siliceous Dust in Relation to Pulmonary Disease, Among Miners in the Joplin District*, U.S. Bureau of Mines, Bulletin No.132 (Washington D.C.: GPO, 1917), 96. See also Alan Derickson, "'To Be His Own Benefactor': The Founding of the Coeur d'Alene Miners' Union Hospital, 1891," in *Dying for Work: Workers' Safety and Health in Twentieth-Century America*, ed. D. Rosner and G. Markowitz (Bloomington: Indiana University Press, 1987), 5. On the disastrous effect of the introduction of power drilling and dynamite on metal miners of the West, see Alan Derickson, *Workers' Health, Workers' Democracy* (Ithaca, NY: Cornell University Press, 1988). See also William J. Cassidy, "The Tri-State Zinc Lead Mining Region: Growth, Problems, and Prospects" (PhD diss., University of Pittsburgh, 1955), 530.

79. Press Committee, District No. 4, IUMMSW, Joplin, Missouri, to James Robinson, May 15, 1935, series 7-0-6-13, Records of the Division of Labor Standards, Department of Labor, National Archives, Record Group 100; James Robinson to Frances Perkins, May 23, 1935, in *"Slaves of the Depression": Workers' Letters About Life on the Job*, ed. Gerald Markowitz and David Rosner (Ithaca, NY: Cornell University Press, 1987), 134–135. In 1932 the International Union of Mine, Mill, and Smelter Workers (IUMMSW) was affiliated with the American Federation of Labor. In 1935 it was one of the unions to form the Committee on Industrial Organization, soon to break away as the Congress of Industrial Organizations (CIO).

80. E. C., Secretary, Cherokee County Central Labor Body, to "Respect Madam" [Eleanor Roosevelt], September 4, 1938, in Markowitz and Rosner, *"Slaves of the Depression,"* 140.

81. Gifford A. Cochran to Perkins, May 26, 1938, series 7-0-6-13, Records of the Division of Labor Standards; Tri-State Survey Committee, *A Preliminary Report on Living, Working, and Health, Conditions in the Tri-State Mining Area (Missouri, Oklahoma and Kansas)*, ed. Anne Couch (New York: Tri-State Survey Committee, 1939).

82. Tri-State Survey Committee, *A Preliminary Report*, 63–65.

83. "Zinc Stink," *Time*, December 4, 1939, 30; "American Plague Spot," *New Republic*, January 1, 1940, 7. See also *New York Times*, November 27, 1939, 19; and "Silicosis," *Survey* 76 (February 1940): 74–75; "Silicosis: Tri-State Dust Storm," *Business Week*, December 9, 1939, 51–52; and Evan Just, "Living and Working Conditions in the Tri-State Mining District," *Mining Congress Journal* 25 (November 1939): 44.

84. V. Zimmer to Perkins, memo, "Meeting in the Tri-State Mining Area," March 2, 1940, series 7-0-4-(3), Records of the Division of Labor Standards. See also Perkins to McTeer, March 28, 1940, Records of the Division of Labor Standards.

85. W. A. Pat Murphy to V. Zimmer, June 3, 1935, series 7-0-6-13, Records of the Division of Labor Standards; Tri-State Conference, *Proceedings*, April 23, 1940, 32, series 7-0-4-(3), Records of the Division of Labor Standards; Zimmer to Perkins, memo, "Tri-State Conference," April 8, 1940, Records of the Division of Labor Standards.

86. Evan Just, "Dust Prevention" in Just to Zimmer, December 6, 1939, National Archives Record Group 100, 7-0-6-13; Evan Just, in Tri-State Conference, *Proceedings*, 13–19.

87. Evan Just, in Tri-State Conference, *Proceedings*, 13–19; Dr. Jesse Douglas, in Tri-State Conference, *Proceedings*, 23. See Zimmer to Perkins, October 25, 1939, series 7-0-6-13, Records of the Division of Labor Standards. Others from the

Tri-State area also placed the responsibility for poor living and working conditions on the independent "American" attitudes of the workers. For example, the Rev. Titus said, "We have a group of laboring men in our state which is all American. . . . They have quite a tradition behind them; they are pretty independent. . . . Most of them own automobiles of some character. They could live, if they wanted to, in some town. . . . Most of them prefer to live down close to the mine, near the chat piles, because they would rather spend their money for something else. They are not so concerned about owning a home or renting a home that might furnish a lot of conveniences." See Rev. Titus, in Tri-State Conference, *Proceedings*, 8–9.

88. See Zimmer to Perkins, October 25, 1939, series 7-0-6-13, Records of the Division of Labor Standards.

89. Notes by R. P. B. [Blake], senior safety engineer, on Just, "Dust Prevention." For an elaboration of management's views, see Evan Just, "Statement to the Honorable Frances Perkins, Secretary of Labor, Representing the Viewpoint of Mine Operators on Living and Working Conditions in the Tri-State District," April 23, 1940, Joplin, Missouri, Office of the Secretary, Records of the Department of Labor.

90. "Silicosis (Some Pertinent Facts About This Occupational Disease for Use by the Secretary at Joplin, Missouri)," April 26, 1940, National Archives, Record Group 174, Joplin, Missouri, Office of the Secretary, Records of the Department of Labor.

91. See New York State, *Second Report of the Factory Investigating Commission*, vol. 1.

92. Frances Perkins, "Oral History," v. 4, part 2, p. 297, Columbia University Oral History Archives; Memorandum, Clara M. Beyer to the Secretary, July 16, 1936, National Archives, Record Group 174, Department of Labor, Office of the Secretary, Folder: "Labor Standards, May–Dec. 1936."

93. "Silicosis (Some Pertinent Facts)"; Frances Perkins, in Tri-State Conference, *Proceedings*, 22–24.

94. Perkins, in Tri-State Conference, *Proceedings*, 22–24.

95. Tri-State Conference, *Proceedings*, 23–24.

96. *St. Louis Post-Dispatch*, April 28, 1940, 1. Perkins's address to the miners, which boosted their morale, was initiated by the miners themselves. See Zimmer to Perkins, memo, "Tri-State Conference," April 8, 1940, series 7-0-4-(3), Records of the Division of Labor Standards; Perkins, in Tri-State Conference, *Proceedings*, 5–7, 40; Tri-State Conference, *Proceedings*, 23–24.

97. Perkins, in Tri-State Conference, *Proceedings*, 22–24.

98. Perkins, in Tri-State Conference, *Proceedings*, 22–24. Alice Hamilton, the noted industrial hygienist, supported Perkins's position in her statement to the conference: "I noticed that one or two people said that this region is thoroughly

'seeded' with tuberculosis. Why should it be? One can understand why an old neglected tenement, a slum area that has been standing in the city for a couple of generations, why those houses should be seeded with tuberculosis, but off here in the country there must be some reason for it. If that is true, then your housing problem really does become quite serious." Tri-State Conference, *Proceedings*, 40.

99. Tony McTeer, "Resume of Conditions in the Tri-State Mining Area," April 23, 1940, Office of the Secretary, Records of the Department of Labor. On labor's position, see also statement by Mr. Reed, in Tri-State Conference, *Proceedings*, 35–36. Hamilton concurred that wet drilling was inadequate to prevent silicosis. Alice Hamilton, "A Mid-American Tragedy," *Survey-Graphic* 29 (August 1940): 435.

100. *Annual Report of the Chief Inspector of Factories and Workshops for the Year 1898: Part II* (London: Her Majesty's Stationery Office, 1899), 171–172.

101. *Annual Report of the Chief Inspector*, 171–172. The following year, the inspectors expanded their observations to the dangers in the "jacketing of pipes." See *Annual Report of the Chief Inspector of Factories and Workshops for the Year 1899* (London: Her Majesty's Stationery Office, 1900). In 1906 again, the factory inspectors identified the problem: "Of all injurious dusty processes of which I have again in 1906 received repeated complaints, some, I believe surpass in injuriousness to the workers the sieving, preparing, carding and spinning processes in manufacture of asbestos." *Annual Report of the Chief Inspector of Factories and Workshops for the Year 1906* (London: Her Majesty's Stationery Office, 1907), 219.

102. Thomas Oliver, ed., *Dangerous Trades: The Historical, Social, and Legal Aspects of Industrial Occupations as Affecting Health, by a Number of Experts* (New York: E. P. Dutton, 1902), 25.

103. F. L. Hoffman, *Mortality from Respiratory Diseases in Dusty Trades (Inorganic Dusts)*, U.S. Bureau of Labor Statistics, Bulletin No. 231 (Washington, DC: Government Printing Office, 1918), 176–180; "News of the Industry," *Asbestos: A Monthly Market Journal Devoted to the Interests of the Asbestos and Magnesia Industries* 6 (October 1924): 42.

104. W. E. Cooke, "Fibrosis of the Lungs Due to the Inhalation of Asbestos Dust," *British Medical Journal* 2, no. 3317 (July 26, 1924): 147; W. E. Cooke and C. F. Hill, "Pneumokoniosis Due to Asbestos Dust," *Journal of the Royal Microscopical Society*, series 3, vol. 7 (1927): 232–238.

105. "Pulmonary Asbestosis," editorial, *Journal of the American Medical Association* 90, no. 2 (January 14, 1928): 119–120; "Pneumoconiosis Caused by Asbestos Dust," *Journal of the American Medical Association* 89 (July 23, 1927): 304, contained reports on a paper presented by Cooke and Hill at a conference of the Royal Microscopical Society.

106. E. R. A. Merewether and C. W. Price, *Report on Effects of Asbestos Dust on the Lungs and Dust Suppression in the Asbestos Industry* (London: Her Majesty's Stationery Office, 1930), 15.

107. Merewether and Price, *Report on Effects of Asbestos Dust*, 5–6.

108. United States Navy Department, Bureau of Medicine and Surgery, *Annual Report of the Surgeon General, U.S. Navy, . . . Concerning Statistics of Diseases and Injuries in the United States Navy for the Calendar Year 1939* (Washington, DC: Government Printing Office, 1941), 24; Walter E. Fleischer, Frederick J. Viles Jr., Robert Gade, and Philip Drinker, "A Health Survey of Pipe Covering Operations in Constructing Naval Vessels," *Journal of Industrial Hygiene and Toxicology* 28 (January 1946): 9–16.

109. *Memorandum on the Industrial Diseases of Silicosis and Asbestosis* (London: Her Majesty's Stationary Office, 1935), 12; William S. Fulton, "Asbestosis," Pennsylvania, Bureau of Industrial Standards, Department of Labor and Industry (Harrisburg, Pa.: Pennsylvania Department of Labor and Industry 1935, 8; S. B. McPheeters, "A Survey of a Group of Employees Exposed to Asbestos Dust," *Journal of Industrial Hygiene and Toxicology* 18 (April 1936): 229–239.

110. Theodore C. Waters, "Legal Aspects of the Dust Diseases," *Pit and Quarry* 30 (December 1937): 59–61.

111. S. Roodhouse Gloyne, "Two Cases of Squamous Carcinoma of the Lung Occurring in Asbestosis," *Tubercle* 17 (October 1935): 5–10; K. M. Lynch and W. Atmar Smith, "Pulmonary Asbestosis III: Carcinoma of Lung in Asbesto-Silicosis," *American Journal of Cancer* 24 (1935): 56–64; Dan S. Egbert and Arthur J. Geiger, "Pulmonary Asbestosis and Carcinoma," *American Review of Tuberculosis* 34 (1936): 143–150; C. S. Anderson and J. Henry Dible, "Silicosis and Carcinoma of the Lung," *Journal of Hygiene* 38 (1938): 185–204.

112. W. C. Hueper, *Occupational Tumours and Allied Diseases* (Springfield, IL: Charles C. Thomas, 1942), 400, 403–404; W. C. Hueper, "Industrial Management and Occupational Cancer," *JAMA* 131 (June 29, 1946): 738–741; W. C. Hueper, "Significance of Industrial Cancer in the Problem of Cancer," *Occupational Medicine* 2 (1946): 190–200; W. C. Hueper, "Cancer in Its Relation to Occupation and Environment," American Society of the Control of Cancer, *Bulletin* 23 (1943): 63–69.

113. Milestone Documents, "President Dwight D. Eisenhower's Farewell Address," National Archives, https://www.archives.gov/milestone-documents/president-dwight-d-eisenhowers-farewell-address, accessed November 14, 2023. See also Kai Bird and Martin Sherwin, *American Prometheus: The Triumph and Tragedy of J. Robert Oppenheimer* (New York: Vintage, 2006), for a vivid description of the different fears the bomb instilled in many Americans.

114. Hibbert Winslow Hill, *The New Public Health* (New York: Macmillan, 1916), 8. See Amy Fairchild, David Rosner, James Colgrove, Ronald Bayer, and Linda Fried, "The Exodus of Public Health: What History Can Tell Us About the Future," *American Journal of Public Health* 100 (January 2010): 54–63, for a fuller account of the transformation of public health in the twentieth century.

115. Susan Reverby, *Examining Tuskegee: The Infamous Syphilis Study and Its Legacy* (Chapel Hill: University of North Carolina Press, 2009); Susan Reverby, *Tuskegee Truths: Rethinking the Tuskegee Syphilis Study* (Chapel Hill: University of North Carolina Press, 2012).

116. Fairchild, Rosner, Colgrove, Bayer, and Fried, "The Exodus of Public Health," 54–63.

6. BETTER LIVING THROUGH CHEMISTRY?

1. E. Vynnycky and P.E.M. Fine, "Interpreting the Decline in Tuberculosis: The Role of Secular Trends in Effective Contact," *International Journal of Epidemiology* 28, no. 2 (1999): 327–334.

2. University of California, "Life Expectancy in the USA, 1900–98," https://u.demog.berkeley.edu/~andrew/1918/figure2.html, accessed October 30, 2023.

3. Centers for Disease Control and Prevention, National Center for Health Statistics, *Health, United States, 2020–2021*, Table 4, "Life Expectancy at Birth, at Age 65, and at Age 75, by Sex, Race, and Hispanic Origin: United States, Selected Years, 1900–2018," https://www.cdc.gov/nchs/hus/data-finder.htm?year=2019&table=Table%20004, accessed July 22, 2023.

4. National Center for Health Statistics, Department of Health Education and Welfare, "Use of Vital and Health Records in Epidemiologic Research," *Vital Health Statistics* 4, no. 7 (March 1968): vi. While it has never been shown that the surgeon general, William Stewart, ever specifically declared infectious diseases in decline, and there are many instances when he affirmed the Public Health Service's attention to them, it is also clear that many subscribed to this general idea of the ascendancy of chronic conditions. See Brad Spellberg and Bonnie Taylor-Blake, "On the Exoneration of Dr. William H. Stewart: Debunking an Urban Legend," *Infectious Diseases of Poverty* 2, no. 1 (2013), https://www.ncbi.nlm.nih.gov/pmc/articles/PMC3707092/#B9, accessed January 9, 2021.

5. "Introduction," in *Vital Statistics of the United States: 1955* (Washington, DC: Government Printing Office, 1957), 1: xlvii.

6. E. R. A. Merewether, "The Pneumokonioses: Developments, Doubts, and Difficulties," *Canadian Medical Journal* 62, no. 2 (February 1950): 169–170.

7. Merewether, "The Pneumokonioses," 170.

8. Richard Doll and A. Bradford Hill, "The Mortality of Doctors in Relation to their Smoking Habits," *British Medical Journal*, June 26, 1954, pp. 1451–1455.

9. See Keith Wailoo, *Pushing Cool: Big Tobacco, Racial Marketing, and the Untold Story of the Menthol Cigarette* (Chicago: University of Chicago Press, 2021), for a detailed discussion of the tobacco industry's targeting of African Americans.

10. Paul Blanc, *Fake Silk: The Lethal History of Viscose Rayon* (New Haven, CT: Yale University Press, 2016), presents a fascinating history of the production of rayon; see also Audra Wolfe, "Nylon: A Revolution in Textiles," *Chemical Heritage*, Fall 2008, 21–23.

11. See Paul Boyer, *By the Bomb's Early Light: American Thought and Culture at the Dawn of the Atomic Age* (Chapel Hill: University of North Carolina Press, 1994).

12. Series P30-133, "Total Capital in Major Branches of Manufacture,"*Historical Statistics of the United States, Colonial Times to 1957*, U.S. Department of Commerce, Bureau of the Census, (Washington: GPO, 1960), 411, 413.

13. Manufacturing Chemists' Association, "Ad Hoc Planning Committee on Environmental Health," Minutes, June 24–25, 1963, 2, MCA Papers in possession of the authors.

14. See, for example, "Duck and Cover—Bert the Turtle" (produced in 1951), https://www.youtube.com/watch?v=IKqXu-5jw60, or "Bombproof," https://www.youtube.com/watch?v=b114xlklDVg, accessed January 9, 2022. Boyer, *By the Bomb's Early Light.*

15. Two industry spokespeople decried "the attitude of smugness which associates atmospheric pollution with industrial prosperity and ignores the desirability of its reduction." W. C. L. Hemeon and T. F. Hatch, "Atmospheric Pollution," *Industrial and Engineering Chemistry* 39 (May 1947): 568. See also Robert E. Swain, "Smoke and Fume Investigations: A Historical Review," *Industrial and Engineering Chemistry* 41, no. 11 (November 1949): 2383–2388.

16. W. Michael McCabe, "Donora Disaster Was Crucible for Clean Air," Pennsylvania Department of Environmental Protection, October 26, 1998, www .dep.state.pa.us/dep/Rachel_Carson/crucible.htm. It was estimated that the air contained between 1,500 and 5,500 micrograms per cubic meter of sulfur dioxide emissions (whereas today's Clean Air Act mandates a maximum average of 80 ug/m³).

17. Erin Peterman, "A Cloud with a Silver Lining: The Killer Smog in Donora, 1948," (Pennsylvania Center for the Book, 2009), Available at: https://pabook .libraries.psu.edu/literary-cultural-heritage-map-pa/feature-articles/cloud -silver-lining-killer-smog-donora-1948, Accessed: March 25, 2024.

18. Paul L. Magill, "The Los Angeles Smog Problem," *Industrial and Engineering Chemistry* 41, no. 11 (November 1949): 2476–2486. See Merlin Chowkwanyun, *All Health Politics Is Local: Community Battles for Medical Care and Environmental Health* (Chapel Hill: University of North Carolina Press, 2022).

19. Robert T. Reinhardt, "West Coast: Smog Ceases to be a Joke to Industrialists Spending Millions of $ for Control of Waste Gases," *Iron Age* 163 (April 14, 1949): 104.

20. See Devra Davis, *When Smoke Ran like Water: Tales of Environmental Deception and the Battle Against Pollution* (New York: Basic Books, 2002), especially 42–48.

21. Manufacturing Chemists' Association, Air Pollution Abatement Committee, "Minutes of Meeting," April 21, 1954, MCA Papers in possession of the authors.

22. John C. Ruddock, "Proceedings," Meeting of the Subcommittee on Atmospheric Pollutants, Medical Advisory Committee, American Petroleum Institute, National Archives, Record Group 90 (Public Health Service), Air Pollution Medical Branch, Project Records, 1955–1960, 241.5, box 6. See also Leon O. Emik, Chief, Laboratory Investigations, Air Pollution Medical Program, to Chief, Air Pollution Medical Program, "Visit with Dr. John C. Ruddock, May 15, 1958," May 29, 1958, National Archives, Record Group 90 (Public Health Service), Air Pollution Medical Branch, Project Records, 1955–1960, 241.5, box 6; John C. Ruddock, "Statement by Chairman, Subcommittee on Atmospheric Pollutants," June 22, 1959, National Archives, Record Group 90 (Public Health Service), Air Pollution Medical Branch, Project Records, 1955–1960, 241.5, box 6.

23. Ruddock, "Proceedings"; see also Emik, "Visit with Dr. John C. Ruddock," and Ruddock, "Statement by Chairman."

24. Jes Fenger, "Air Pollution in the Last 50 Years—From Local to Global," *Atmospheric Environment* 43, no. 1 (January 2009): 14.

25. Chowkwanyun, *All Health Politics Is Local*; Davis, *When Smoke Ran like Water*, 80–84.

26. Manufacturing Chemists' Association, Public Relations Advisory Committee, "Report of Glen Perry, Chairman," "Minutes of the 115th Meeting of the Directors of the MCA," February 13, 1962, MCA Papers.

27. Manufacturing Chemists' Association, Air Pollution Abatement Committee, "Minutes of Meeting," February 7–8, 1962, MCA Papers.

28. Dan Pontefract, "What's Good for Our Country Was Good for General Motors," *Forbes*, November 26, 2018, https://www.forbes.com/sites/danpontefract/2018/11/26/whats-good-for-our-country-was-good-for-general-motors/?sh=43a0cf2b2075.

29. Linda Lear, *Rachel Carson: Witness for Nature* (New York: Henry Holt, 1997), 429.

30. Rachel Carson, *Silent Spring* (New York: Houghton Mifflin, 1962), 5–6.

31. Rachel Carson, *Silent Spring*, 10. The National Agricultural Chemicals Association, the trade association for pesticide manufacturers, and the Manufacturing Chemists' Association, which led the attack on Carson and her writings, sent "out a steady stream of brochures and bulletins denouncing things that Carson had never said and circulating 'fact kits' to members." See Lear, *Rachel Carson*, 431.

32. David Rosner and Gerald Markowitz, "Persistent Pollutants: A Brief History of the Discovery of the Widespread Toxicity of Chlorinated Hydrocarbons," *Environmental Research* 120 (January 2013): 126–133.

33. Manufacturing Chemists' Association, Minutes, Environmental Health Council, "Chart of Proposed Organization," v, vi, attached to MCA, "Recommendations of the Ad-Hoc Planning Committee on Environmental Health" draft, August 13, 1963.

34. James Sterner, Chair, Environmental Health Advisory Committee, "Report to the Board of Directors of the Manufacturing Chemists' Association, Inc.," March 14, 1967, MCA Papers.

35. J. Brooks Flippen, *Nixon and the Environment* (Albuquerque: University of New Mexico Press, 2000), 46.

36. Flippen, *Nixon and the Environment*, 85.

37. Flippen, *Nixon and the Environment*, 25.

38. George Best to Environmental Health Committee, January 20, 1970, MCA Papers.

39. See David Vogel, *Fluctuating Fortunes: The Political Power of Business in America* (New York: Basic Books, 1989), 69.

40. Riley E. Dunlap, "Trends in Public Opinion Toward Environmental Issues: 1965–1990," in *American Environmentalism: The U.S. Environmental Movement, 1970–1990*, ed. Riley E. Dunlap and Angela G. Mertig (Philadelphia: Taylor and Francis, 1992), 92.

41. Robert Gottlieb, *Forcing the Spring: The Transformation of the American Environmental Movement* (Washington, DC: Island Press, 1993), 96.

42. In fact, David Vogel argues that the strong "performance of the economy" was critical to the "upsurge of citizen activism during the late 1960s and early 1970s." See Vogel, *Fluctuating Fortunes*, 96.

43. Flippen, *Nixon and the Environment*, 5. David Vogel points out that between 1966 and 1968 eight significant pieces of consumer legislation were enacted, including the Truth in Lending Act, the Flammable Fabrics Act, the Fair Packaging and Labeling Act, and the Child Protection Act. See Vogel, *Fluctuating Fortunes*, 38; Samuel Hays, *Beauty, Health, and Permanence: Environmental Politics in the United States, 1955–1985* (Cambridge: Cambridge University Press, 1987); Martin V. Melosi, "Lyndon Johnson and Environmental Policy," in *The Johnson Years*, vol. 2: *Vietnam, the Environment, and Science* (Lawrence:

University Press of Kansas, 1987), 115–117; and Hal K. Rothman, *The Greening of a Nation? Environmentalism in the United States Since 1945* (Fort Worth, TX: Harcourt Brace, 1998), 101–103.

44. Hays, *Beauty, Health, and Permanence*; Melosi, "Lyndon Johnson and Environmental Policy," 115–117.

45. Charles Noble, *Liberalism at Work: The Rise and Fall of OSHA* (Philadelphia: Temple University Press, 1986), 70. Coal miners working with the Black Lung Association and physicians such as Loren Kerr also demanded improvements in working conditions, and compensation was perhaps the most important action around safety and health in the decade.

46. Noble, *Liberalism at Work*, 70.

47. Interview with Anthony Mazzocchi, January 25, 2001.

48. Tony Mazzocchi, "Introduction," in *A Collection of Documents from the OCAW Struggle for Worker Health and Safety* (Washington, DC: Alice Hamilton College, 1998).

49. Tony Mazzocchi, "Foreword," in *Hazards of the Industrial Environment*, proceedings of conference sponsored by District 8 Council, Oil, Chemical and Atomic Workers International Union, Holiday Inn, Kenilworth, NJ, March 29, 1969, 2.

50. Mazzocchi, "Foreword," 2.

51. Interview with Tony Mazzocchi, January 26, 2001, New York City.

52. Ray Davidson, *Peril on the Job: A Study of Hazards in the Chemical Industries* (Washington, DC: Public Affairs Press, 1970), 184–185.

53. See Laura Pulido, *Environmentalism and Economic Justice: Two Chicano Struggles in the Southwest* (Tuscon: University of Arizona Press, 1996), especially chap. 3.

54. Erik Wallenberg, "Staging Nature: Environmental Crises in War, Housing, and Labor" (PhD diss., City University of New York, 2023), 355.

55. Linda Nash, *Inescapable Ecologies: A History of Environment, Disease, and Knowledge* (Berkeley: University of California Press, 2007), 128.

56. CBS News, Edward R. Murrow, narrator, *Harvest of Shame*, documentary, 1960, Youtube.com/results?search_query=harvest+of +shame, accessed February 20, 2023.

57. Linda Nash, "The Fruits of Ill-Health: Pesticides and Workers' Bodies in Post-World War II California," *Osiris*, 2nd series, 19 (2004): 203–219. We thank Erik Wallenberg for this and other references to the farmworkers' struggle.

58. Lori A. Flores, *Grounds for Dreaming: Mexican Americans, Mexican Immigrants, and the California Farmworkers Movement*, (New Haven: Yale University Press, 2016), 194-195.

59. Nash, *Inescapable Ecologies*, 164, 166, 167.

60. Quoted in Chad Montrie, *Making a Living: Work and Environment in the United States* (Chapel Hill: University of North Carolina Press, 2008), 124.

61. Nash, *Inescapable Ecologies*, 164, 166, 167.

62. Montrie, *Making a Living*; Wallenberg, "Staging Nature."

63. Montrie, *Making a Living*, 125.

64. Nash, *Inescapable Ecologies*, 164, 166, 167.

65. Noble, *Liberalism at Work*, 93–96. The section referred to is 6B[5].

66. Paul Brodeur, "The Magic Mineral," *New Yorker*, October 12, 1968, 117–165.

67. See, for example, the extensive literature on the history of asbestos, including David Rosner, Gerald Markowitz, and Merlin Chowkwanyun, "'Nondetected': The Politics of Measurement of Asbestos in Talc, 1971–1976," *American Journal of Public Health* 109, no. 7 (July 2019): 969–974; David Rosner and Gerald Markowitz, "'Unleashed on an Unsuspecting World': The Asbestos Information Association and Its Role in Perpetuating a National Epidemic," *American Journal of Public Health* 106, no. 5 (May 2016): 834–840; and Barry Castleman, *Asbestos: Medical and Legal Aspects*, 5th ed. (Boston: Aspen, 2004).

68. See Gerald Markowitz and David Rosner, *Deadly Dust: Silicosis and the Politics of Industrial Disease* (Princeton, NJ: Princeton University Press, 1991), for an extensive review of its history.

69. See Gerald Markowitz and David Rosner, *Lead Wars: The Politics of Science and the Fate of America's Children* (Berkeley: University of California Press, 2014), for a full account of the growing attention to lead poisoning in the 1960s–1990s; and Gerald Markowitz and David Rosner, *Deceit and Denial: The Deadly Politics of Industrial Pollution* (Berkeley: University of California Press /Milbank Memorial Fund, 2002).

70. See Markowitz and Rosner, *Deceit and Denial*, for an extended discussion of the 1960s and 1970s controversy.

71. Still others, particularly young physicians, joined groups like the Medical Committee for Human Rights or read the newly emerging progressive health-focused publications like *Health PAC Bulletin*, or *Science for the People* and saw in OSHA and NIOSH opportunities to fulfill their goals as both scientists and socially progressive citizens.

72. During the Obama administration, he was appointed to the President's Advisory Board on Radiation and Worker Health. See "President Obama Appoints Hunter Professor Emeritus Kotelchuck to Key Post," *Hunter College News*, https://www.hunter.cuny.edu/communications/news/top-featured-stories/president-obama-appoints-hunter-professor-emeritus-kotelchuck-to-key-post, accessed August 24, 2023. See also http://www.davidkotelchuck.net/pages/aboutdavid.html.

73. See Stellman's substantial contributions to women and work: *Women's Work, Women's Health: Myths and Realities* (New York: Pantheon, 1977); *Office Work Can Be Dangerous to Your Health: A Handbook of Office Health and Safety Hazards and What You Can Do About Them* (New York: Pantheon, 1984); *Too Little, Too Late: Dealing with the Health Needs of Women in Poverty* (New York: Routledge, 1989); and *Work Is Dangerous to Your Health: A Handbook of Health Hazards in the Workplace and What You Can Do About Them* (New York: Pantheon, 1973); and others.

74. Victor Cohn, "Occupational Safety, Health Chief Fired," *Washington Post*, March 6, 1981, https://www.washingtonpost.com/archive/politics/1981/03/06/occupational-safety-health-chief-fired/76c96b05-cac5-43c0-97e3-94f93fb52eef/, accessed December 26, 2022. Robbins was fired at the start of the Reagan administration's reign.

75. Dennis C. Williams, "The Guardian: EPA's Formative Years, 1970–1973," U.S. Environmental Protection Agency, September 1993, https://www.epa.gov/archive/epa/aboutepa/guardian-epas-formative-years-1970-1973.html, accessed July 22, 2023.

76. Charles Reich, "Reflections: The Greening of America," *New Yorker*, September 26, 1970, 42; See also Charles Reich, *The Greening of America* (New York: Random House, 1970).

77. Reich, "Reflections," 44.

78. Reich, "Reflections," 42.

79. Reich, "Reflections," 42.

80. Reich, "Reflections," 79–80.

81. Reich, "Reflections," 42.

82. Lewis Powell to Eugene Sydnor, "Confidential Memorandum—Attack on American Free Enterprise System," August 23, 1971, https://www.historyisaweapon.com/defcon1/powellmemo.html, accessed January 15, 2023. See also Sheldon Whitehouse, *The Scheme: How the Right Wing Used Dark Money to Capture the Supreme Court* (New York: New Press, 2022), 39–43, which places this memo in the context of the contemporary capture of SCOTUS today.

83. Powell to Sydnor, "Confidential Memorandum."

84. Powell to Sydnor, "Confidential Memorandum."

85. Powell to Sydnor, "Confidential Memorandum."

86. Powell to Sydnor, "Confidential Memorandum."

87. Powell to Sydnor, "Confidential Memorandum."

88. Powell to Sydnor, "Confidential Memorandum."

89. Among them were the following: The *CATO Institute*, founded 1974, is a libertarian think tank dedicated to "the traditional American principles of limited government, individual liberty, free markets, and peace"; see https://www.cato.org/about. The *Alexander Hamilton Society* is dedicated "to identify, educate,

and launch young men and women into foreign policy and national security careers" in part because "American universities are not providing our young people with an education that allows them to understand what they are defending and why"; its principles include that "America's greatness is the result of its commitment to individual liberty, limited government, economic freedom, the rule of law, human dignity, and democracy"; see Alexander Hamilton Society, "What We Believe," https://www.alexanderhamiltonsociety.org/what-we-believe, accessed February 13, 2023. The *Heritage Foundation*, founded in 1973, promotes "public policies based on the principles of free enterprise, limited government, individual freedom, traditional American values, and a strong national defense"; it prides itself on being a home to Friedrich Hayek and Milton Friedman; see https://www.heritage.org/about-heritage/mission. The *Manhattan Institute*, founded in 1977, considers itself "a leading free-market think tank" focusing on "Economic Growth, Education, Energy and Environment, Health Care, Legal Reform, Public Sector, Race, & Urban Policy." The *Free Congress Foundation*, founded in 1977, is a conservative think tank founded by Paul Weyrich, a "religious conservative political activist." The *Ethics and Public Policy Center*, founded in 1976, considers itself the "premier institute working to apply the riches of the Judeo-Christian tradition to contemporary questions of law, culture and politics"; see eppc.org, accessed February 13, 2023. The *Heartland Institute*'s mission is "to discover, develop, and promote free-market solutions to social and economic problems"; see Heartland.org, accessed February 13, 2023. The *American Enterprise Institute* is among the few conservative think tanks founded earlier, in 1938; see AEI, "Koch Brothers," https://www.aei.org/tag/koch-brothers/, accessed February 13, 2023.

90. Whitehouse, *The Scheme*.

91. Paul Brodeur, "The Magic Mineral," *New Yorker*, October 12, 1968, 117–165. In 1971, OSHA lowered the "permissible exposure limit," or PEL (the average exposure of a workers over an eight-hour day), substantially and lowered it further the next year.

92. U.S. Department of Labor, Occupational Safety and Health Administration, "Occupational Exposure to Asbestos," August 10, 1994, https://www.osha.gov/laws-regs/federalregister/1994-08-10, accessed December 24, 2022.

93. Matthew Swetonic, "Presentation," Asbestos Textile Institute, June 7, 1973 Available at: at: https://www.toxicdocs.org/d/4LwXVawbaOOOvNO24mg RZ7Bx?lightbox=1, accessed: March 25, 2024. For extended discussions of the role of Hill & Knowlton in developing strategies for toxic industries, see Allan Brandt, *The Cigarette Century: The Rise, Fall, and Deadly Persistence of the Product That Defined America* (New York: Basic Books,

2007); and Robert Proctor, *Golden Holocaust: The Origins of the Cigarette Catastrophe and the Case for Abolition* (Berkeley: University of California Press, 2011).

94. M. Swetonic, "Presentation, Asbestos Textile Institute," typescript, June 7, 1973, https://www.toxicdocs.org/d/rpow6N87j9jBLvzJpNpoqDzpV?lightbox=1, accessed January 28, 2023.

95. See Altria Group, "Reduce the Harm of Tobacco Products," marketing material, https://www.altria.com/en/moving-beyond-smoking/reduce-the-harm-of-to-bacco-products, accessed November 15, 2023.

96. Elmer Wheeler, "Interview with Elmer Wheeler on May 12, 1972," https://www.toxicdocs.org/d/p22BG1LowaJY6xQZMMXdrboD6?lightbox=1, accessed May 11, 2022.

97. Ira Katznelson, *Fear Itself: The New Deal and the Origins of Our Time* (New York: Liveright, 2013).

98. American Petroleum Institute, *API Toxicological Review: Benzene*, September 1948, 2–6, https://www.documentcloud.org/documents/1373098-00010795.

99. American Petroleum Institute, *API Toxicological Review: Benzene*, 3.

100. A few examples of references to the dangers during the 1930s include the following: F. B. Flinn and N. E. Jarvik, "Action of Certain Chlorinated Naphthalenes on the Liver," *Proceedings of the Society for Experimental Biology and Medicine* 35, no. 1 (1936): 118–120; William B. Fulton and Julia L. Matthews, *A Preliminary Report of the Dermatological and Systemic Effects of Exposure to Hexachloro-Naphthalene and Chloro-Diphenyl*, Special Bulletin No. 43 (Harrisburg: Bureau of Industrial Standards, Pennsylvania Department of Labor and Industry, 1936); Jack W. Jones and Herbert S. Alden, "An Acneform Dermatergosis," *Archives of Dermatology and Syphilology* 33 (1936): 1022–1034; Louis Schwartz, "Dermatitis from Synthetic Resins and Waxes," *American Journal of Public Health* 26 (June 1936): 586–591; Monsanto Manuscripts, *Diphenyl and Chlorinated Diphenyl Derivatives*, June 1935, https://cdn.toxicdocs.org/ba/baaaYyD2zXZ2ednN3rMpo2q16/baaaYyD2zXZ2ednN3rMpo2q16.pdf.

101. Monsanto Manuscripts, *Diphenyl*.

102. Cecil K. Drinker, Madeline Field Warren, and Granville A. Bennett, "The Problem of Possible Systemic Effects from Certain Chlorinated Hydrocarbons," *Journal of Industrial Hygiene and Toxicology* 19 (September 1937): 283–311; Granville A. Bennett, Cecil Drinker, and Madeleine Field Warren, "Morphological Changes in the Livers of Rats Resulting from Exposure to Certain Chlorinated Hydrocarbons," *Journal of Industrial Hygiene and Toxicology* 20 (February 1938): 97–123; Cecil Drinker, "Report to the Monsanto Chemical Company," September 15, 1938, in possession of the authors; Leonard Greenburg, May R.

Mayers, and Adelaide Ross Smith, "The Systemic Effects Resulting from Exposure to Certain Chlorinated Hydrocarbons," *Journal of Industrial Hygiene and Toxicology* 21 (February 1939): 29–38.

103. K. Herxheimer, "Chloracne," *Munshener Medizinische Wochenschrift* 47 (1899): 278, as noted in J. R. Allen, L. J. Abrahamson, and D. H. Norback, "Biological Effects of Polychlorinated Biphenyls and Triphenyls on the Subhuman Primate," *Environmental Research* 6, no. 3 (September 1973): 344–354.

104. See Gerald Markowitz and David Rosner, "Monsanto, PCBs, and the Creation of a 'World-wide Ecological Problem,'" *Journal of Public Health Policy* 39, no. 4 (November 2018): 463–540, for more detailed descriptions of Monsanto and PCB pollution.

105. David Rosner and Gerald Markowitz, "A 'Gift of God'? The Public Health Controversy over Leaded Gasoline During the 1920s," *American Journal of Public Health* 75, no. 4 (April 1985): 344–352; David Rosner and Gerald Markowitz, "Safety and Health on the Job as a Class Issue: The Workers' Health Bureau of America in the 1920s," *Science and Society* 48, no. 4 (Winter 1984–1985): 466–482.

106. See Paul Blanc, *Fake Silk: The Lethal History of Viscose Rayon* (New Haven, CT: Yale University Press, 2016).

107. Wilhelm Hueper, *Occupational Tumours and Allied Diseases* (Springfield, IL: Charles Thomas, 1942), 347. In 1948 Hueper became the director of the National Cancer Institute's Environmental Cancer Section and remained in that position until the early 1960s.

108. "Found! Three Industries That Can't Use Aroclors," *Saturday Evening Post*, 1946.

109. See ads for "electrical living": https://www.youtube.com/watch?v=7Fwramn5U3M.

110. Alice Hamilton, "The Toxicity of the Chlorinated Hydrocarbons," *Yale Journal of Biology and Medicine* 15, no. 6 (July 1943): 787–801. Robert Proctor, *Cancer Wars: How Politics Shape What We Know About Cancer* (New York: Basic Books, 1995), 46; Hueper, *Occupational Tumours*.

111. "Paul Müller: Biographical," Nobelprize.org, Official Website of the Nobel Prize, http://www.nobelprize.org/nobel_prizes/medicine/laureates/1948/muller-bio .htmlS, accessed July 24, 2012.

112. O. G. Fitzhugh and A. A. Nelson, "The Chronic Oral Toxicity of DDT," *Journal of Pharmacology and Experimental Therapeutics* 89, no. 1 (January 1947): 18–30.

113. Franklin C. Bing, "Chemicals Introduced in Foods," *American Journal of Public Health* 45, no. 5 (May 1955): 681–682; H. B. Haag, J. K. Finnegan, P. S. Larson, M. L. Dreyfuss, R. T. J. Main, and W. Riese, "Comparative Chronic Toxicity for Warm-Blooded Animals," *Industrial Medicine and Surgery* 17, no. 12 (December 1948): 477–484.

114. "Chemicals in Food Products," *Hearings Before the House Select Committee to Investigate the Use of Chemicals in Food Products*, 81st Cong. (1951) (testimony

of Dr. James O. Clarke, Director, Division of Program Research, Food and Drug Administration), 65.

115. "Chemicals in Food Products," *Hearings* (testimony of Dr. Paul A. Neal, Director, Public Health Service).

116. "Chemicals in Food Products," *Hearings* (testimony of Dr. Morton S. Biskind), 700–701, 713.

117. "Chemicals in Food Products," *Hearings* (testimony of Dr. Morton S. Biskind), 335.

118. "Chemicals in Food Products," *Hearings* (testimony of Dr. Morton S. Biskind), 337.

119. J. M. Barnes, "Toxic Hazards of Certain Pesticides to Man," *Bulletin of the World Health Organization* 8 (1953): 466. Monsanto had reason to worry that the link of DDT to other chlorinated hydrocarbons would easily be made. As early as 1948, Monsanto officials were suggesting the "possible use of liquid Aroclors as an auxiliary solvent for DDT and other insecticides in various formulations." See Benignus to E. W. Leake, U.S. Department of Agriculture, "Aroclors and MB-40," June 17, 1948, Available at: https://www.toxicdocs.org/d/qmajxOg5vmqr5j3Y3Ea5domo5?lightbox=1, Accessed: March 24, 2024.

120. H. Stilwell, "Farm Fallout Can Kill You!," *True* (March 1960). Quoted in A. P. Davies, American Meat Institute, to E. L. Peterson, Assistant Secretary, USDA, March 4, 1960, National Archives, Record Group 16, Records of the Office of the Secretary of Agriculture, General Correspondence, box 3455; Mrs. A. J. Jr. to E. L. Peterson, Assistant Secretary, USDA, March 4, 1960, National Archives, Record Group 16, Records of the Office of the Secretary of Agriculture, General Correspondence, box 3455.

121. See Markowitz and Rosner, "Monsanto, PCBs," 463–540; and Rosner and Markowitz, "Persistent Pollutants," 126–133, for fuller accounts of these issues.

122. P. G. Benignus, memo, "Aroclor Use to Increase the Insecticidal Life of Lindane," August 9, 1957, https://cdn.toxicdocs.org/jm/jmR3VMwvoxnVovaKqzLMMNmyQ/jmR3VMwvoxnVovaKqzLMMNmyQ.pdf; L. V. Sherwood to P. G. Benignus, "Re: 'Aroclor Use to Increase the Insecticidal Life of Lindane,'" August 30, 1957.

123. Markowitz and Rosner, "Monsanto, PCBs," 463–540.

124. "The Desolate Year," *Monsanto Magazine*, October 1962, 4–9.

125. Soren Jensen and Gunner Widmark, "Presence of Polychlorinated Biphenyls at Residue of Biological Samples," September 1, 1966, Available at: https://www.toxicdocs.org/d/kmabGzY6J6KM576mZJNZbVjrO?lightbox=1, Accesssed: March 24, 2024; D. V. N. Hardy to Benignus et al., "Aroclor—Sweden," January 12, 1967, Available at: https://www.toxicdocs.org/d/gb57aK1abE5mBE oVYw6wLGLYL?lightbox=1, Accessed: March 24, 2024; Henry Strand, Rising and Strand, Sweden, to David Wood, Monsanto, Brussels, November 28, 1966,

https://www.toxicdocs.org/d/aJR6mQe7gX3Yn5VLgrmgKdbYR?lightbox=1, accessed November 4, 2021.

126. D. H. Hardy to Kelly, February 21, 1967, Available at: https://www.toxicdocs .org/d/4aK0E4K49XaxbovyBk5vYb5Vj?lightbox=1 Accessed: March 24, 2024; Strand to Wood, November 28, 1966, Available at: https://www.toxicdocs .org/d/bygGLLJDODkv1de4qVv4yyOo6?lightbox=1, Accessed: March 24, 2024.

127. David Perlman, "A Menacing New Pollutant," *San Francisco Chronicle*, February 24, 1969, 1, 20.

128. Joan H. Rivers to Charles Sommer Jr., February 26, 1969, https://www.toxicdocs .org/d/NK78DEvKKyQQZVyb8ZR25yD8?lightbox=1, accessed November 5, 2021.

129. Memo, P. G. Benignus and N. T. Johnson to various employees, "Pollution Studies," March 3, 1969 Available at: https://www.toxicdocs.org/d/XMMNQBxx71QX7 xxd9zOQEpqw?lightbox=1, Accessed: March 24, 2024 .

130. PCB Committee, August 25, 1969, handwritten notes, https://www.toxicdocs .org/d/X7JKvqo1ExZb77QZ857rM8y7d?lightbox=1, accessed November 13, 2021.

131. "Production and Sales: Polychlorinated Biphenyls (PCB): Monsanto Industrial Chemicals Company (Short Tons)," table, https://www.toxicdocs.org/d/JDGjnm D3DzKD22vmBV5k8ZKO?lightbox=1, accessed November 13, 2021.

132. "Possible Customers' Questions on PCBs' Publicity," Q and A for sales reps, https://www.toxicdocs.org/d/zbovDwKrZ1LgExZVr9e1j30da?lightbox=1, accessed November 13, 2021.

133. See Robert Metcalf, "Report and Comments on Meeting on Chlorinated Biphenyls in the Environment at Industrial Biotest Laboratories," Chicago, March 21, 1969, https://www.toxicdocs.org/d/2JqOqNKQJDM8xMogejnbDepeg?lightbox=1, accessed June 15, 2022.

134. William Boyd, "Making Meat: Science, Technology, and American Poultry Production," *Technology and Culture* 42, no. 4 (October 2001): 635.

135. William Boyd, Michael Watts, and D. Goodman, "Agro-Industrial Just-in-Time: The Chicken Industry and Postwar American Capitalism," in *Globalizing Food: Agrarian Questions and Global Restructuring*, ed. David Goodman and Michael Watts (London: Routledge, 1997), 145.

136. Jack D. Early, Monsanto, to G. Papageorge, February 2, 1971, https://www .toxicdocs.org/d/mpx8bNqz5nR8qEoq9YKm78n3B?lightbox=1, accessed: February 21, 2021.

137. Early to Papageorge.

138. Early to Papageorge.

139. Early to Papageorge.

140. Gossage to Fallon, "Therminol FR Fluids," July 16, 1971, Available at: https:// www.toxicdo143cs.org/d/MG53edYoN653VDMe2ereEQbEM?lightbox=1, Accessed: March 24, 2024.

141. "Farm Unit, Producers Hunt for Chickens Tied to Contaminated Feed," *Wall Street Journal*, July 26, 1971, https://www.toxicdocs.org/d/zdmo30oryyZJbD zdwkB3Xq4Ga?lightbox=1, accessed June 15, 2022.

142. "The Menace of PCB," *Time*, October 11, 1971, https://www.toxicdocs.org/d /J39VG4MB1q0ONgwEVvpaBb97B?lightbox=1, accessed June 16, 2022.

143. William Blase Company Confidential, "Confidential Legal Opinion," *PCB Legal Review*, December 6, 1971, 1–39.

144. "Background Statement by Environmental Protection Agency Administrator, Russell E. Train, at a Press Conference on PCBs," December 22, 1975, https://www.toxicdocs.org/d/pe8qv17NDZK7zqYnzBLwdB52E, accessed January 9, 2022.

145. Train to Hanley, December 22, 1975, https://www.toxicdocs.org/d/rEJvvvmR8 Lo9JZmyYVdnOdNr?lightbox=1, accessed January 9, 2022.

146. D. R. Bishop, "EPA/PCB Press Conference," December 22, 1975, https://www .toxicdocs.org/d/85XxDg2beZbar4LmveLaKEzOa?lightbox=1, accessed January 9, 2022.

146. Environmental Protection Agency, "Summary of the Toxic Substances Control Act," https://www.epa.gov/laws-regulations/summary-toxic-substances-control -act, accessed July 24, 2023.

148. Robert D. Bullard, *Dumping in Dixie: Race, Class, and Environmental Quality* (Boulder, CO: Westview, 1990), 30.

149. Bullard, *Dumping in Dixie*, 32.

150. Bullard, *Dumping in Dixie*, 40–45.

151. Jordon Kleiman, "Love Canal: A Brief History," Geneseo.edu/history/love_canal _history; see also Robert Thomas, *Salt and Water, Power and People: A Short History of Hooker Electrochemical Company* (Niagara Falls: Hooker Chemical Co., 1955), https://babel.hathitrust.org/cgi/pt?id=mdp. 39015070160174&view=1up&seq=11, accessed January 28, 2023.

152. Eckardt Beck, "The Love Canal Tragedy," *EPA Journal*, January 1979, https:// www.epa.gov/archive/epa/aboutepa/love-canal-tragedy.html, accessed January 28, 2023; EPA, "Superfund Site: Love Canal Niagara Falls, NY Cleanup Activities," https://cumulis.epa.gov/supercpad/SiteProfiles/index.cfm?fuseaction=second .cleanup&id=0201290, accessed January 28, 2023.

153. EPA, "Superfund: CERCLA Overview," January 24, 2023, https://www.epa.gov /superfund/superfund-cercla-overview, accessed February 10, 2023.

154. See Markowitz and Rosner, *Deceit and Denial*, 260–286, for an extended discussion of the story of Cancer Alley and the chemical industry.

155. Centers for Disease Control, *National Report on Human Exposure to Environmental Chemicals*, December 15, 2022, https://www.cdc.gov/exposurereport /index.html, accessed February 4, 2023.

156. David Rosner and Gerald Markowitz, "Baby Powders and the Precautionary Principle," *American Journal of Public Health* 110, no. 9 (September 2020): 1378–1379; Rosner, Markowitz, and Chowkwanyun, "'Nondetected.'"

157. Sarah Vogel, "The Politics of Plastics: The Making and Unmaking of Bisphenol A 'Safety,'" *American Journal of Public Health* 99, Supplement 3 (November 2009): S559–S566, https://www.ncbi.nlm.nih.gov/pmc/articles/PMC2774166/, accessed July 24, 2023.

7. DARKEST BEFORE THE DAWN?

1. See, for example, Frederick Engels, *The Condition of the Working-Class in England* (New York: Oxford World Classics, 1993), originally published in 1845.

2. N. Eberstadt, "The Health Crisis in the USSR," *New York Review of Books*, February 19, 1981, 23–31.

3. Albert Szymanski and Nick Eberstadt, "The Health Crisis in the USSR: An Exchange," *New York Review of Books*, November 5, 1981, http://www.nybooks.com/articles/archives/1981/nov/05/the-health-crisis-in-the-ussr-an-exchange/, accessed January 12, 2022.

4. Mara Mordecai and Aidan Connaughton, "Public Opinion About Coronavirus Is More Politically Divided in U.S. than in Other Advanced Economies," Pew Research Center, October 28, 2020, https://www.pewresearch.org/fact-tank/2020/10/28/public-opinion-about-coronavirus-is-more-politically-divided-in-u-s-than-in-other-advanced-economies/, accessed March 17, 2022.

5. Steven Woolf, "The Growing Influence of State Governments on Population Health in the United States," *JAMA* 327, no. 14 (March 11, 2022): 1331–1332; Jennifer Rubin, "Opinion: Living in Red America Can Be Life-Threatening," *Washington Post*, March 17, 2022, https://www.washingtonpost.com/opinions/2022/03/17/living-in-red-states-can-be-life-threatening/.

6. Anne Case and Angus Deaton, "Rising Morbidity and Mortality in Midlife Among White Non-Hispanic Americans in the 21st Century," *Proceedings of the National Academy of Sciences* 112, no. 49 (November 2, 2015): https://www.pnas.org/content/112/49/15078, accessed January 15, 2022.

7. David Michaels, "Adding Inequality to Injury: The Costs of Failing to Protect Workers on the Job," Washington, DC: U.S. Department of Labor, Occupational Safety and Health Administration, June 2015, https://www.dol.gov/osha/report/20150304-inequality.pdf, accessed January 15, 2022; J. Cassidy, "Why Did the Death Rate Rise Among Middle-Aged White Americans?," *New Yorker*, November 9, 2015, http://www.newyorker.com/news/john-cassidy/why-is-the-death-rate-rising-among-middle-aged-white-americans, accessed January 15, 2022.

8. Mary Bassett, "An Unbroken Thread: Epidemiology and Advocacy," Zena Stein Lecture, HIV Center, Columbia University, September 7, 2023.

9. Case and Deaton, "Rising Morbidity and Mortality," 2.

10. Tara Gomes, Mina Tadrous, Muhammad Mamdani, J. Patterson, and David Juurlink, "The Burden of Opioid-Related Mortality in the United States," *JAMA Network Open* 1, no. 2 (June 1, 2018), https://jamanetwork.com/journals/jama networkopen/fullarticle/2682878, accessed January 27, 2022. Recent data indicate that this downward trend may have reversed in the past several years. See National Institutes of Health, National Institute on Drug Abuse, "Drug Overdose Death Rates," https://nida.nih.gov/research-topics/trends-statistics /overdose-death-rates, accessed July 24, 2023.

11. American Lung Association, State of the Air, "Key Findings," https://www.lung .org/research/sota/key-findings, accessed January 27, 2022.

12. Centers for Disease Control, National Center for Health Statistics, "Life Expectancy in the U.S. Dropped for the Second Year in a Row in 2021," August 31, 2022, https://www.cdc.gov/nchs/pressroom/nchs_press_releases/2022/20220831 .htm, accessed February 10, 2023.

13. CDC, National Center for Health Statistics, "Life Expectancy in the U.S. Declined a Year and a Half in 2020," July 21, 2021.

14. Donna L. Hoyert, "Maternal Mortality Rates in the United States, 2021," National Center for Health Statistics, https://www.cdc.gov/nchs/data/hestat /maternal-mortality/2021/maternal-mortality-rates-2021.htm#:~:text=In%20 2021%2C%20the%20maternal%20mortality,for%20White%20and%20Hispanic %20women, accessed July 23, 2023.

15. Latoya Hill, Nambi Ndugga, and Samanaha Artiga, "Key Data on Health and Health Care by Race and Ethnicity," Kaiser Family Foundation, March 15, 2023, https://www.kff.org/racial-equity-and-health-policy/report/key-data-on -health-and-health-care-by-race-and-ethnicity/, accessed July 24, 2023.

16. Gerald Markowitz and David Rosner, *Deceit and Denial: The Deadly Politics of Industrial Pollution* (Berkeley: University of California Press/Milbank Fund, 2002).

17. Leah Aronowsky, "Unruly Life: The History of the Biosphere in the Environment, 1945–90" (PhD diss., Harvard University, 2020); James Lovelock, *Gaia: A New Look at Life on Earth* (New York: Oxford University Press, 1979); see, for example, a variety of Exxon Mobil ads and op-eds, including "Science: What We Know and Don't Know," *New York Times*, November 6, 1997; and "Unsettled Science," *New York Times*, March 23, 2000.

18. William Boyd and Michael Watts, "Agro-Industrial Just-in-Time: The Chicken Industry and Postwar American Capitalism," in *Globalizing Food: Agrarian Questions and Global Restructuring*, ed. David Goodman and Michael Watts (London: Routledge, 1997), 139–140.

19. Maryn McKenna, as quoted in Terry Gross, "'Big Chicken' Connects Poultry Farming to Antibiotic-Resistant Bacteria," National Public Radio, *Fresh Air*, November 2, 2017, https://www.npr.org/sections/thesalt/2017/11/02/561584723 /big-chicken-connects-poultry-farming-to-antibiotic-resistant-bacteria, accessed June 22, 2022; USDA, Economic Research Service, "Per Capita Availability of Chickens Higher than That of Beef," January 14, 2021, https://www .ers.usda.gov/data-products/chart-gallery/gallery/chart-detail/?chartId=58312, accessed June 23, 2022.

20. Nicholas Freudenberg, *Lethal but Legal: Corporations, Consumption, and Protecting Public Health* (New York: Oxford University Press, 2014), 3–19; Nina Lakhani, Aliya Uteuova, and Alvin Chang, "Revealed: The True Extent of America's Food Monopolies, and Who Pays the Price," *The Guardian*, July 14, 2021, https:// www.theguardian.com/environment/ng-interactive/2021/jul/14/food-monopoly -meals-profits-data-investigation, accessed June 22, 2022.

21. See updated tables in "National Report on Human Exposure to Environmental Chemicals," U.S. Department of Health and Human Services, Centers for Disease Control and Prevention, January 2019, https://www.cdc.gov/exposurereport /index.html, accessed June 20, 2022.

22. Centers for Disease Control and Prevention, "Fourth National Report on Human Exposure to Environmental Chemicals, Updated Tables, March 2021," https:// www.cdc.gov/exposurereport/pdf/FourthReport_UpdatedTables_Volume3 _Mar2021-508.pdf, accessed January 3, 2022.

23. U.S. Department of Health and Human Services, *ATSDR Case Studies in Environmental Medicine, Polychlorinated Biphenyl (PCBs) Toxicity*, May 14, 2018, https://www.atsdr.cdc.gov/csem/pcb/docs/pcb.pdf, accessed January 3, 2022.

24. World Health Organization, *Polychlorinated Biphenyls and Polybrominated Biphenyls*, IARC Monographs on the Evaluation of Carcinogenic Risks to Humans, Volume 107, https://publications.iarc.fr/131, accessed June 19, 2022.

25. Markowitz and Rosner, *Deceit and Denial*.

26. Laurie Garrett, *The Coming Plague: Newly Emerging Diseases in a World Out of Balance* (New York: Farrar Straus, 1994).

27. Laurie Garrett, "How HIV and COVID-19 Variants Are Connected," *Foreign Policy*, December 2, 2021.

28. International Energy Agency, Global EV Outlook, "Trends in Electric Light-Duty Vehicles," https://www.iea.org/reports/global-ev-outlook-2022/trends-in-electric -light-duty-vehicles, accessed February 10, 2023; Jack Ewing, "Sales of Electric Vehicles Surpass Diesel in Europe, a First," *New York Times*, January 17, 2022.

29. David Gelles, Brad Plumer, Jim Tankersley, and Jack Ewing, "The Clean Energy Future Is Arriving Faster Than You Think," *New York Times*, August 17, 2023,

https://www.nytimes.com/interactive/2023/08/12/climate/clean-energy-us -fossil-fuels.html, accessed August 18, 2023.

30. Centers for Disease Control and Prevention, "Multidrug-Resistant Organisms (MDRO) Management in Healthcare Settings," 2006, https://www.cdc.gov /infectioncontrol/guidelines/mdro/index.html, accessed January 21, 2022.

31. Nadja Popovich, Livia Albveck-Ripka, and Kendra Pierre-Louis, "The Trump Administration Rolled Back More than 100 Environmental Rules. Here's the List," *New York Times*, January 20, 2021, https://www.nytimes.com/interactive /2020/climate/trump-environment-rollbacks-list.html.

32. Coral Davenport, "Republican Drive to Tilt Courts Against Climate Action Reaches a Crucial Moment," *New York Times*, June 19, 2022, 1, https://www .nytimes.com/2022/06/19/climate/supreme-court-climate-epa.html, accessed June 22, 2022.

33. Supreme Court of the United States, *West Virginia et al. v. Environmental Protection Agency et al.*, June 30, 2022, https://www.supremecourt.gov/opinions /21pdf/20-1530_n758.pdf.

34. U.S. Department of Labor, OSHA, "Permissible Exposure Limits—Annotated Tables," https://www.osha.gov/annotated-pels, accessed December 24, 2022.

35. Sharon Lerner, "As Workers Battle Cancer, the Government Admits Its Limit for a Deadly Chemical Is Too High," *ProPublica*, December 15, 2022, https:// www.propublica.org/article/goodyear-niagara-rubber-plant-ortho-toluidine, accessed December 15, 2022; Sharon Lerner, "Why Government Fails to Limit Many Dangerous Chemicals in the Workplace," National Public Radio, December 15, 2022, https://www.npr.org/sections/health-shots/2022/12/15/1142915184 /ortho-toluidine-exposure-workplace-osha, accessed December 24, 2022.

36. Victoria Rome, National Resources Defense Council, "Ten New Environmental Laws in California," November 30, 2021, nrdc.org/experts/Victoria-rome/ten -new-environmental-laws-california, accessed June 21, 2022.

37. Maaz Gardezi, Carrie Chenault, and Hannah Dankbar, "Climate Change and Environmental Justice: A Conversation with Dr. Robert D. Bullard," chrome-extension://efaidnbmnnnibpcajpcglclefindmkaj/https://iastatedigital press.com/jctp/article/566/galley/446/view/, accessed January 17, 2022.

38. Ross Geredien, "Post-Mountaintop Removal Reclamation of Mountain Summits for Economic Development in Appalachia," prepared for the Natural Resources Defense Council, December 7, 2009, 3.

39. Gregory J. Pond et al, "Downstream Effects of Mountaintop Coal Mining: Comparing Biological Conditions Using Family- and Genus-Level Macroinvertebrate Bioassessment Tools," *Journal of the North American Benthological Society* 27, no. 3 (2008): 717–737; Geredien, "Post-Mountaintop Removal Reclamation," 3.

40. M. M. Ahern et al., "The Association Between Mountaintop Mining and Birth Defects Among Live Births in Central Appalachia, 1996–2003," *Environmental Research* 111, no. 6 (2011): 838–846.

41. "Human Health Impacts," Appalachian Voices, https://appvoices.org/end -mountaintop-removal/health-impacts/#1, accessed June 22, 2022; Michael Hendryx, Leah Wolfe, Juhua Luo, and Bo Webb, "Self-Reported Cancer Rates in Two Rural Areas of West Virginia with and Without Mountaintop Coal Mining," *Journal of Community Health* 37 (April 2012): 320–327. "Mountaintop Removal Maps and GIS Resources," http://ilovemountains.org/maps, accessed August 20, 2014. For an extraordinary discussion, see Merlin Chowkwanyun, "Dilemmas of Community Health Medical Care and Environmental Health in Postwar America" (PhD diss., University of Pennsylvania, 2013).

42. Jay Lau, "Why Are We Seeing New Malaria Cases in the U.S.?," *Harvard T. H. Chan School of Public Health, News*, July 12, 2023, https://www.hsph.harvard .edu/news/features/new-malaria-cases-in-the-u-s-manoj-duraisingh/, accessed August 13, 2023.

43. Alejandra Vorunda, Lauren Sommer, and Rebecca Hersher, "Climate Change Affects Your Life in 3 Big Ways, a New Report Warns," National Public Radio, *Morning Edition*, November 14, 2023, https://www.npr.org/2023/11/14/1206506962 /climate-change-affects-your-life-in-3-big-ways-a-new-report-warns, accessed November 17, 2023. See also *The Fifth National Climate Assessment*, ed. A. R. Crimmins et al. (Washington, DC: U.S. Global Change Research Program, 2023), https://doi.org/10.7930/NCA5.2023.

44. Emily Anthes, "U.S. Sees First Cases of Local Malaria Transmission in Two Decades," *New York Times*, June 27, 2023, https://www.nytimes.com/2023/06/27 /health/us-malaria-mosquitoes.html, accessed July 25, 2023.

45. Damian Carrington, "World Close to 'Irreversible' Climate Breakdown, Warn Major Studies," *The Guardian*, October 27, 2022, https://www.theguardian.com /environment/2022/oct/27/world-close-to-irreversible-climate-breakdown -warn-major-studies, accessed February 24, 2023. See Intergovernmental Panel on Climate Change (IPCC), "Climate Change 2022: Mitigation of Climate Change," https://www.ipcc.ch/report/ar6/wg3/, accessed February 24, 2023.

46. United Nations, "UN Climate Report: It's 'Now or Never' to Limit Global Warming to 1.5 Degrees," *UN News*, April 4, 2022, https://news.un.org/en/story /2022/04/1115452#:~:text=A%20new%20flagship%20UN%20report,limit%20 global%20warming%20to%201.5, accessed June 22, 2022.

47. "World Energy Outlook 2019," International Energy Agency, November 13, 2019, https://www.iea.org/reports/world-energy-outlook-2019.

48. Nadja Popovich and Denise Lu, "The Most Detailed Map of Auto Emissions in America," *New York Times*, October 10, 2019, https://www.nytimes.com

/interactive/2019/10/10/climate/driving-emissions-map.html, accessed November 27, 2019.

49. United Nations, Press Release, "Cut Global Emissions by 7.6 Percent Every Year for Next Decade to meet 1.5°C Paris Target—UN Report," November 26, 2019, https://unfccc.int/news/cut-global-emissions-by-76-percent-every-year -for-next-decade-to-meet-15degc-paris-target-un-report#:~:text=The %20report%20finds%20that%20greenhouse,55.3%20gigatonnes%20of %20CO2%20equivalent, accessed June 22, 2022.

50. Scott Kulp and Benjamin Strauss, "New Elevation Data Triple Estimates of Global Vulnerability to Sea-Level Rise and Coastal Flooding," *Nature Communications* 10, no. 4844 (October 29, 2019), https://www.nature.com/articles /s41467-019-12808-z, accessed November 27, 2019.

51. Brad Plumer, "5 Global Trends Shaping Our Climate Future," *New York Times*, November 26, 2019, A-7, https://www.nytimes.com/2019/11/12/climate/energy -trends-climate-change.html, accessed November 27, 2019.

52. Lisa Friedman and Coral Davenport, "Senate Ratifies Pact to Curb a Broad Category of Potent Greenhouse Gases," *New York Times*, September 21, 2022, https://www.nytimes.com/2022/09/21/climate/hydrofluorocarbons-hfcs-kigali -amendment.html, accessed February 24, 2023.

53. David Rosner, "Webs of Denial: Climate Change and the Challenge to Public Health," *Milbank Quarterly* 94, no. 4 (December 2016): 733–735; David Rosner, "Climate Denial and a (Hopeful) Lesson from History," *Milbank Quarterly* 96 (September 2018): 430–433; David Rosner, "Health, Climate Change, and the Descent of Science-Based Policy," *Milbank Quarterly* 95, no. 1 (March 2017): 36–39; David Rosner and Gerald Markowitz, "An Enormous Victory for Public Health in California," *American Journal of Public Health* 109, no. 2 (February 2019): 211–212; David Rosner, "Sophie's Choice on the Nation's Health," *Milbank Quarterly* 95, no. 3 (September 2017): 482–485.

54. Philip Landrigan et al., "The *Lancet* Commission on Pollution and Health," *Lancet Commissions* 391, no. 10119 (February 3, 2018): 462. See also Frederica Perera, "Multiple Threats to Child Health from Fossil Fuel Combustion: Impacts of Air Pollution and Climate Change," *Environmental Health Perspectives* 125, no. 2 (2017): 141–148. See "GAHP is improving health by addressing all forms of toxic pollution," Available at: https://www.gahp.org/, Accessed: March 22, 2024.

55. Nadia Sam-Agudu, Boghuma Titanji, Fredos Okumu, and Madhukar Pai, "The Pandemic Is Following a Very Predictable and Depressing Pattern," *The Atlantic*, March 4, 2022, https://www.theatlantic.com/health/archive/2022/03/pandemic -global-south-disease-health-crisis/624179/, accessed March 8, 2022.

56. Wolfgang Streeck, *How Will Capitalism End? Essays on a Failing System* (New York: Verso, 2016).

57. John Elflein, "Total Number of Cases and Deaths from COVID-19 in the United States as of April 26, 2023," Statista, https://www.statista.com/statistics/1101932/coronavirus-covid19-cases-and-deaths-number-us-americans/, accessed February 23, 2023.

58. Ari Shapiro, "President Trump Wants to Reopen Economy Despite CDC Warnings," National Public Radio, May 6, 2020, https://www.npr.org/2020/05/06/851631806/president-trump-wants-to-reopen-economy-despite-cdc-warnings, accessed May 28, 2020.

59. Ali Velshi, "Fmr. OSHA Chief After SCOTUS Shuts Down Vaxx Requirement: 'I Believe in My Heart That They Don't Care,'" January 16, 2022, https://www.msnbc.com/ali-velshi/watch/fmr-osha-chief-after-scotus-shuts-down-vaxx-requirement-i-believe-in-my-heart-that-they-don-t-care-130990149775, accessed January 18, 2022.

Index

carbon disulfide, 261

Caribbean islands, 21, 38, 76, 311n56; diseases on, 33, 48, 55, 56, 71, 93; slave plantations on, 7, 28, 40, 44, 45–48, 58, 71, 79, 93; trade with, 28, 29, 58

Carnegie, Andrew, 129, 168, 181

Carson, Rachel, 239–240, 246, 266–267. See also *Silent Spring*

Carter, Jimmy, 251

Case, Anne, 281–282

Cato Institute, 256, 360n91

cellulites (St. Anthony's fire), 109

Centers for Disease Control and Prevention (CDC), 18, 283, 290; on dangerous chemicals, 277, 287; on racial disparities in health, 5, 283

Chadwick, Edwin, 61, 70, 125, 280

Chapin, Charles, 141

charities, 108, 128–131

Charleston, S.C., 39, 42, 44, 48, 82, 92

Chavez, Cesar, 244

chemical industry, 232, 235–236, 237, 238, 250, 259; growing criticism of, 239–242, 247, 276; public relations efforts of, 236, 237–239, 240–241, 256, 277–278, 356n33. *See also* petrochemical industry

Cherniack, Martin, 204

Cherokee Indians, 80

Cherry, Ill., 182

chicken broiler industry, 271–273, 286

child labor, 65, 93, 102–103, 105, 172, 182; in Britain, 61, 65; movement against, 104, 211; on slave plantations, 81, 87

Chinese Americans, 124–125

Chinese Exclusion Act (1882), 125

chloracne, 261, 287

chlorinated hydrocarbons, 232, 258–260, 261–269, 287; growing concern about, 262, 264–268 (see also *Silent Spring*). *See also* Aldrin; Lindane; DDT; PCBs; polyvinyl chloride

cholera, 4, 33; declining incidence of, 9, 113–114, 139, 145, 224, 226, 299

—in nineteenth century, 58, 70, 74, 97–99, 113, 120, 152, 299; in cities, 3–4, 14, 120–121, 128; among slaves, 88–89

chronic conditions, 16; growing recognition of, 187, 201, 205, 223, 235; long latency of 201, 209, 227; and new chemicals and products, 225–227, 264–265, 286–287

cigarettes, 29, 230; production of, 177–181, 225. *See also* tobacco products

Clark, Claudia, 184

Clark, William Mansfield, 196

Clean Air Act (1970), 251, 355n18

Cleveland, Ohio, 5, 95, 100

climate change, 285, 291, 293, 295–298, *See also* global warming

coal, 237, 290, 291–292, 297; greenhouse gases from, 291, 297. *See also* coal dust; coal industry

coal dust, 182, 188, 227–228. *See also* black lung disease

coal industry, 95, 182–183, 294–295; in Britain, 61, 68, 70; fracking by, 293; labor conflict in, 103, 169, 357n47; and mountaintop removal, 294–295

—hazards in, 189, 243, 294–295; from coal dust, 187, 188, 205, 227–228; from mining accidents, 156, 166, 182–183

Coal Mine Safety and Health Act (1969), 243

"Collins, Dr." (pseud.), 45–48